Breast Cancer

Rose Kushner

BREAST CANCER

A Personal History
and an Investigative Report

FOREWORD BY THOMAS L. DAO, M.D.

NEW YORK AND LONDON
Harcourt Brace Jovanovich

The quotations from *Early Detection,* by Dr. Philip Strax, are used by permission of Harper & Row, Publishers.

Library of Congress Cataloging in Publication Data

Kushner, Rose.
Breast cancer: a personal history and
an investigative report.

Bibliography: p.
Includes index.
1. Breast—Cancer. I. Title. [DNLM: 1. Breast neoplasms—Personal narra-
tives. WP870 K97c]
RC280.B8K87   616.9′94′49   75-17688
ISBN 0-15-122569-9

B C D E

In memory of Ann London Scott and the hundreds of thousands of other women who have died—too soon—from breast cancer

To Harvey . . . for everything he has done. And to Gantt, Todd, and Lesley . . . for helping him.

Contents

Foreword

When Rose Kushner first told me she wanted to write a book on breast cancer, my reaction was quick and primitive. I was dubious and responded negatively. "Rose, you know I have been asked to write such a book for the last ten years and have always turned such requests down. Do you really understand what you are getting into? It's an enormous job, and I cannot give you much, if any, help." The idea of her book was truly inconceivable to me. A touch of male chauvinism? Perhaps. But Rose Kushner is her own woman, and in the relatively short period of less than a year her idea has become a reality. Amazing! As soon as she recovered from her mastectomy, she found a publisher and was on her way to Europe, to visit various institutions and interview numerous experts for her book. This demonstration of energy and zest for life after a mastectomy should be an inspiration to women everywhere.

The author tells the story of her own encounter with breast cancer and then skillfully guides the reader through the complexities of scientific, medical, socioeconomic, and psychological aspects of breast cancer. No aspect of the disease—epidemiology, causation, diagnosis, treatment, rehabilitation—is left out. The research involved has been enormous.

Mrs. Kushner makes an exceptional effort to deal with the subject of oral contraceptives and breast cancer. Her concern over the lack of warning about the risk of breast cancer in users of oral contraceptives is both reasonable and justifiable. She correctly stresses the importance of early detection and the absolute necessity for women to learn and practice breast self-examination (BSE). Where surgery is necessary, as it so often is, she confronts the major controversial issue in breast-cancer treatment squarely. The issue is freedom of choice in surgery, and the controversy it has aroused will not soon be stilled. The issue is inevitably an emotional one, since no one can deny the mutilating effect of radical surgery and its aftermath for women young or old. Mrs. Kushner so rightly stresses the necessity of proper staging to determine the extent of cancer before any operation is contemplated. Her explanation of the various kinds of mastectomy operations and their comparative value and risk is invaluable. In postoperative care, she is right to emphasize the necessity of fitting a good prosthesis, a very important point often neglected by both patients and physicians.

Mrs. Kushner and I do not agree on every detail of her argument—she is harder on general surgeons than I would be, and what she says about the "economic incentive" in the diagnosis and treatment of breast cancer is not what I would say—but the value of her discussion far outweighs any differences we may have.

As Mrs. Kushner knows, it is difficult to find a discussion on breast cancer for lay people that tells them all they need to know, and impossible to find one in which the disease and the prospects for its cure are adequately described and which, at the same time, recounts one full human response to it from an actual patient's point of view. That is what Rose Kushner has done in *Breast Cancer*.

Women who read this book will be better informed consumers of medical services. They will be given the facts about the disease, its possible causes, potential cures, and what constitutes proper care—and follow-up care—when the diagnosis of cancer is made.

The author draws every woman reader into the sisterhood of fear and suffering. She exhorts women to protect themselves by regular breast self-examination, education, and critical evaluation of what they are told. Moreover, she does not shrink from

confrontation with the medical profession, should such be unavoidable.

Some of the responsibility for the health care we receive rests
squarely on our own shoulders. Every woman in the United
States should read this book. Medical and paramedical profes-
sionals would do well to add a copy to their working libraries.

THOMAS L. DAO, M.D.

Director
Department of Breast Surgery and
   Breast Cancer Research Unit
Roswell Park Memorial Institute

Professor of Surgery and Physiology
State University of New York at Buffalo

Buffalo, New York
April 7, 1975

Breast Cancer

1

What Happened to Me

It was Saturday night, June 15, 1974, when I found the tiny bulge on the edge of my left nipple. The date will probably stay with me forever. Like all outstanding anniversaries, the precise time a malignant tumor is found has a way of sticking in one's memory.

I was in the tub, luxuriating in an unexpected reprieve from a business dinner party. The children were out, and Harvey and I had the house and the television all to ourselves. I wondered if there was a good movie on that night.

"Don't take too long," I remember his shouting from the living room. "It's a great night to be home—Archie Bunker, *M*A*S*H*, and a Humphrey Bogart oldie."

And then I found it.

I was not examining myself for suspected cancer. All I was doing was shaving under my arm.

Somehow the little finger of the hand that held the razor leap-frogged over something irregular, a minute hemisphere that curved ever so slightly above the firm strand of muscle. It was so small that I was not sure there was really anything different about the spot. But if my head pretended for a moment that nothing was there, my stomach knew immediately something was wrong. It coiled into a tight ball and stayed that way for weeks.

Until I was struck by cancer myself, the only women I had

ever known personally who had the disease were all dead: several relatives on my husband's side of the family (no one on mine, so far as I knew), a dear friend, and friends of friends. Of course, everyone in Washington knew about Alice Longworth, Theodore Roosevelt's astonishing daughter. She had had both her breasts removed for cancer almost a half century ago and billed herself as "the flattest-chested woman in the capital." Sometimes she joked that she was the only really topless woman in town.

But former presidents' daughters are legends; that's why she survived. Mere mortal women died from breast cancer.

I also knew about Senator Birch Bayh's wife, Marvella, Shirley Temple Black, and Mrs. William Fulbright. But they were all recent victims, not long-term cures a woman could hang her hopes on.

Betty Ford and Happy Rockefeller had not yet discovered their tumors. The flood of information and optimistic facts that filled newspapers and magazines after their operations had not yet appeared. There was nothing I had ever come across to show me anything but the shadow of imminent death.

On that awful Saturday night when I discovered the bump, I knew a great deal more about the history of the Arabs on the West Bank in Israel than I did about breast cancer. All I was sure of were the seven danger signals of cancer, and a lump in the breast was definitely one of them.

I can't remember how long I stayed rigid with fear in the tub. Finally Harvey came to remind me that Archie Bunker was about to begin. He opened the bathroom door and poked his head around it.

"What's keeping you?" he asked, annoyed. "Dinner is—"

I must have looked strange, because he stopped in midsentence. He came in, shut the door behind him, and forgot dinner and the Bunkers.

"It's cold in here." He reprimanded me gently. "You'll catch pneumonia."

I waved my hand in a weak shrug.

"Is anything wrong?"

"Feel this place," I said, pointing to the suspicious spot.

He leaned over. "I don't feel anything."

"Nothing much could hide in me, could it?" I smiled at our old family joke.

I reached for the bar of soap. "Try feeling the place with some soap on your finger," I said. "See if you can find it now."

Without a question, he did as I asked.

"There's something there," he said in a flat monotone. "You'd better call the doctor first thing Monday morning. Don't put it off."

The rest of the evening and all day Sunday stand out in my memory as hours of bizarre charades. I tried to read the *Washington Post*, cooked breakfast, and even had friends over for an early-summer barbecue—all done automatically. How did I do it?

What else was there to do? The children, of course, knew nothing, and I was reluctant to talk to Harvey about the possibility of having breast cancer. The epidemic that had flared through his family in recent years had claimed a cousin and two aunts. In his family, the disease was synonymous with death.

On Monday morning, I began calling my internist's office long before his secretary arrived. I was her first caller.

"I have a lump in my left breast," I told her.

Usually, to be squeezed into his busy schedule required at least a massive hemorrhage or a minimum temperature of 106. Perhaps it was his normal policy to examine breast lumps without delay, or maybe it was something urgent in my voice. There was no waiting this time.

"Can you be here at ten?" the secretary asked immediately.

"I'll be there, don't worry."

An hour to wait.

I had read somewhere about a new breast-cancer detection machine, the thermograph, that was being installed at a Washington hospital. I called the hospital and was referred to the American Cancer Society.

"This screening is a joint project of the American Cancer Society and the National Cancer Institute," I was told by a clerk there. "It is for women who have no symptoms at all. I'm afraid—"

"I am not interested in being part of the project," I explained. "I don't need anything to tell me if I have a lump. I can feel it.

I just need to know if it's malignant or benign. Can the thermo-graph do that?"

"That's the whole point of the project," she answered impa-tiently. "This is what must be evaluated."

Giving up on the American Cancer Society, I called the hospital back. Couldn't they just slip me in? Yes, I'd come in as an outpatient. Yes, I'd be happy to be billed. No, I didn't need anything else.

"Come in Friday, June 21, at 10:00 A.M.," I was finally told. "But you will not be part of the ACS-NCI demonstration project."

That done, I drove off to my internist's office. Although the waiting room was crowded, his nurse escorted me into an exam-ining room as soon as I arrived. Normally, when my doctor looked me over, his face was an expressionless mask that told me nothing. This time I read his signals loud and clear; he didn't like what he was feeling.

"You've never had lumps before, have you?" he queried.

"Never."

"Let's try to get some light on the subject," he joked feebly, turning off the switch. In the darkened room, he flashed a beam of powerful light in the direction of my lump.

"What's that?" I asked.

"Transillumination," he replied. "If it's a fluid-filled cyst or anything hollow, it will show up as a shadow."

"Is it?"

He shook his head. "It looks pretty solid to me."

The knot in my belly tightened and cramped. "What next? I've already made an appointment to get a thermogram at—"

He waved away any thought of the new detection machine. "That's not reliable enough. I'd like you to get a xeromammo-gram."

"A what?"

"A xeromammogram. It's a new way to take mammograms—pictures of the breasts. They've just installed the equipment at the hospital." Dr. Heckman explained that the full, official name of this new X-ray technique is xeroradiomammography. "But that's a mouthful to say. So most of us just call it xeromammog-raphy and xeromammograms. Some even cut it down more—to xerographs and xerograms."

He told me that the basic picture is taken by conventional X-ray machinery, but that the configuration of the breast is then reproduced on paper, instead of on film.

"Is it better than plain X-rays?"

"That's what I've been told," he answered matter-of-factly. "According to what radiologists say, it's more detailed and easier to read."

"Is it accurate?"

He shrugged. "Probably about as accurate as any picture can be. You know," he warned, "even if the reading is negative—which means the lump isn't malignant—the only way to be certain is to cut the thing out and look at it under a microscope."

I nodded.

"No matter what the pictures say, you've got something in that breast that doesn't belong there. It will have to come out."

Again I nodded, this time more numbly.

The radiology department tried to set my appointment for three weeks ahead, but a magic word from Dr. Heckman and I had a slot at one o'clock that afternoon for a mammogram.

He led me to a chair in his office. "It will have to be biopsied," he said gently.

"I guess so."

"Is there anyone you have in mind for the surgery?"

"Just that I want a breast specialist."

"I don't know of anybody in this area who specializes in breasts," he said, surprised.

"I don't want any ordinary surgeon cutting into a possible cancer," I insisted. "It's got to be an oncologist."

He stared at me, amazed that I knew a cancer specialist is called an oncologist.

"I don't know of any oncologist in this area who specializes in breasts," he told me.

"I don't want any ordinary surgeon cutting into a possible cancer," I repeated. "It's got to be an oncologist."

"Why?"

"Well," I reminded him, "I use you—an internist—and not just a general practitioner. You must have learned something more in your two extra years of residency in internal medicine to make you a better doctor than just a GP. No?"

"Sure," he answered emphatically. "But any—"

"No, not *any* general surgeon can do a mastectomy, if I need one. It's got to be an oncologist. How can a person who knows a little bit about cutting everything know as much as someone who does only cancer surgery?"

"I guess you've got a point there," he conceded.

"After all"—I smiled weakly—"if I had a detached retina, you'd send me to an ophthalmologist, wouldn't you?"

"Naturally. I don't know a damned thing about detached retinas, except to recognize one when I see it."

"Then why send me to a general surgeon for cancer?"

He had no answer. For a minute or two, he said nothing. "I know a head, neck, and chest man in town, but no one who works only with breasts."

"There's a whole breast-cancer clinic out at NIH—the National Institutes of Health," I said. "There must be a specialist in breast cancer there."

"If you like a research setup . . ."

"What do you mean?"

"You might wind up being a random sample in some experiment."

"I don't believe that would happen at all," I argued. "I've seen enough clinical trials at Johns Hopkins, when I worked there in psychiatry, to know there's such a thing as 'informed consent.'"

"That's what they say. But some patient has to get the experimental treatment."

"I'll debate all that with you some other time." I waved my hand impatiently. "Right now, all I can say is that a research hospital is the best place for me. They've got the best."

Clearly, he didn't agree. "It's your body," he said. "Whatever you say."

"I'll need a letter to the National Institutes of Health," I told him, not even remembering how I knew. "The law says I'll have to be referred."

"If you know where to find a breast-cancer specialist, I'll write whatever letter you need," he promised.

"I'll find one, don't worry."

"First of all, you have to get that mammogram."

"All right."

"Then we'll worry about the surgeon. If the radiologist is sure it's nothing, all you need is a good general man."

It had been only about a half hour between the time I got to his office and the time I left, but it seemed as if a week had gone by.

The hospital was not far away; it made no sense to go all the way home and back for the xeromammogram. Stiff as a robot, not seeing or hearing anything along the route, I drove to Harvey's office to wait. Several of the people he works with told me afterward that I saw them in the elevator or the corridor without even nodding hello. I'm not surprised; I don't even remember getting there. Somehow, suddenly, I was standing in front of his desk.

"What did Bernie say?"

"He wants to do a xeromammogram."

"A what?"

As accurately as I could, I recited the definition of the new technique.

"What time?"

"One."

"Do you want to go out for some lunch?"

I shook my head. "I don't think anything would stay down— not even Maalox."

Harvey tried his best to be cheerful and nonchalant. "Well, it will just be nothing like everybody else's has been, and that'll be the end."

"No. Whatever the result is, the lump will have to come out."

"So why get the X-ray taken in the first place?"

"It's something to go on, I guess. And Bernie says it's right about 85 per cent of the time. So I'd have some idea in advance about what I want to do."

"What do you mean, what you want to do?"

It was good to talk. I sat down on his visitor's chair and lit a cigarette. "Well, if it shows up a definite positive, I'm certainly not going to have any hack general surgeon operate on me. How can somebody who knows how to do hernias and gall bladders be an expert in breast cancer?"

After twenty-three years of marriage, Harvey knew my prejudices in favor of specialists well enough not even to bother to ask for logic. We had already gone 'round that mulberry bush with miscellaneous children's crises; he had become a convert to specialization.

"It's probably nothing," he insisted. "Remember Joan? And Nan, and Gloria? They all went through the same scare, and it was just a cyst or something."

"But remember that they didn't know it in advance. Every one of them went to sleep on the operating table not knowing whether she'd wake up with one or two. It's only afterward that everything's—"

"Why do you always have to look at the worst side?" Harvey exploded angrily.

"The lump still has got to come out." I almost shouted across the desk. "You're the one who's always telling me about the unreliability of machinery. You're the one who keeps arguing about contingency planning. That's all I'm doing—trying to decide what to do *if*."

Harvey waved his reluctant concession to my attitude. "Okay, what if?"

"First of all, I've scheduled an appointment to have a thermogram."

I described what little I knew about this detection machine, which measures heat patterns in the breast. Harvey, an engineer, who had had lots of courses in thermodynamics, needed only a sketchy explanation.

"If that's either positive or negative, and if it agrees with the Xerox pictures from the mammogram, the statistics say the diagnosis would be 95 per cent reliable."

"Then?"

I took a deep breath. "Well, if they are both negative, I'll go to that guy who did your hernias. He can do the biopsy."

"And if it's positive on both?"

I took a deeper breath. "I'll go to the National Cancer Institute. What's the point of living ten minutes from NIH—the top government medical-research center in the country—and not using the place?"

"Can you get in?"

"With all the friends we've got who work there, somebody will have some influence."

"When do you get the thermogram?"

"Friday."

"That's a long time to wait."

"That's okay. There's a lot I've got to learn about breast cancer. I need the time."

Harvey's secretary came in. "There's a call from—"

"Is there a typewriter I can borrow somewhere?" I asked her, assembling myself to leave the room.

She nodded. "Sure. Ev is in New York. You can use hers."

I turned back to Harvey. "One thing you can be sure of. Nobody's hacking off my breast while I'm unconscious unless I'm convinced that that's the only thing there is to do."

He smiled weakly and picked up his telephone as I left.

In Ev's office, I called some friends, who gave me the names of their friends in the higher echelons of NCI—the cancer *I* of the National Institutes of Health. It was all set. Friday, June 21, at 2:00 P.M., I had an appointment in the breast-tumor clinic. Someone told me what had to be included in my doctor's referral letter, and I typed it out for his signature. I was as efficient and unemotional as the IBM computer clattering at the end of the hall.

"I've got an appointment at NCI right after the thermogram on Friday," I told Harvey. "It'll be a busy day."

"What are you going to do now?" he asked.

"I'm going to ride over and get Bernie Heckman to sign this referral letter," I told him, waving the paper. "Then I'm going to the X-ray clinic, and then to the library."

"You'll call me as soon as the thing is done?" he asked.

I smiled. "I doubt that I'll know anything today, but I'll call."

I felt much better. Now that there were things to be done, the knot in my belly had relaxed somewhat. For me, nothing is worse than being pushed or pulled by events, with no gas pedal or brake I can operate myself. With appointments scheduled, a glimmer of plans made, books to read, at least I had my forefinger in my own destiny. I would be no slab of silly-putty to be manipulated helplessly by a pack of doctors.

The referral was signed in minutes, and I was soon waiting in the radiology department of the hospital. The technician was a round, jolly comedian.

"You should have seen the patient before you," she joked. "Hers were so huge I needed to use two plates for each one. It cost her, or her insurance company, twice as much as the regular price."

Her macabre humor was contagious. "Do I get a discount?" I wisecracked. "You're not even using half of each plate."

She thought I was hilarious. "I'll have to remember you, too," she roared. "Between the two of you, I'll have a great story to tell in the staff dining room."

I watched her process the photographs of my breasts in the huge, conventional-looking Xerox machine in the corridor. The technique of taking the pictures in the darkened X-ray chamber had not seemed to be any different from old-fashioned mammography, but the rest of the procedure was new to me. The plates are treated with certain chemicals, I learned later, and are put into a specially built photocopier. The result is a carefully detailed blue-and-white image of the breast, showing the delicate network of blood vessels, ducts, and glands, as well as muscle and fat.

To the trained eye, both kinds of mammograms can predict the presence of cancer in about 85 per cent of cases. However, the xeromammogram, according to experts in the detection field, has several advantages. There is more detailed illustration of the structure, and a more objective opinion can be given; the previous experience of the "reader" in interpreting shadows, hollows, and densities is not as vital. Also, the processing takes much less time, and xeromammograms can be available quickly, if needed.

"But is the thing accurate?"

She was defensive about her machine toy. "It's every bit as good as film," she lectured, "and a heck of a lot faster and easier to read. You don't have to wait hours for these things to dry."

Pictures of my breast were sliding from the slot, as quickly as copies of an ordinary letter. I stared at my innards. On one marked with an *L*, I noticed an odd bluish spot that seemed to coincide with my lump's geography. But there was also an odd bluish spot on one marked *R*. There were lots of funny bluish spots on both.

"How does the left one look to you?" I asked anxiously. "I can't see much of a difference."

"That's the boss's job." She grinned, getting back her good humor. "If I could do it, he'd be out of work."

"How long does it take?"

"He usually comes in about two every day to read them," she said. "I'll put yours up front, so he'll be sure to get to it today. Tell your doctor to call about ten tomorrow morning."

"Thanks," I said gratefully. "It's hard to wait."

"Well, you're the only one with a real symptom today. The rest are just routine examinations. They're not as worried."

The session over, I drove to our public library and looked up breast cancer in the card catalogue. There was a listing for just one book—*What Women Should Know About the Breast Cancer Controversy,* by Dr. George Crile, Jr.

I hadn't even known, then, that there *was* a breast-cancer controversy!

Back home, I still had an hour or so before I had to face the chores of dinner. I scooped a hole for myself in my favorite bean-bag chair and had finished the book before the dogs began to whimper for their chow. Harvey found me at the can opener.

"You didn't call," he scolded.

"I'm sorry. I guess I forgot, because there was nothing to say except to tell you about the new machine they're using." Knowing his consuming interest in any and all gadgetry, I described the Xerox technique.

"Amazing!" he said, and paused. "But what about you?"

"The technician said to tell Bernie to call about ten tomorrow morning."

"Did you find anything in the library?"

"Mainly that there's a big fight going on over what to do about breast cancer," I told him. "What was done to everybody we know is not necessarily the only way to go."

"There never is an only way to go with anything," he said scientifically. "Everything has an alternative if you look for it."

"I've never heard of doing anything but cutting off the breast and then drying yourself out with X-ray," I replied. "But now there's this Dr. Crile, in Cleveland, who says that sometimes taking out the lump is enough. He's also violently against having X-ray treatments afterward. Besides that, there's more than one operation for taking off—"

"Now, wait a minute, honey," cautioned Harvey, always the scientist. "*His* way may be no good, either. You're going from one extreme to the other. There must be things in the middle. There always are."

By then it was time to eat. We had decided still not to say anything to the children, and the subject was dropped. Later, while I cleaned up the kitchen, Harvey skimmed through Crile.

"He's got a great pedigree," he commented, after everyone had disappeared from the immediate vicinity of the kitchen sink. "But he doesn't write like a scientist. He sounds as if he's on some kind of a vendetta because his wife died even though she had her breast taken off."

"He does sound bitter about that," I agreed, "because it was done for nothing. She went through all the pain and mutilation of a mastectomy, and the cancer had already been spreading."

"But when they operated there was no way to know that," he reminded me. "It took five years. Maybe she could have been saved. Maybe it was a freak. You really have got to find out more about it, and not go by one man's opinion."

I nodded. "I'll go over to the NIH medical library tomorrow. This is all there was in the public library."

The next day, as soon as the family had left, I drove to the National Institutes of Health and installed myself in a quiet corner of the library (which is open to the public), on a comfortable leather couch piled high with everything I thought I could decipher on mammary carcinoma—the medical term for breast cancer.

Before leaving, I had called my internist with the message from the X-ray technician, and I read with one eye on the clock. My first question was answered right away: the thing had to come out. Every scientist was emphatic that even if every possible external test indicates a lump is nothing to worry about, the only way to know for sure is to cut it out and look at it under a microscope. While eighty-five out of every hundred diagnoses of mammograms are accurate, the other fifteen are not. How could I know I wasn't one of those fifteen?

I took time out to call about my result. "Everything is fine," Dr. Heckman's nurse told me. "The radiology department says it's just benign fibrocystic disease—nothing to worry about."

With the information about "false negatives" fresh in my mind, however, the news did not fill me with optimism. I was convinced by now that I would have to undergo a biopsy no matter what the mammography result was. (As it turned out, I was indeed one of the fifteen—a "false negative." "It happens," the radiologist told me casually afterward. "Nothing's perfect. The only way to be sure is on biopsy.")

According to the literature I was reading, two kinds of biopsies are most popular in the United States. One is the excisional biopsy. The entire lump, or tumor, is removed intact, surrounded by some insulating tissue. The other is the incisional biopsy. Only a part of the tumor is removed. Most surgeons routinely cut out the whole mass, unless it is very large.

Afterward, the common practice here is to send everything to the pathology laboratory for fast-freezing—the procedure called a frozen section—while the patient is unconscious on the operating table. A slice of the lump is put under the microscope, and within minutes the surgeon is given the diagnosis. If the tumor is benign, the incision is closed, and the patient is up and around in a few hours. However, if it is malignant, most surgeons in the United States perform a radical mastectomy then and there.

So, in most instances, a woman going to sleep for a simple biopsy does not know whether she will wake up with two breasts or one.

(Incidentally, I also learned that the plural—breasts—is not strictly accurate. The breast is actually a single organ with an internal crossover between its two segments. For the sake of clarity, however, I have decided not to pay too much attention to this nicety of medical syntax.)

Sometimes, of course, for medical reasons, the biopsy and mastectomy as a single procedure is imperative. If a general anesthetic is to be used and the patient has something else wrong that makes her a high surgical risk, one operation is better than two. In addition, sometimes tumors are so big, so irregularly shaped, or so widespread that they cannot be removed intact. In these cases, an incisional biopsy is the only alternative. Then, should the frozen section show the growth is malignant, the breast has to be removed right away. Everything I read agreed that an open, oozing cancer should not be left in the body.

Under ordinary circumstances, however, there are advantages to the patient in having a two-stage procedure instead of the one-stage. To me, at that time, the psychological part was the most important. Not to know beforehand what was going to happen was unthinkable. Needing to have a mastectomy would be bad enough, but not to have time to adjust to the idea in advance seemed absolutely barbaric!

And separating the biopsy from the mastectomy has benefits for the patient in addition to preventing psychic trauma. The surgeon does not have to make the critical decision on the basis of the quick-frozen section, but can wait for the more trustworthy permanent section. Although it is rare for the fast method to be inaccurate, it has happened.

Also, the patient can do some research into the various alternatives and decide for herself what she wants to do about the tumor. While anything short of mastectomy is considered very risky, why should the doctor, husband, father, brother, or whoever make the choice? It is, after all, the woman's life—not someone else's.

Once a decision is made, the woman can shop around for a surgeon. Although a competent general surgeon may do a beautiful biopsy, this skill does not mean he will do a beautiful—and thorough—piece of cancer surgery. Someone who performs ten mastectomies in the course of a year cannot, understandably, be as experienced as a surgeon who does the operation every day.

Later, after my mastectomy, as I learned more and more about "the breast-cancer controversy," I also learned more and more reasons for separating the diagnostic procedure from the surgery for the removal of the breast. But that is getting ahead of my story.

What I already had learned made it easy for me to decide about the one-stage versus the two-stage procedure. My lump was tiny, and I was no surgical risk. I made up my mind to have the biopsy first and then wait. After all, the one diagnostic test I had had said it was benign anyhow. At the time, I was naïve enough to believe that any surgeon would do as I asked. This, I discovered, was more naïve than to believe a radiologist's report is always accurate.

I read on, anxious to know what oncologists think about the opinions of their colleague Dr. George Crile.

Apparently, not too much—for some reasons that made sense to me and others that did not. First, there is what is called the multicentricity of breast cancer. Pathologists, specialists in the study of cells and tissues, have proven that many breasts with a cancerous tumor that can be felt or seen also have microscopic malignancies that will grow into big ones sooner or later. This condition was found in Happy Rockefeller's right breast, for example.

Therefore, oncologists argue, how can Dr. Crile or any surgeon following his theories know that the single lump he removes is all the cancer there is in the breast without examining the organ under a microscope? How can he be sure no cancerous "centricles" are hiding in the hundreds of lobules that make up the breast? How can he tell that no stray cancer cells have escaped from the primary tumor to metastasize, or spread, into other glands?

There is no way.

Opponents of mastectomy argue that there are ways to detect an *in situ* cancer—a tumor that is positively self-contained and in a single spot. But what about those possible microscopic "centricles"? Even if the lump itself is *in situ* without any question, how can anyone be sure about other malignant spots? Later I learned, from new data gathered by the National Cancer Institute, that even *in situ* cancers almost always become invasive, and begin to spread and grow within ten years.

Another of Dr. Crile's arguments against mastectomy is his theory that the lymph nodes of the armpit—a part of the body's first line of defense against infection and other diseases—must not be removed. In the most common surgical procedure used in the United States, the radical mastectomy, about twenty-five to thirty of these dime-sized arsenals are removed, along with the breast and, usually, certain chest muscles. Pathological examination of

the nodes tells the doctor whether the disease was confined to
the mammary gland alone or whether it has already conquered
parts of this defensive line. Future treatments for the patient depend on the state of her nodes. If none are malignant, she is
declared "localized" and is often told she is "as good as cured."
The chance of cure is reduced in proportion to the number of
nodes involved.

Unfortunately, despite efforts around the world, no technique
has been found to examine the axillary (underarm) nodes without taking them out and putting them under a microscope.

Dr. Crile argues that if the cancerous lump alone is removed,
the apparatus of the nodal system is set free to fight multicentricles, stray cells, and even the invasion of a fellow node or two.
He feels that, in some patients with early cancer, leaving these
immunological factories in place may permit the woman's own
body to fight any remnants of the cancer that might still be there.

A growing body of evidence indicates that the immunological
system does indeed play a major role in preventing cancer and
stopping its spread, and perhaps even in causing cancer (by
breaking down or becoming weak). But so far this evidence is
based on animal models and not humans. Therefore, Dr. Crile's
thesis that removing the nodes may do harm to the immune system is not generally accepted. Moreover, some immunologists
believe that, as with veins and arteries, the hundreds of other
nodes throughout the body begin to work harder—within a matter
of hours—to compensate for the ones removed from the armpit.
However, this also has been shown only in animal models.

Of course, these were "preliminary opinions." But all the opinions, including Dr. Crile's, were too preliminary for me to risk
my life on. Trusting the immune system to kill off hidden "centricles" seemed too unreliable.

And even if I had wanted to go along with his "lumpectomy,"
I discovered, this kind of surgery was out for me; Dr. Crile himself would not recommend it. He wrote: "Cancers that are large
in relation to the size of the breast, cancers that are located near
the center of the breast . . . are *not* well adapted to treatment
by partial mastectomy." Since my unwanted lump bordered the
nipple of my left breast, I could not be a candidate for less than
total removal, should the diagnosis be cancer.

The problem I would have to face then was not whether to have a mastectomy or not, but what kind of mastectomy.

There are several types of "lesser surgeries"—lesser, that is, than mastectomy, or complete removal of the breast. Lumpectomy, tylectomy, and local excision are nothing but other names for an excisional biopsy—the tumor is removed, along with a bit of surrounding tissue.

Partial mastectomies, segmental resections, and wedge resections, on the other hand, are the removal of somewhat more than the growth itself and a little tissue. Depending on the size of the tumor and its location, the surgeon also excises a considerable part of the breast, the overlying skin, and the underlying fascia, or membrane. The breast is left smaller, but still a breast. Obviously, there is not much sense in using this procedure if the nipple is involved, since the remaining curve minus the nipple would not look very breastlike.

There is also a plastic-surgery breast operation—mammoplasty —called subcutaneous mastectomy. Here, the nipple and skin of the mammary gland are preserved intact, but the contents are scooped out and replaced with a silicone-pad insert (*not* an injection). The incision is then closed with fine, almost invisible stitches. Axillary nodes may or may not be removed. Plastic surgeons have developed many of these ingenious reconstructive surgeries, which enable women, under certain circumstances, to have everything that is malignant removed internally, while to outward appearances a normal breast remains. Such surgery has added risks, but many women are willing to take them.

Except for these operations, however, all mastectomies involve the amputation of that part of our bodies we women know as our breasts. In the one called the simple, or—as doctors now prefer—the total, mastectomy, only the breast is removed, leaving the nodes intact.

The radical mastectomy is more extensive. In one kind of radical mastectomy, known as the Halsted, the pectoral muscles of the chest are also removed. In the modified radical mastectomy, these are left in place. There are several ways to accomplish this so that any nodes lying under the pectorals can be seen and removed. In the standard modified radical, both of the pectoral muscles, the pectoralis major and minor, are retracted (held back by special instruments); another version, the Patey modified radical, developed in England, requires the muscles to be cut and restitched, if necessary. *All* radical mastectomies require that the nodes in the armpit be cut out.

I absorbed all this with what seems now to have been an almost insane clearheadedness I never could muster while cramming for final exams during my college days.

As I have said, I recognized immediately that anything less than removing the entire breast was out for me if the lump was malignant.

Frankly, I could not understand why there was so much medical fuss about leaving the nodes, via the simple (or total) mastectomy, if there was any chance that some of them might be cancerous. I thought the important parts of me were the external breast and the internal chest muscles—in that order —yet surgeons and researchers kept arguing about taking out or leaving in the axillary lymph nodes. To me, looking as normal as possible minus the breast, having as little scarring as possible, and getting out all of the cancer were the important issues—not the invisible nodes. Later, I was to learn about the importance of the nodes.

After reading the literature and telephoning some friends at the National Cancer Institute, I made my choice: a modified radical mastectomy, if my lump turned out to be cancer. My breast and lymph nodes would be removed; the chest muscles controlling my left arm would stay with me.

Although I knew that 90 per cent of the surgeons in the United States who perform mastectomies do the Halsted radical, I found no cancer expert—in books or by personal questioning—who thought it was necessary to take out the pectoral muscles.

"But it depends on what the surgeon learned in school and during his training," a friend warned. "Don't let any inexperienced guy do you a favor by leaving your muscles alone if all he's ever done in his life are Halsteds. You don't want to be his guinea pig."

Another friend at the NCI agreed. "The Halsted's easier. It's like being a barber. You don't need to be as expert just to shave all the hair off as to give somebody a good-looking cut. And if a surgeon is used to having a clear field of vision, with no muscles in his way," he continued, "he could easily miss a couple of positive nodes."

Nevertheless, it was to be a modified radical mastectomy for me, provided I needed one, even if I had to go to Timbuktu to find an experienced surgeon to do it.

Friday morning came, and the thermogram was taken. In spite of my pleas of urgency, I could get no promise of an early reading. When the result was finally called in to Dr. Heckman weeks later—while I was already recuperating from the mastectomy— it was: "Mildly suspicious neovascularization of the left breast around the areola." This was a bit more accurate than the mammogram, I agree. But my cancerous tumor had been no microscopic "centricle"; it had been a full-blown, palpable lump. The diagnosis from the thermogram had not been something that could be trusted, either.

I spent the time between the thermogram and my two-o'clock appointment at the breast-tumor clinic of the National Cancer Institute shopping for a new wardrobe of underwear. I had no premonition; I just had two hours to kill, with Lord & Taylor on my way from the Georgetown University Hospital to NIH. Besides, even an overnight stay in the hospital for a biopsy deserved better than the raggedy old nightgowns I had been wearing. Some wild bikini panties also went into my shopping bag. And I bought two new-style bras that latched in the front, for easier opening and closing.

I repeat, I had no superstitious premonition! I just needed new underwear.

After a long wait in the breast clinic, I unhappily discovered that becoming a patient in a federal facility means a lot of rigmarole and red tape—even when you have friends working there. Because of certain inflexible laws, no surgeon could put a scalpel to my lump unless and until I underwent considerable preoperative testing and examination, which took about ten days to two weeks.

"I thought we weren't supposed to wait," I complained to the doctor who examined my lump. "They always say, 'Rush to your physician.'"

He smiled. "Don't wait six months," he said. "But ten days

won't matter. The tests and scans have to be done in advance."

He explained that if all the preoperative tests were negative, then an operation would be scheduled. However, if they turned up any sign of existing spread of a malignancy into bones, stomach, or other organs, there was no point in operating at all. "A mastectomy is done to arrest the carcinoma," he said. "If the disease has already metastasized beyond the regional nodes—in your case, the ones in the left axilla—there's no reason to put you through the ordeal at all. We'd go right to chemotherapy."

"But I don't even know that it *is* cancer," I wailed. "The mammogram said benign fibrocystic disease. Do the biopsy, and then we'll worry about your scans and tests."

"What you say makes a lot of sense from an ordinary medical point of view," he conceded. "But this is a research hospital, established by law to conduct clinical trials under certain rather rigid rules. One of these is that every patient must have a complete work-up before anything at all is done, so that we have base-line data on everything." He smiled apologetically. "A good many of the tests might be helpful in other areas of NIH research."

Maybe this was what Dr. Heckman had meant when he said "if you like a research setup" so scornfully.

"I don't know if my mind can stand the wait, even if my body can," I said now.

The doctor nodded his agreement. "I understand. If it were my wife, I'd tell her to have the tumor biopsied immediately. Then, if it was diagnosed as carcinoma, she could have the mastectomy without worrying about being in a protocol. That's what we call a clinical trial," he explained, "a protocol. Every one has its own guidelines and requirements here."

Suddenly the almost forgotten cramp in my belly was back. His face, his tone of voice, his attitude, all shouted that, negative mammogram or not, his fingers told him a mastectomy would be needed. For two days I had been unpanicked; now I was again gripped by dread.

"Do you have any friends in private practice?" I asked him.

He took a pad and wrote down the names of some surgeons he knew in the area who had had considerable cancer training.

"I don't know if they're involved with breasts," he said. "But

I've trained with them all in oncology in various places around the country."

My clothes flew on, and I cashed two dollars into dimes. Locking myself into a public phone booth, I started on his list.

"No patient is going to tell me how to do my surgery," one of them growled when I asked for a two-stage operation—biopsy now, mastectomy later. "I've never heard of such a thing."

"You're absolutely ridiculous!" another exploded. "If the diagnosis is positive on frozen section, the breast must come off immediately."

And so it went.

Frantically, I called Dr. Heckman at 4:50 and outlined what had happened.

"Calm down," he urged. "If you want just the biopsy without a mastectomy, you don't need a cancer specialist. I told you before, any competent surgeon can do that. What about the man who did Harvey's herniorrhaphy?"

He was right, of course. And I had a better chance of getting things done my way with a long-time family surgeon, who had stitched many a child's cut in addition to that hernia.

"Don't be so pessimistic," the surgeon soothed, when I reached him by phone. "You're probably making a mountain out of a molehill. After all, eight out of ten breast tumors are benign. Take it easy." He did want to know why I was so insistent on having the operation done in two stages.

"If the thing is cancer," I told him honestly, "I'm going to NCI or to Sloan-Kettering, in New York, to find a breast-cancer specialist."

"But the mammogram diagnosed it as benign?"

"Yes," I said. "Otherwise I'd be on a plane up there for the biopsy, too."

He sounded offended. "What do you mean?"

"I'd feel like an idiot, running off to a cancer hospital when the only test there is says it's nothing."

"I think you're being unnecessarily gloomy," he said. "But I'll go along with you. I'm sure it's probably a cyst or something benign."

He kindly met me long after his regular office hours, examined the tumor, tried to aspirate the contents with a hypodermic

needle (nothing aspirated), and said he would schedule the biopsy as soon as possible, because hospital beds were in short
supply.

"Fine," I agreed.

With the help of a lawyer, I drafted a legalistic document, to
be countersigned by the surgeon before my operation, refusing
to authorize him or the hospital to do anything more than a
biopsy.

24 June, 1974

Under no circumstance is   or anyone else in the
operating room of   to perform
the procedure known as mastectomy (removal of either breast).

I hereby release   and all other parties connected with the above consented-to procedure from any liability
for damage sustained by me due to my refusal to consent to the
performance of mastectomy (removal of either breast).

ROSE KUSHNER

On admission to the hospital the following Tuesday, I scratched
lines through the part of the routine form every new patient must
sign that gives blanket permission to the doctor and the hospital
to do anything "deemed necessary." I also blacked out the part
that gives permission to dispose of "the tissue removed." Nobody
objected at the time. My surgeon treated the contract as a huge
joke, signing it with a flourish as I watched from my stretcher.

"Ready to be put to sleep now, worrywart?" he scolded when
I finished rereading it.

Afterward, he was not so flippant. He seemed to take my refusal to let him do the mastectomy as a personal insult, although
I had told him more than once that I planned to find a breast-
cancer specialist to do it. He must have forgotten; or perhaps
he hadn't understood me in the first place.

I was still drifting in and out of anesthetic euphoria when his
face appeared, grim and angry, over the rail of my crib.

"I've got bad news," he said. "It's cancer."

Without another word, my noble healer turned away and

went to the anteroom with the same message for my worried husband.

One of the nurses told me I had hurt his feelings badly. "He's considered one of the best general surgeons around," she explained.

"I know," I recall telling her sleepily. "But for cancer I want more than a general surgeon."

She patted my hand. "I'd do the same thing in your shoes, Mrs. Kushner," she assured me. "Exactly the same thing."

Since I had not entered a protocol at the National Cancer Institute for the biopsy, it would have taken the intervention of friends to have the mastectomy done there. Besides, July 1 (and the beginning of a new medical and fiscal year) was only a week away, and not even the most influential of friends could get space for me on an operating-room schedule upset by vacations, rotating staffs, and new budgets.

"The end of June is no time to expect any action from any government agency," one of them told me sadly. "There's nothing I can do now until July 1." Because the biopsy had already been performed, he suggested I not wait. "Nobody's sure about anything, you understand," he explained. "But most experts think a woman shouldn't play around once the tumor is cut out. It could have been nicked or something."

I needed no encouragement from anyone. I was ready to run. The day after the biopsy, Harvey and I left for New York, pathology slides and tumor (pickled in sauce) in hand.

Unlike the National Cancer Institute, Memorial Sloan-Kettering Cancer Center is a private institution. A friend at NIH had arranged an appointment for me that same afternoon with one of its top breast-cancer specialists, and before any surgery could be scheduled, I first had to be examined by him in his office. Of course, I already knew the diagnosis was carcinoma. I was still groggy from the general anesthetic and shock as I listened to the surgeon tell me what he would do.

"There will be a vertical incision. I'll excise the breast, axillary nodes, pectoral muscles, and pectoral nodes," he said in a monotone. "You will have some numbness for a variable period of time. There will be some temporary muscular disability, which can be overcome with proper exercise, but some permanent disability in your left arm may remain. There may also be some permanent swelling. This varies."

The room was quiet and his voice was soft. In the state I was in, his words barely penetrated. The only things I remember hearing were "Fourth of July . . . shortage of staff . . . new interns and residents . . . no beds."

The important words, "Halsted radical," were never mentioned, and so I never heard them.

We left the office, with the nurse promising to get me a bed as soon as possible. It was not until I had had two sips of a very strong Scotch, back in our hotel, that the full meaning of what the doctor had said entered my befuddled brain.

"He wants to do a Halsted," I told Harvey weakly. "That's what he meant by the pectoral muscles and permanent disability. It didn't sink in."

"I've been calling all over to see if anybody I know has influence with Sloan-Kettering, so we can get you in right away," he said.

"Forget it! I'm not having a Halsted. We've got to find out where I can get a modified."

I was so terrified by the surgeon's quiet description of the Halsted he proposed to do that it never occurred to me to ask if someone at Sloan-Kettering would do a modified radical mastectomy instead. In my panicky state, I assumed it was standard hospital policy to do Halsteds, not a matter of a surgeon's personal preference.

After some frantic telephoning, a business associate in the New York office of Harvey's firm gave me the name of an internist in Manhattan, who referred me to Roswell Park Memorial Institute, in Buffalo, where, he told me, Halsteds are never done. Roswell Park, a New York State hospital, is the oldest cancer hospital in the world, dating back to 1895—and, as I was to learn, is one of the best there is. We flew up to Buffalo that same evening, and I was examined the next morning by Dr. Thomas L. Dao.

Under the direction of Dr. Dao, who is chief of both breast-cancer surgery and breast-cancer research, I was X-rayed and tested in advance, as the National Cancer Institute surgeon had told me I should be. That took two days. By the time Dr. Dao came in to announce that I "could be scheduled for surgery," that "everything was clear and clean," being a suitable candidate for mastectomy was the best news anyone could have given me.

As I had learned all too well by then, breast-cancer experts do not perform any mastectomy if there are signs that the malignancy has metastasized beyond the regional nodes, since it is pointless to put a woman through major surgery when the cancer has already spread. So my good test results meant that—as far as any mortal could determine in advance—the little centimeter-long tumor removed in the biopsy had been all there was. It had been caught in time. But the mastectomy still had to be done, in the event I had any multicentricles—those microscopic scattered cancers that often grow, along with the big one, in other parts of the breast. And the radical part of the mastectomy—removing the lymph nodes in the armpit—was necessary, to know if the nodes had been invaded.

Suddenly, surprisingly, hilariously, being able to have a mastectomy had become good news! As they say, everything is relative.

The operation was long and tedious for Dr. Dao, but uneventful for the rest of the twelve-man team. None of my nodes was malignant on gross examination—to the naked eye, without a microscope—and there weren't any visible pieces of tumor that could be retrieved for an experiment Dr. Dao's laboratory was working on. Pretending to be disappointed, Dr. Dao came into my room grinning as I woke up. "I couldn't even find a little bit. There was absolutely nothing. If anything has spread to the nodes, it was microscopic."

My physical recovery is described in another chapter, and the psychological details are elsewhere, too. But I am going to talk here about one aspect of my experience as a cancer patient, because going to a research hospital is so frowned upon by many doctors, and because these institutions so often are thought of as last resorts for hopeless cases.

I admit that my first half day in Roswell Park was a difficult adjustment. All I could think of was Alexander Solzhenitsyn's *Cancer Ward;* I didn't belong with all these people. Although few had any visible signs of being cancerous, *I* knew they were. Why was I here?

It took a while to accept the fact that I did belong. In retro-
spect, it was only a few hours before I began to realize the
benefits of being in a cancer ward. The first advantage was the
incredibly sensitive care everyone gave every patient. From
the cleaning staff up to the top physicians, all are specially trained
to deal with patients who have a potentially fatal disease. The
treatment is a combination of intensive attention to the most insignificant symptom and the almost pitiless realism of "Everyone
has to die sometime." The entire staff has been taught how to
live with the prospect of death, and the patients are the bene-
ficiaries.

Second, I had the support and comfort of people who had lived
with cancer as long as twelve years. A plumber who had been
brought in as terminal years before puffed on his cigar while he
described the advanced treatments available only at places like
this, treatments that had kept him alive, reasonably well, and
still plumbing after that diagnosis of terminal. In the course of
his more than a decade of intermittent care at Roswell Park,
he told me, he had developed and regressed at least sixteen cancerous tumors throughout his body.

It is a very personal decision whether to go to a research hospital. Institutions like Roswell Park do make certain demands on
patients that non-research hospitals do not make. Physicians,
nurses, psychologists, and social workers often interview and
question patients. Members of the medical staff may want to
examine their wounds; many people object to being handled by
anyone but their private physicians, except for emergency care.
As for being part of a random sample, I may have been, for all
I know. My operation may have been done using a new type of
scalpel, while a sample of other women were cut by an older
instrument. I honestly don't know. But what difference does it
make?

If anything untried and unproven—and with possibly serious
consequences—is to be done, patients or their families must give
what is called "informed consent." The experimental procedure
must be explained, as well as the reasons the physician feels it
should be done. Papers are signed by the patient or the family
to authorize any extraordinary treatments. This was not necessary
in my case; the mastectomy was quite humdrum.

I also want to stress the value of breast self-examination (BSE) and the value of mammography. Although the technique did not diagnose my own cancer accurately, the mammogram (xero- or conventional) is the best external detection technique available today. Thermography, while not nearly as reliable yet, will undoubtedly be perfected.

Even the best mammography can give a "false negative" diagnosis, and that is why I say—as strongly as possible—that all strange lumps should be removed, no matter what the tests show. (A woman who is constantly "lumpy" or "cysty" is one of the few exceptions to this rule.)

Last, I do not doubt that there may be surgical treatments for breast cancer equally as effective—by current standards—as the modified radical mastectomy. I had, for instance, read in advance about the Edinburgh and Cardiff clinical trials of simple (or total) mastectomy along with irradiation of the nodes, but I decided against that route for me. While the "end results"—the survival rates—were not much different from the results of other treatments, I felt that my own temperament and my status in life could not tolerate the uncertainty about the condition of my nodes.

I mention status in life because I have found that age, marital status, and family enter into every decision about breast cancer. No one can put herself in another woman's place. In my own case, being almost forty-five, with my youngest child reaching sixteen, and being guaranteed an operation with minimal physical aftereffects, I simply did not want the worry and the inevitable side effects I would have if the axillary nodes were left in and irradiated. Other women may feel differently—and, as far as I can find out, the outcome is pretty much the same after ten years or so. The important thing is that what I chose was my own decision.

I must add here, for women's liberationists who see an evil plot to mutilate women by mastectomy, that I found none—anywhere. There has definitely been male chauvinism—enough to warrant a separate chapter later. But I found no one like Dr. Towers, the sadistic surgeon Henry Bellaman describes in his novel *King's Row* (the role played in the movie by Claude Raines). I found no surgeons, male or female, who have any doubts that radical mastectomy offers women their best chance to survive breast cancer. This—not male chauvinism—is why mastectomies are recommended.

The controversial issues are separating the diagnostic biopsy from mastectomy, what kind of mastectomy should be performed, and who should decide. In my case, the choices were my own.

Again, my ideas may differ from those of other women. But the point of this book is to show that we women should be free, knowledgeable, and completely conscious when the time comes for a decision, so that we can make it for ourselves. *Our* lives are at stake, not a surgeon's.

My experience is no model of what to do or not to do. It is only one example of what women can do—if they have some information to go on.

It also does no harm to have a streak of stubbornness, and a loud voice as well.

2

What Is Cancer?
What Is Breast Cancer?

Vung Tau, South Vietnam, October 22, 1967: The short, square-faced Vietnamese major, wearing the black pajamas of the Revolutionary Development Cadre, was briefing the press (me).

"Mao Tse-tung has written that the insurgent guerrilla is a fish, and the people are the water that nourishes the fish," Major Nguyen Bé chanted. "I would like to change Chairman Mao's quotation." He smiled.

"To me, an insurgent is like a fragment of cancer in a healthy body—invading, destroying, and drawing its nourishment from the healthy organs around it. The goal of this fragment of cancer is not to live peacefully side by side; its goal is to replace all the healthy organs with the disease. Its aim is the total destruction of the body—in the case of a nation, the government."

It was hot and the small room was not air-conditioned. To keep out Vung Tau's gargantuan mosquitoes, the windows were tightly closed. The ancient French ceiling fan droned lazily around, so slowly that each of its four blades could be clearly defined. I was the only reporter to attend the briefing that beautiful Sunday afternoon; everyone else was romping on the silken white sands of the resort's famous beach.

Major Bé doggedly pursued his analogy. "A healthy stomach, for example, does not voluntarily give to the fragment of cancer the vitamins, minerals, and other substances it needs to live,"

31

he explained. "The malignancy takes these materials from the healthy stomach against its will. The cancer forces the healthy stomach to bring about its own death."

His physiology was bad, but his English was excellent. And his parallel between what he thought the rebellious insurgents were doing in Vietnam and what a cancer does when it invades an organ was a novel approach to me. I made a note to remember it when I tried to describe the Vietnam war to my readers back home. Everybody, of course, knows what cancer is, I thought to myself. That will make it easier to describe what this crazy civil war in Vietnam is all about.

The idea that within a few years I would be trying to define cancer via the Vietnam-war analogy never occurred to me. But here I am doing exactly that.

A human body invaded by cancer is like a country battling a small guerrilla insurgency. If the government (the body) is strong and healthy, if there are no weak spots in its economy (possible genetic predisposing factors), if there are no traitors within the government to help the enemy (chemical, viral, or radiation carcinogens), and if the defense machinery (the immunological system) is strong, then the insurgency can be put down with a minimum of over-all damage. However, bodies and governments are rarely fault-free. A microscopic cancerous rebellion, started in the proper environment and supported and nourished by various contributing factors, can grow and grow, until—like the war in Vietnam—it endangers the very life of the whole body. Without the right kind of outside treatment, the malignancy will inevitably cause the body's death.

To understand cancer, it is important to know a little about a normal cell and how it works. Cells—all cells—are microscopic bits of a jellolike material called protoplasm. Inside the cell is a structure called the nucleus, and around the outside of the cell is a membrane that filters certain materials in and others out. Scattered through the cell are various microscopic factories that extract whatever they need from the nutrients that are sieved through the membrane from the blood stream. The most important work of cells is to produce energy to support the functions of the particular organ in which a cell is situated and—except for muscle and nerve cells—to reproduce themselves, by mitosis, or division. (Nerve and muscle cells—including those of the heart—do not reproduce; when we are born, we have all of them we will ever have.)

Cells reproduce at different intervals. Those of the blood and skin, for example, reproduce rapidly, liver cells very slowly. But they all reproduce by the same technique—mitosis.

Inside the nucleus of every cell of every animal is a certain number of chromosomes, arranged in strands. Every organism has a different number; humans normally have forty-six, twenty-three inherited from each parent. At specified, regulated periods in every cell's life, the strands of chromosomes begin to duplicate themselves, in a process called twinning. When a double set of "daughter" chromosomes has developed, the two strands separate from each other and move toward opposite sides of the cell. The two sets of daughter chromosomes will be parts of the nuclei of two new daughter cells by the time the cell division is completed.

Meanwhile, the outer membrane of the cell has developed a barely perceptible waistline, which indents quickly into a wasp waist once the daughter chromosomes are in place. The "cleavage"—the last stage of mitosis—occurs when the parent cell breaks apart at the waistline into two daughter cells.

After resting for whatever length of time their biological stop clock has decreed they should, the daughter cells begin the reproductive cycle again.

Until the electron microscope was invented, the existence of this stop clock was theory, not fact. How a cell knew what to do, and when, was one of the big mysteries of life. Now scientists have unraveled enough about the computer-tape-like chromosomes to know that they are winding strips of complex molecules called deoxyribonucleic acid—DNA, or "genes." Everyone knew about genes, those bits of matter on the chromosomes that somehow pass along parental traits and characteristics. But it took the electron microscope to show that the bits are not just passengers on the chains, but are actually segments of DNA, hooked together in two linked spirals—the "double helix."

If all goes well, and the chromosomes duplicate and split identically, without an error, or mutation, the daughter cells will look and behave exactly like the parent—down to having the same stop clock, for instance.

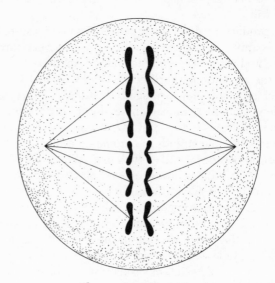

Chromosomes Twinning

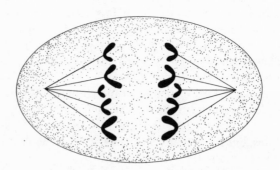

"Daughter" Chromosomes Moving Apart

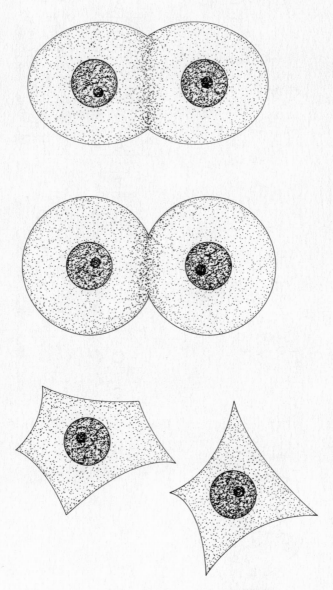

Cleavage of a Cell into Two New "Daughter" Cells

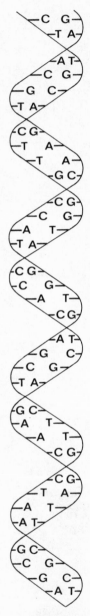

DNA Helix

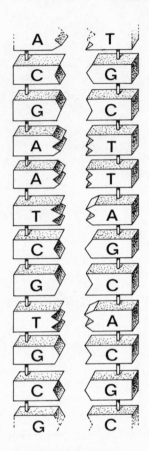

Diagram of Part of a DNA Molecule

But there are those mutations.

Serious mutations happen rarely. Considering that DNA consists of thousands of units of four different substances, arranged in a very precise order, it is a marvel that mistakes are not more frequent. For example, the same two substances must always be paired directly opposite each other on the twisting chains. If for some reason just two units on a chain are switched, this pairing would not occur. In addition, adjacent pairings of the other two substances would also be mutated.

Sometimes the mutation is so damaging that the cell dies altogether. But most errors are not so severe; they just change the way one particular gene behaves. If the mutation is in the gene that regulates iron absorption, say, that one cell's daughter cells and their descendants will not use this mineral normally. However, the end result of this kind of mutation is unlikely to affect the over-all functioning of the organ very seriously.

On the other hand, if the mutation is in the gene that regulates the growth and reproduction of the cell itself, the result could be cancer. This is how all cancers begin: one cell loses control over its own reproductive machinery, and a neoplasm—a malignant tumor—is born.

Before going on, I must emphasize that the cellular reproduction under discussion here is *not* the kind of reproduction that results in a baby. Gamete reproduction—both the sperm and the egg are gametes—is a unique and different process. (Mutations can occur in the genes of the sperm or the egg, or in the developing baby during pregnancy—mutations that could cause albinism, a different color in each eye, physical malformation, and some diseases. Also, there are some neonatal cancers—for example, Wilms' tumor, a kidney malignancy.)

Most of us think of genes only in relation to babies. Genes are actually present in every cell of every organ in the body from fertilization onward and are constantly being duplicated by mitosis throughout the organism's lifetime. In humans, by the way, it is a random half of the forty-six chromosomes that makes up the twenty-three each parent gives to the sperm or the egg. Each sperm and each egg hold a different selection of chromosomes from the father and mother. (Only identical twins, the result of a freakish separation of the fertilized egg, have the same sets of chromosomes.)

Returning to mutations that affect cellular reproduction, one way this function can be altered is by a chance or accidental disarrangement in the gene governing growth and reproduction. Other suspects are chemicals that get into our tissues one way or another. In the case of some neoplasms—including some of the breast cancers—viruses may be the causative agents. Irradiation from the sun's rays, from X-rays, and from nuclear particles can also affect that important dot of DNA and cause a cell to "transform" from being healthy to being cancerous.

So far, nothing has been targeted as a single cause of malignancy in the cells of the breast, although there are many theories. The process is known, however. For a healthy cell to become malignant, its growth-and-reproduction gene must be changed during the brief period when the chromosomes are twinning. Whatever the cause of the cancer may be, the basic mechanism is the same: a foul-up during the duplication of the gene that computer-programs how much a cell will grow, how rapidly it will divide, and how long it will continue to reproduce.

Just think, if the cells of the body did not have such a preordained brake on their growth and reproduction, we would have a world filled with giants; all of us would be eternally growing children who never reached adulthood. Luckily, there is a built-in stop light, and cells eventually reach a point at which they reproduce exactly the number required to replace those that die off, but no more.

If they are normal cells, that is. Cancer cells never stop reproducing.

Understanding the role of DNA and mutations clarified how cancer begins, but it did not help me understand the step-by-step transformation of a normal cell to a malignant one. I asked a research professor I was interviewing for a simple explanation.

"Something occurs in the growth gene during the twinning process," he explained. "This can best be described by showing you a very simplified diagram of the life cycle of a cell."

I studied the diagram while he continued his professorial lecture. "The life cycle of a normal cell can be divided into four periods. There is D—it stands for division—the period during

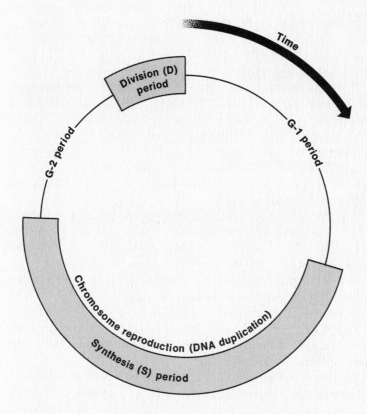

Life Cycle of a Cell

which actual separation into two cells occurs.* This is followed by a stage called the G-1—meaning Gap 1—period, which begins as soon as the previous mitosis has been completed and lasts until the beginning of the next cycle of DNA duplication. That is the S—for synthesis—period, when the DNA molecules—those forty-six chromosomes in the human—manufacture their identical twins. The G-2 period is the interval during which the two sets of chromosomes move apart and the parent cell prepares to break into two daughter cells.

---

* Many scientists call this the M period—for mitosis, the technical term for cell division.

"While the length of the G-1 period varies from organ to organ, the other phases are the same in all cells. The G-2 period lasts two hours, D takes forty minutes, and S seven hours." He seemed to be enjoying himself.

"The single gene, or segment of DNA, in every cell that is preprogramed to control growth and reproduction knows exactly how frequently that particular cell should divide," the professor went on. "The gene also knows when the cell should stop reproducing altogether and just stay dormant, remaining so until the tissue of which it is a part needs new cells to replace those that have died. This resting phase occurs during the G-1 period in every healthy cell, but different kinds of cells have different dormant times."

He reminded me that nerve and muscle cells are arrested in the G-1 period when the organism is born and never reproduce again. Blood and skin cells, on the other hand, have very short G-1 periods, and are always making new daughters.

Then the professor gave me a list of books to read for more information about transformation—the process by which a normal cell becomes malignant.

Using as my mental guide an accidental switch in the arrangement of the substances of the growth gene, transformation was not too hard to understand.

During the S period of the cell, while the chromosomes are twinning, that accidental switch will be duplicated, too. The chromosome carrying the altered gene will make two new chromosomes with the same mutation built into them. The two resulting daughter cells will be different from their parent cell.

Their built-in brake has been changed, and it no longer tells them when to stop growing and go into G-1 sleep, as their healthy sisters do. Instead, the mutated daughter cells keep dividing and making new daughters quite madly, on their own new preprogramed schedule.

In normal breast tissue, for example, cells generally go to sleep after twenty or thirty divisions and stay in G-1 until the breast signals that it needs some replacement parts. The cells then wake up and go through just enough "passages" to fill the order, before they return again to their dormant G-1 period. Their transformed sisters, however, keep on reproducing themselves long after the need for new cells has passed. They have become cancer.

Cancer cells do absolutely nothing to benefit the body. They do not supply energy or support the functions of the tissues or organs they are part of; they only use up nutrients to make more and more cancer cells. As Major Bé said, in comparing them with the Vietcong guerrillas, they help themselves to what they need from surrounding healthy tissue, turning an entire organ—if unchecked—into a cancerous one.

Cancer is also very species-specific. That is, each type has an affinity only for certain animals. The mouse gets almost every kind of cancer there is; the monkey gets few. Injecting a monkey with tissue taken from a cancerous cat would probably not give the monkey the disease. Dogs get breast cancer, but not the same kind that thrives in mice or in humans.

This selectivity of cancer is one of the major obstacles to research. Experimentation cannot be done on humans, of course, but with many diseases it is often possible to extrapolate, or apply to humans, information from experiments on lower animals. The species-specificity of cancer, according to many authorities, makes extrapolation unreliable for investigating this disease.

These, then, are the characteristics that all kinds of cancers have in common: They are caused by something that upsets the segment of DNA in a particular cell that controls its growth and reproduction. They never stop growing, but appear to proliferate wildly and invade other parts of the body helter-skelter. They contribute nothing whatsoever toward the functioning of the organism. The disease is highly species-specific.

Here the nature of cancer changes, and every kind seems to go its own way.

Cancer is actually a blanket term that covers more than a hundred different types of invasive diseases, which are very different from each other except for the factors just mentioned. For example, if a breast cancer metastasizes to the lung, this secondary tumor will be composed of the same kind of cell as those in the breast growth. But a primary lung cancer—one originating in the lung—will be composed of a different kind of cell.

Some cancers, particularly the leukemias, afflict young people; prostatic carcinoma mainly attacks older men. Some organs are seldom, if ever, invaded; cancer of the heart is a medical rarity. In other words, while anything that is malignant and invasive can be called cancer, "cancer" is really many different diseases, with different causes, victims, and treatments.

When scientists speak of cancer's "wild, uncontrolled proliferation," they are comparing the malignant cells with the normal ones around them. In fact, the disease's growth is rigidly controlled by certain rules that are seldom broken.

Neoplastic cells reproduce rapidly or slowly, depending on the reproduction rate of the normal cells of the same organ. Healthy liver cells reproduce slowly, and so do cancerous ones; healthy blood cells reproduce rapidly, and so do cancerous ones.

Of course, if an organ is damaged or injured, the trauma triggers the dormant growth gene back into immediate reproduction. If one kidney is removed, for example, the normally slow-growing cells in the remaining organ begin reproduction to take over the work of its missing twin. A damaged liver—whose cells normally reproduce slowly—will regenerate quickly. Adults whose bones have stopped growing will suddenly get new bone cells if a limb is broken and needs repair. Also, once a malignant invasion begins in a slow-reproducing organ like the liver, the presence of cancer cells can itself foul up the growth genes of neighboring normal cells and trigger cancer, just as trauma does. This phenomenon is not well understood, but it does occur.

The important thing, though, is that cancerous cells never *stop* reproducing and soon outstrip the growth of the healthy tissue surrounding them.

The second rule that governs cancer growth is more complicated, but when it is explained, one of the puzzles of cancer becomes easier to understand. This is the phenomenon of doubling time.

Often a person with cancer will say, "I just had a checkup a couple of months ago, and then the lump was only a little thing to keep an eye on. It is the size of a marble now." The reason is doubling time.

By the time any neoplasm—not only one in the breast—is large enough to be palpable, or felt, it has gone through at least thirty "generations" of doubling in size. (This assumes that a lump can be palpated when it weighs one gram.) Thirty doublings can take anywhere from weeks to many years; the length of time depends on the kind of cell it is. Doubling is not haphazard, but is a steady, exponential growth that one writer has described as obeying "the compound-interest law": each increase in size is added in before the next increase is calculated.

There is a big difference between cancer and a bank account, however. An especially high-yield bank might pay a depositor 10 per cent in interest every year. Cancer's interest rate is 100 per cent, compounded more frequently. One cell becomes two, two become four, then eight, sixteen, thirty-two, and so on, until after some twenty generations there are about 1 million cells, weighing approximately one milligram (one-thousandth of a gram). The tumor is still in its "preclinical" stage, invisible to the human eye and not palpable by even very sensitive and experienced fingers.

Then the compound-interest law that brought a single cell to 1 million cells in twenty generations will take the milligram of cancer and multiply it by a thousand in just ten more generations. After thirty doublings, there will be 1 billion cells, weighing one gram. A tumor this size can easily be palpated.

Bear in mind that it grew a thousand times larger in half the time required for it to reach a thousandth of a gram. If the gram-size cancer is not detected and removed at this stage, one more generation will increase it to two grams. Another single generation will make it four grams. (Of course, cancer cells, like other cells, do die. Unfortunately, their death rates are far lower than their birth rates.)

To put doubling into another kind of time frame, a tumor having a 100-day cycle, which took nine years to grow from a single cell to a one-gram lump—the size at which it can be felt—would take only about fifteen months longer to become a tumor weighing about sixteen grams—about half an ounce. In just another fifteen months, it would weigh about a pound. Thus, in exactly the same length of time, the size of the neoplasm would increase thirty-two times!

The same exponential rules of doubling apply to metastases. If, when a primary cancer is discovered, a secondary one is also

Doubling Time "Atomic Explosion"

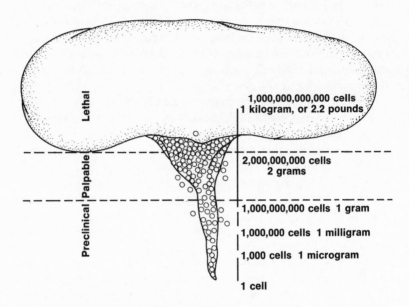

1,000,000,000,000 cells
1 kilogram, or 2.2 pounds

2,000,000,000 cells
2 grams

1,000,000,000 cells 1 gram

1,000,000 cells 1 milligram

1,000 cells 1 microgram

1 cell

Lethal

Palpable

Preclinical

Reproduced with permission from *Scientific Foundations
of Oncology* by T. Symington and R. L. Carter.
William Heinemann Medical Books Ltd., London.

found somewhere else in the body, it is a sign that the metastasis
began very early in the life of the first malignancy. Otherwise,
it would not be palpable.

President Gerald Ford, in an announcement about his wife's
breast cancer, wondered aloud how a tumor an inch in diameter
could have developed in the seven months since her last physical
examination. Cancer's laws of proliferation and doubling time
are the explanation. It almost seems like an optical illusion, this
business of having nothing and then something relatively enormous within a few short months. But that is the nature of the
growth of cancer. It is very important to understand this dou-
bling-time rule, because the best hope of curing breast cancer
today is to find ways to diagnose it during those first twenty
generations of preclinical life—before a lump can be felt.

Although doubling time applies to all cancers, palpability of a
mass is useless as a test for tumors of the ovary, pancreas, liver,

or other deep-seated organs. By the time such cancers are symptomatic, it is usually too late for anything.

Benign tumors, by the way, are caused by somewhat the same kind of disturbance of the growth gene that makes a cell cancerous. The difference is that benign tumors usually grow more slowly and in due course stop growing; they remain localized, *do not metastasize,* and do not destroy normal cells while they are growing. Benign-tumor cells live peacefully side by side with healthy ones. Many people believe—wrongly—that a benign tumor, if ignored, will become malignant, but this seldom happens. A benign growth in the breast, for example, is usually not dangerous in itself. The reason it should be removed (and the same reasoning applies to benign tumors elsewhere) is that it could mask or hide a cancerous growth, either by growing around the neoplasm or by shielding it from the diagnostic eye of the mammograph.

I once met a veteran sports reporter who constantly griped about the trials and tribulations of having to deal with athletes. "Why in the world did you decide to be a sportswriter, then?" I asked him. "You don't seem to like the people you have to cover."

"I'll tell you why, honey." The old man grinned. His eyes crinkled closed and he chuckled. "It's the only kind of journalism there is where a guy doesn't have to start every new piece by saying, 'Baseball is a game with nine players on each side. One is the pitcher, a second the catcher. The other seven are field men. The game is played with two teams on a field shaped like a diamond.' And so on and so on, the way everybody else has to do in a regular news piece."

I have a similar advantage now. I certainly do not have to say, "Female breasts are two globular organs located on a woman's chest in the area between her shoulders and her waistline." But it may well be necessary to add the reminder that the primary function of the breasts, the reason they are there, is to make milk for feeding the young. Although they have been sex symbols from the beginning of time, the mammary glands were *not* created for the purpose of attracting males.

From the day a teen-age girl begins to menstruate, her breasts regularly prepare themselves, month after month, for a possible pregnancy. Organs like the heart and lungs may work harder twenty-four hours a day, but the breasts have many more, and more varied, jobs to perform. Their continual cyclical change of function is accompanied by changes in the tissues and cells, and this is the main reason the female breast is especially vulnerable to cellular damage. Any routine that is constantly being upset by one interruption or another—even if it is perfectly natural for it to be upset—is subject to a greater risk of errors. The overworked breast cell is always being bathed in some hormone that orders, "Stop doing that. Start doing this." No wonder so many of the daughter cells go haywire.

The largest number of breast cancers occurs in the milk ducts, where the cells are most subject to being annoyed by hormonal or chemical agitators. Relatively few start in the fatty tissues, which have considerably less work to do.

Not only does the breast perform an enormous number of jobs; it also contains every kind of tissue to be found anywhere in the body, except for bone. And each tissue—skin, duct, fiber, fat, and the rest—has a different vulnerability. As if this were not enough, cancers of the nipple, in or between the lobes, of the smooth muscle, and so on, all have their own doubling times and other individual peculiarities.

All the apparatus of the mammary gland is enclosed by a membrane called the fascia. The fascia immediately under the skin and over the breast tissue is the superficial fascia; the membrane that separates the breast tissue from the muscles of the chest wall is the deep fascia. There are two muscles under the breast, the pectoralis major and the pectoralis minor, which cover the ribs and control much of the mobility of the arms. The Cooper's ligaments (named for the anatomist-surgeon who discovered them) are attached to the pectoral muscles, and these are what keep the breasts attractively tilted upward. (So all those pectoral-muscle exercises we do are absolutely no good for improving up-lift; it's the Cooper's ligaments that count.)

In each breast, scattered within, among, and beneath protective layers of fat, are twenty or more lobes, further subdivided into lobules, ending finally in tiny bulbs called acini. These are the milk-producing factories, and they are all connected to the nipple by a network of very fine ductules, leading into larger ducts, which finally merge as they enter the nipple into a single main tube, the lactiferous sinus. The external opening of the tube consists of a number of pin-sized holes in the nipple that secrete milk when it is needed.

The nipple is made of a sturdy, pigmented, corrugated kind of skin tissue and is filled with tiny glands that lubricate the area during breast feeding. It is surrounded by the areola, a pink or brownish circle of skin. The nipple and areola also contain many nerve endings and blood vessels, which come from larger connections in the breast itself.

Along with an extensive network of arteries, veins, and their capillary subdivisions, each breast has a network of lymphatic vessels that drain into the lymph nodes in the armpit. Each breast also has an internal mammary chain of nodes, which runs down the center of the chest alongside the breastbone. Knowing something about what the lymphatic system and axillary lymph nodes do is especially important to an understanding of breast cancer.

The lymphatic vessels, which are found throughout the body, are primarily involved in removing wastes from the tissues. But they also carry many of the components of the immune system. Every organism is endowed with a self-defense force to keep it healthy and help it fight off any invaders that might injure or destroy it. This immunological system is so sophisticated and complex that scientists—even with today's technical know-how—have barely begun to penetrate its mysteries. (Immunology is one of the youngest of the medical sciences.)

The regional lymph nodes are the first defense outposts in the human immunological system. These vital little fortresses, often misnamed glands, are scattered in critical spots throughout the body. The nodes under the cheeks in the upper neck are the ones we are most familiar with; they ward off and destroy harmful substances that enter the body through the nose or mouth. When these nodes are busy attacking an invader, a case of "swollen glands" results. All the nodes in the body are constantly manufacturing lymphocytes—cells that go out into the blood stream and attack anything that doesn't belong there. Usually they succeed. But sometimes they need help from other elements of the immune system, which will be described in more detail later.

The nodes and the lymphatic vessels—the channels connecting the nodes—play a part in the metastasis of cancer from a single

localized spot to another organ of the body. The lymphatics are
the usual invasion route a cancer cell takes when it breaks away
from the primary tumor. Luckily, it is not an express route. The
highways have many barricades—those trusty guardians, the
lymph nodes—which block the channels and try to filter out and
destroy the wandering malignant invader. But sometimes the
nodes themselves are conquered. The danger of having breast
cancer spread to the axillary lymph nodes in this way explains
why most doctors feel it is imperative to perform the "radical"
part of a mastectomy—excising them as well as the breast itself.

Most women have between twenty-five and thirty nodes in
each axilla, and when they are removed, each one is carefully
examined under the microscope by a pathologist, who is looking
for a sign that the node has been invaded. If a node is cancerous,
it is diagnosed as "positive"; if it is normal, it is called "negative."
With more than a century of experience to rely on, surgeons and
statisticians have been able to compute the relative risk of
metastasis elsewhere in the body based on the number of involved nodes found.

The very best report a pathologist can give, of course, is that
all the nodes are negative. This means that the disease has been
caught while still localized in the breast itself—even if, as in
Happy Rockefeller's case, there was not one but multiple tumors
in both breasts. Doctors have different rules of thumb regarding
what to do about how many positive nodes. Nodal status and its
implications for further therapies of all kinds will be treated elsewhere in this book.

Some surgeons believe that the internal mammary chain of
nodes, the ones lying along the breastbone, should also be removed during a mastectomy. However, it has been found that
these nodes are rarely involved if the primary cancer is in the
outer half of the breast. Since that is where most of the tumors
do appear, removing the internal mammary chain is usually unnecessary. There is some argument about this, but the consensus
seems to be that the surgery required is too extensive to be performed routinely.

Cancer cells trapped in the lymph system are more likely to be
destroyed than those in the blood stream, which lacks the nodal
filters and screens. The blood stream, however, does have its own

kinds of cancer killers floating around in it, as will be made clear in the later discussion of the immune system.

The location of a tumor can affect its seriousness and potential invasiveness. A relatively slow-growing neoplasm can metastasize quickly if it is near a lymph channel or near a blood vessel. Cases have been recorded in which a stray cell floating in the lymphatic system caused a cancer to grow to palpable size in the axillary nodes, although the original malignancy in the breast itself remained microscopic. No examination of the breast, by palpation, mammography, or thermography, would be able to detect such a cancer.

Furthermore, the lymphatic system links the two breasts, under the breastbone. That is why, if a breast cancer reappears, the most frequent site for the recurrence is in the other breast.

The terms metastasis and recurrence are not synonymous, by the way, though both refer to second cancers. Metastases are tumors that have spread to other—often quite distant—parts of the body via the blood stream or lymphatic system. Recurrences are new cancers that appear in the immediate area of the first—in the second breast, for instance. Metastases are more dangerous and insidious, because there is no way to know where a circulating cancer cell may decide to stop and colonize. The lungs, liver, and bone are the most common sites for breast-cancer metastases, but they can begin to grow anywhere and be far advanced before their discovery by even the most careful examination after surgery. Recurrences are more likely to be found early, when treatment can be effective, since even a superficial follow-up includes careful scrutiny of the operative area, the second breast, and the axillas.

The cyclical changes in the breasts and the nature of the regional nodes are enough to show how breast cancer spreads, but pregnancy and lactation (breast feeding) worsen a woman's condition if she has cancer.

During ovulation, the breasts begin to get ready for the conception of a baby. They become enlarged and engorged as the milk glands grow. If there is no pregnancy, the swelling disappears, and for the rest of the cycle the breasts are in their normal state. This is the reason for the periodic lumpiness and soreness every woman experiences—they are perfectly normal.

However, if pregnancy does occur, the glandular system keeps on growing, so that it will be able to provide a good milk supply; more lobules are produced and the duct system expands. Then, if the mother breast-feeds her baby, all these additional assets continue to be used to make milk. If she does not breast-feed, or as her milk supply dries up, the breasts gradually return to their prepregancy state.

All of these changes are triggered by a variety of hormones, some of which aid and abet neoplastic growth. More about these later.

The work of the hormones leaves permanent changes in the mammary gland after a pregnancy. It will never again be a "virgin" breast. Even though external shapeliness might not have been affected, the breasts have undergone changes of internal structure, which will remain forever. The changes may not be visible to the eye, but they often show on mammograms as areas of less density, leaving light spaces and gaps on the film. Nulliparous—never pregnant—breasts have a dark, compact firmness.

There are many different kinds of breast cancers, all blanketed under the label mammary carcinoma. The specific name of each generally identifies the kind of breast tissue that has become malignant. A favorite starting place for a cancer—about half of all— is in one of the hundreds of milk ducts, and these are known as intraductal carcinomas.

Although all breast cancers are technically classified as soft-tissue tumors, some feel hard and can assume various shapes; others are gelatinous and mushy. Still others feel fibrous. Some cancers of the breast have no lump or thickening at all.

The uncommon Paget's disease (named after the doctor who first described it) is one of these. At the beginning the nipple and areola look as if they had a slight case of eczema. Then the nipple begins to crack, and to leak what sometimes looks like milk and sometimes is a greenish or bluish fluid. Even though there is no lump, Paget's disease is a cancer, and a mastectomy must be performed. However, when Paget's disease spreads and invades a duct, there is a lump.

Another one of these is a generalized (in medical parlance, the opposite of localized) breast cancer, a relatively rare type that gives as its first symptom only pain and soreness, no lump that can be seen or felt. Since a certain amount of breast tenderness is a regular part of every woman's life, this cancer can be very dangerous—especially in premenopausal women—because the symptoms may be ignored and the cancer go undetected until after it has already metastasized. However, it can be caught in time if the woman is alert and not bashful about seeing her doctor for what could turn out to be an insignificant symptom (and about insisting that he do an examination and order a mammogram). When it is found early, the outlook for this kind of nonlumpy, nonthickening cancer is as good as for any other malignancy diagnosed at an early stage. But it must be found early for successful treatment, because it may be the onset of inflammatory carcinoma.

Inflammatory carcinoma is very virulent, and usually by the time it is diagnosed the skin and lymphatics are severely inflamed, and the breast is swollen, hot, red, puffy, and excruciatingly painful. Experience has made surgeons pessimistic about the outlook for this kind of cancer, and many of them simply pronounce it inoperable. Others will do a mastectomy, but the results have not been good. I think the decision should be the woman's, not the surgeon's, because doing nothing means certain—not probable —death.

A rare kind of breast cancer—mammary sarcoma—attacks the connective tissue of the muscles, ligaments, and tendons that back up and support the breasts. For a variety of reasons, connective tissues are among the last parts of the body to be invaded by cancer. In other words, the pectoral muscles—routinely cut out during the Halsted radical mastectomy—are very low-risk targets of malignant invasion. Many experts, in fact, have told me that by the time a woman's pectorals are invaded, she probably has so many other metastases in her body that any kind of mastectomy would be an unnecessary ordeal.

Cancers in the large milk glands are called lobular carcinomas, and they are often found *in situ*. This is the term used to describe a noninvasive, microscopic cancer that may stay in the same spot, without spreading. When looking at a biopsy specimen under the microscope, the pathologist looks for a band of healthy cells completely circumscribing and insulating the cancerous ones, and also for membranes with solid, unbroken perimeters enclosing the cancerous cells. If both these conditions exist, the pathologist

will diagnose it as an *in situ* cancer and will predict that metastasis to the axillary nodes is highly unlikely.

Some surgeons do a mastectomy in such cases, and some do not.
Whether the breast should be amputated for an *in situ* cancer is,
I think, also a decision the woman really must make for herself.
To do so, however, she should know that follow-up studies have
shown that a large proportion of these carcinomas do change and
become invasive within ten years.

Each of these mammary carcinomas, then, is quite different
from the others. Doubling times for human breast cancers vary
widely, too, ranging from twenty-three days to 209 days. Depending on the kind, it can take anywhere from two years to seventeen
years for the cancer to reach a size that can be felt. Stated another way, the twenty-three-day carcinoma—the one with the
shortest doubling time—could not be palpated for two years at
the earliest.

Actually, the doubling times of the various breast cancers follow no known hard-and-fast rules. The interval varies with the
reproductive rate of the part of the breast from which the cancerous tumor came, since the proliferating malignant cells follow
the same relative speed of division as the tissue from which they
grew. Skin, blood, and other fast-growing tissues, for example,
would have faster-growing malignancies; connective tissue, slow
ones; nerve and muscle cells would never become malignant.

This explains why there are no cancers of the heart, an organ
composed almost entirely of muscle cells. If these cancers exist
at all, they are so rare I could find no one who had ever heard or
read of one. Muscle sarcomas are suspected of arising from epi-
thelial or other cells nearby, not from the muscle cells themselves,
which never divide, and brain tumors such as gliomas are thought
to develop in the same way. The reason scientists hedge by saying
"suspected" or "thought to" is that once a cell becomes malignant,
its cellular origin cannot always be determined. Therefore, these
are assumptions based on the firm knowledge that nerve and
muscle cells never reproduce and should, theoretically, never
have an S period during which they can be transformed.

All the tissues found in the breast, except for those of the
nipple, are scattered throughout the organ. Therefore the various

kinds of cancers, aside from Paget's disease and others of the nipple, can begin anywhere. Statistically, however, the upper outer quadrant—the quarter of the breast closest to the armpit— is the birthplace of about half of all breast cancers. Another one-fourth begin in the nipple. The other three quadrants account for the remaining 25 per cent.

For reasons unknown, it is far more common for breast cancers to develop in the left breast first.

An interesting opinion I learned during a tour of European cancer centers is that premenopausal and postmenopausal breast cancer are two completely different diseases, having different causes and requiring different treatments. This theory has been supported by recent studies in the United States, and it explains many age-related differences and paradoxes about breast cancer that had puzzled me throughout my research. For example, I had learned that breast-cancer statistics show a very distinctive pattern of incidence according to age groups, and statisticians told me that this kind of age-specific incidence rate is uncommon in cancers of other organs. I will go into this in greater detail later, and just say now that the many opinions about the reasons for this phenomenon all revolve around the menopause and the reduction of estrogens in the body of an older woman.

A word must be said about breast cancer in men. Although it is extremely rare—less than 1 per cent of all breast cancers—it does exist. It is by and large a disease that hits men who are in middle and old age and who, in the United States, are predominantly white and foreign-born or of Jewish background. Another interesting aspect of the male disease is that older men being treated for prostatic cancer with estrogens have developed breast cancers from taking the female hormones. However, many of these are also metastases from the prostatic cancer.

One oddity of masculine breast cancer might someday help in finding the cause of breast cancer in women. Men who have Klinefelter's syndrome—a rare genetic defect that gives their sex-bearing chromosome two X genes and a single Y gene, rather than the normal X and Y—have a much higher incidence of breast cancer than do men in the rest of the population. Many scientists believe this is evidence that breast cancer is genetic, and that the technical know-how to find a specific breast-cancer gene on a chromosome has just not been developed yet.

Whatever the cause, cancer of the breast in men is treated in the same way as it is in women: by mastectomy, preferably a modified radical, which leaves the muscles intact. Also, if the tumor developed from taking female hormones, they would probably be discontinued. Since the disease usually occurs in older men, and since it makes up such a tiny percentage of all breast cancers, male mastectomy is not a burning issue. When the day comes that female breast cancer can be cured, male breast cancer will also disappear.

That day may not be as far off as many fear. Although it is likely that breast cancer has been around since man first scratched on the wall of his cave, the real thrust of organized research in this country began only in 1970. In October of that year, as a result of a 1966 congressional recommendation that the National Cancer Institute create a Breast Cancer Task Force, a group was formed to concentrate on the disease. Members of the task force and its various committees meet about twice a year, and they include not only Americans, but specialists from all over the world. More has undoubtedly been learned and accomplished since October 1970 than in all the earlier centuries.

I hope so.

I and millions of other women have an absolute stake in their success.

3

History, Myths, and Quackery

HISTORY

Breast cancer has probably existed since at least the time of Eve. But the first known reference to it in medical history is found in the "Edwin Smith Surgical Papyrus," written during the time of the Old Kingdom in Egypt, which extended from around 3000 to 2500 B.C. (No one knows who wrote these ancient scrolls; Smith was the archeologist who discovered them.)

I was curious about the omission of breast cancer from the cave and wall scratchings of primitive man, and most of the authorities I asked about this said that it was probably because women died of other causes long before they reached the vulnerable breast-cancer age. "Few women lived past thirty in those days," one expert at the National Cancer Institute told me. "They just didn't live long enough to get breast cancer." Another specialist suggested that early man wouldn't have known it was the actual cause of death. "A woman doesn't die of the breast disease itself," he explained, "but from its spread to a vital organ. So if a woman died of metastatic liver or lung disease, who would think the problem had originated in the breast?"

For whatever reason, the Smith papyrus has the earliest known mention of breast cancer—male or female—in medical history. Even the eight cases the papyrus describes are called not breast cancer, but cases of "bulging tumors," and all were found in males. This first doctors' manual says, with straightforward honesty, "There is no treatment." In another Egyptian medical papyrus, written about 1,500 years later (this one named for Georg Ebers), no cases of "bulging tumors" are mentioned, but prescriptions are given for healing fatty tumors and abscesses "with the knife" and by fire.

There are also recorded references to breast cancer in ancient Mesopotamia. Here (where poppyheads were used to relieve pain), cutting out breast tumors was routine procedure—and presumably the noble poppy was used as a painkiller during the surgery.

Then, in the chronicles of ancient Greece, the historian Herodotus tells the case history of Atossa, the daughter of the Persian king Cyrus the Great and the wife of Darius I. She had a breast tumor, which she attempted to conceal from everyone, until finally, according to Herodotus, it ulcerated and spread, and she could no longer hide the problem. Atossa then sent for the court physician, Democedes, and he cured her. No details are given about this legendary successful treatment. However, one thing hasn't changed much: even in those long-ago days, women delayed before seeing a doctor.

As a matter of fact, Dr. Edward Lewison, of the Johns Hopkins Hospital, in his textbook *Breast Cancer and Its Diagnosis and Treatment,* complains that Atossa's attitude is typical of all women through the ages everywhere.

It is a revealing commentary to note that throughout the annals of history women have never outlived their vanity. Cosmetic considerations and false modesty have hindered the early diagnosis and timely treatment of breast cancer from the dawn of humanity until today. Since the breast has always been an esthetic symbol of fertility and womanhood, amputation of the breast provoked mutilation of the mind as well as the body. Women have taken great pride in their breasts and formerly wore décolleté dresses with disarming propriety. Indeed, it was a customary and respectful form of salutation up until the seventeenth century to touch the breasts in a warm and friendly greeting. Thus, through the ages, vanity has always been the death-trap of reason in the struggle toward the early diagnosis and treatment of breast cancer.

So much for critics who say American culture is mammary-mad.

Hippocrates, the "Father of Medicine," who was born about 460 B.C. and was roughly a contemporary of Herodotus, made his opinion about all cancers perfectly clear: they were incurable. In his monumental seventy-volume medical encyclopedia, he wrote, "Those diseases that medicines do not cure are cured by the knife. Those that the knife does not cure are cured by fire. Those that fire does not cure must be considered incurable." The extreme nature of the cures is probably why Hippocrates did not try to do much for his cancer patients. As he said, "It is better to omit treatment altogether: for, if treated, the patients soon die, whereas if let alone, they may last a long time."

In defense of Hippocrates, it must be remembered that he had no anesthesias (apparently, he knew nothing about the Mesopotamian use of the poppy), no antiseptics, and no effective way to stop hemorrhage except by searing the wound with fire (called then, as now, cautery).

For 500 years Hippocrates' theories reigned supreme and unchallenged in the known medical world. Then, in the first century A.D., a Roman dilettante, Aulus Cornelius Celsus, switched his attention from agriculture, military science, law, and philosophy to medicine, particularly the study of cancer. According to his contemporaries, Celsus wrote many volumes about medicine, although only eight are still in existence. But those few indicate that he may have known more about the natural history of cancer than Hippocrates did. Celsus's writings also imply that not all of Hippocrates' successors had followed their master's warning to leave cancers alone; some of them must have been performing surgery, including breast amputations, because Celsus emphasized that "irritation of cancer by the imprudent intervention of a physician could put the patient into danger."

Interestingly, almost 2,000 years ago Celsus came out strongly against removing the pectoral muscles if a mastectomy was attempted. His influence apparently was great enough that throughout the so-called "dark ages of medicine" surgeons left the pectoral muscles intact. It took the bright age of modern medicine to make excision of these chest muscles a routine practice. By and large, Celsus was against treating any but very early cases of

breast cancer. He felt that to use "caustics . . . burning irons
. . . or [to] remove the growth with the scalpel never cured a
patient." In particular, "burning exasperates and the growth
spreads rapidly until it proves fatal."

Not that Celsus believed in doing nothing. His treatment seems
to have been based on the idea—one still wrongly held by many
—that there is some turning point after which benign tumors
(which he called *cacoethe*) become malignant. Since he had
no way to know exactly when the change would occur, Celsus's
rule of thumb was to put caustic, burning medications on the
breast as soon as a symptom was noticed. If the symptom disappeared and the patient's condition improved, he assumed that
the *cacoethe* had been caught in time. He then proceeded to do
whatever surgery or cautery he felt was indicated. However, if
there was no change or if the patient's condition worsened,
Celsus believed this meant that the tumor had already become
malignant, and he did nothing more.

A century after Celsus, the famous Roman physician Galen
(who was born in Greece) appeared on the scene and captured
the imaginations of his colleagues with his four-humor theory
of health and disease.

The human body, he said, was governed by the four humors of
black bile, yellow bile, phlegm, and blood, and in a person who
was healthy all four were in perfect balance. Minor imbalances
shaped temperament and personality. Too much black bile produced melancholia or depression; excitable people had a shade
too much yellow bile, lazy folk suffered from an excess of phlegm,
and nice people inclined toward too much blood. The presence
of a disease, however, meant that the humors were seriously out
of kilter—the implication being that all physical ailments were
generalized diseases of the whole body, with none confined to a
single organ.

And what did the great Galen have to say about cancer? That
the disease was caused by an overload of black bile and should
be treated by special diets and purges. But there were exceptions. A breast tumor, for example, was usually cut out if it moved
around easily and was not in a fixed position. In addition to
surgery, a variety of medicines was used during that period. The
most common were caustics, which, it was hoped, would burn

out the cancer. It was Galen, by the way, who named the disease *cancer*—the Latin for "crab"—because most malignant tumors looked so much like this crustacean.

There were also prayers and incantations, for medicine then was as much religion, superstition, and mysticism as empirical knowledge. Indeed, such practitioners might be considered the forerunners of today's quacks. Even in those far-off times, victims of cancer were exploited by healers who promised a sure cure for a fast fee. Along with feminine vanity, crooks and quacks seem to permeate the entire history of breast cancer.

Of all cancers.

Although Galen's humoral theory traveled only as far as the borders of the Roman world, this was a considerable realm. His opinions were also perpetuated for centuries. In medieval times, Galen's views were accepted everywhere as "God-ordained," and his own words became his epitaph. "Never as yet have I gone astray," he wrote, "whether in treatment or in prognosis." For his apostles, he prophesied, "If anyone wishes to gain fame . . . all that he needs is to accept what I have been able to establish."

Galen was certainly ahead of his time, but not ahead by more than a thousand years. Yet his authority, supported by the Roman Catholic church, was so incredible that it was not challenged until 1543, by a young anatomist, Andreas Vesalius. In that year, he proved, by the dissection of cadavers, that the human thigh bone was straight, not curved, as Galen had stated—and he was severely attacked for contradicting medical doctrine. "To question Galen was unorthodox heresy," medical historians have written, in describing these dark ages of medicine.

In the age we live in now, when every new medical theory has to be experimentally and clinically verified by independent researchers before it becomes scientific gospel, it is hard to believe that Galen's ideas, however brilliant they might have been, could still have controlled medicine so completely in the sixteenth century. Yet Vesalius was told that, in spite of what his cadavers showed about straight thigh bones, Galen had been right. The femur had changed, because since his time men had begun wearing tight-fitting clothes instead of togas!

We really should not be too hard on Galen. He was, after all, far ahead of his time as a physician. Until the first microscope was put together, about 1590, it was impossible to know much about the actual nature of health or disease. All that could be done was to observe, classify, and theorize. Treatment was the repetition of what had worked before in a similar case, sheer guesswork, or, more likely, the combination of both.

This was especially true for cancer. By definition, it is a disorder that involves cellular growth and reproduction, and no one could begin to understand it until the microscope permitted scientists to peer into the mysteries of cells and learn something of how they worked. Quite literally, all progress in learning about cancer has been directly related to the development of better microscopes. In the last quarter of the twentieth century, this is still the story I frequently hear from frustrated cancer researchers: "We don't have the technical know-how to see that yet."

I don't mean to imply that there were no changes in the way breast cancer was managed between Galen's time and that of Vesalius. When tumors were small, cutting them out and cauterizing were often successful. Leading physicians and surgeons began to believe, correctly, that if the cancer could be caught before it had spread into the armpit, there was a good chance of a cure. There were medical as well as surgical attacks, including the use of arsenic, zinc-chloride pastes, and other caustics to try to burn out the tumor; doctors thought that if the skin over the growth began to corrode or blister, it would somehow pop out of the diseased breast.

Even without anesthesia or antiseptics, enough mastectomies were apparently being done to justify a section in a medical book giving detailed instructions for performing the operation. Except for the poppyheads of ancient Mesopotamia, I found no mention of a painkiller for any surgery. Split-second speed seems to have been the only way agony could be alleviated. Organs were pinched, sawed, or hacked off, and burning irons were put directly on the wounds to stop the bleeding. There are no data on the mortality rates from infection and massive hemorrhage, but these, like the torment, must have been horrendous.

By the mid-1500s, Galen's medical authority was clearly on the wane. Vesalius had been the first to undermine that authority, and his *De Humani Corporis Fabrica* is considered to mark the beginning of the modern study of anatomy. Soon a wholesale exodus from Galen's dark ages into a medical renaissance was under way. One of the foremost leaders of the movement was William Harvey, who in the early 1600s discovered the principles of the circulation of blood. Between laboratory advances in the study of the nature of cells, courtesy of the microscope, and advances in the knowledge of anatomy and physiology, a great deal was soon learned about cancer in general, as well as about breast cancer.

Unfortunately, all the new knowledge did not make much difference in the outcome. Breast cancer was almost invariably fatal. But now doctors understood why. Once the malignancy had reached into and beyond the lymph nodes of the armpit, it was no longer breast cancer; it was spreading through the whole body. For successful treatment, the malignancy had to be cut out before this happened.

The most thoughtful surgeons of those early centuries of modern medicine theorized, accurately, that careful removal of the entire breast and the lymph nodes gave the best chance for a cure. But who could bear such excruciating, lengthy surgery while remaining fully conscious? Also, any kind of surgery was perilous. Although techniques had been developed to ligate—tie off—arteries and veins, so that massive hemorrhage could be controlled, there was still infection to battle. So, even though by at least 1800 it was known that the breast should be removed and the armpit cleared of nodes, medicine lacked the technical know-how to do this safely and without hours of wakeful agony.

Then, in 1846, a dentist named William Morton successfully used a painkilling drug during an operation at Massachusetts General Hospital, in Boston. His creation was an early chloroform. In 1865, Dr. Louis Pasteur developed his germ theory of disease, and soon afterward Joseph Lister presented the world with a compound he named an antiseptic. These advances changed the nature of surgery almost overnight, and a new era opened up for breast-cancer patients.

At the time, a long-term cancer survivor was a clinical curiosity. But in 1867, Mr. Charles H. Moore, a surgeon at the Middlesex

Hospital in England,* began to perform, with a good deal of success, what we would now consider a very extended radical mastectomy. (He removed the breast, neck, chest, and axillary nodes, some muscles, and even rib-cage bones.) More important than his survival rate, however, was what he learned—and wrote —regarding the nature of breast cancer. "Local recurrence of cancer is due to the continuous growth of fragments of the principal tumor," he said. "It is not sufficient to remove the tumor, or any portion only of the breast in which it is situated; mammary cancer requires the careful extrication of the entire organ." Moore also insisted that the surgeon must not cut into the tumor at all and should be careful to remove the axillary nodes in a single, continuous operation with the breast itself.

Before anesthesia or antiseptics, surgeons tore into a woman's chest with all the precision of an amateur demolition freak planting dynamite. They had no choice—if they didn't work as fast as possible, she would die on the operating table. According to Moore's lectures to his colleagues, even after anesthesia was introduced, these practices were still going on. He called them "barbarous, not to mention dangerous," and his operations and his statistics were convincing. By 1889, Moore's technique had been refined into the operation that remains more or less the standard procedure in the United States today—the Halsted radical mastectomy. It was first performed, in Baltimore, by one of the Johns Hopkins Hospital's greats, William Stewart Halsted.

Halsted was one of the first surgeons in the world to use gloves and a mask routinely. By the time he did his first mastectomy he already had an international reputation as a skillful surgeon, inventive genius, and inspiring teacher. His original radical mastectomy removed a great deal: the breast, the lymph nodes and all their surrounding tissue in the armpit, a lot of skin, and the large pectoral muscle with all its connecting ligaments and tendons. He grafted skin to cover the resulting hole in the chest wall. It was a mutilating operation, but it seemed to give survival rates that surpassed anything else ever done.

The frozen-section technique for quick pathological examina-

* In Great Britain, then as now, surgeons are called not "doctor," but just plain "mister"—perhaps a leftover from the day when barbers did all surgery.

tion of a biopsied specimen had been introduced in 1818 by a Dutch physician, Pieter de Riemer, and, after anesthetics came into use, it became a godsend in treating breast cancer. (A biopsy diagnostic technique had long been used for uterine and cervical cancers, but it was not too helpful for breast tumors, since the microscope slide took about a week to prepare.) Now, being able to freeze a bit of tissue and examine it within minutes meant that the tissue specimen could be diagnosed while the patient waited unconscious on the operating table. (Though surgeons doubtless applaud this as a clear advance, I see it as a mixed blessing. Without the frozen sections, they would have to delay their mastectomies, giving their patients time to think.)

After 1889, the technological know-how began to come quickly. X-ray was discovered, and it did not take long for doctors to realize that this strange, powerful, but invisible force was lethal to cancer cells. By 1913, it was routine to give a "shot" of X-ray after cancer surgery, just to be sure any remaining stray malignant patches were destroyed.

Surgical pioneers—Dr. George Crile, Sr., in the United States and David Patey in England—developed mastectomies that did not require the disfiguring and disabling excision of the pectoral muscles. The Patey modified radical became popular in Europe after its introduction in 1930. Unfortunately, Dr. Crile was not as successful in defeating the Halsted in this country, and it is still most surgeons' first choice here.

In the late 1800s, a search had begun for a drug that would kill cancer. Talk—and hope—intensified after Dr. Paul Ehrlich developed his "magic bullet" against syphilis. But nothing came of it then.

It took World War II and the research that produced nitrogen mustard to bring on the era of chemotherapy. Mustard gas was known in World War I, but it was outlawed by international agreement after the war because it was so poisonous. However, because it poisoned cells, research chemists quickly recognized that this quality might make mustards effective anti-cancer drugs. Thus the "alkylating" mustards became the first important members of medicine's arsenal of chemical weapons against the disease, and trials with various combinations of such compounds went on for years. Some were so potent that they killed the pa-

tients before their cancers were affected; others had hardly any
effect. Finally, during World War II, a nitrogen-mustard combination was developed, which proved to be both effective and
relatively safe.

Another big advance in cancer research resulted from that war.
Part of the fallout from the atomic bombs dropped on Hiroshima
and Nagasaki, which released an intensely powerful X-ray-like
force, was new knowledge of the relationship between irradiation and cancer. While it was already known that the mysterious
force could cure or arrest cancer, the A-bomb also caused much
malignant disease.

The high incidence of cancer, especially leukemia, in the
Japanese survivors was proof that "shots" of X-ray could not be
used indiscriminately as treatment. The technical know-how accumulated in developing the bomb was now applied to the invention of high-dosage, higher-precision equipment that would
destroy neoplastic tissue but avoid healthy cells. Then came
another surprise: not only were large numbers of abnormal and
deformed infants being born to A-bomb survivors, but also many
members of the second generation were developing cancer. The
irradiation had apparently done something to the chromosomes
of the parents, and the mutation had been passed on. But what?

As in the sixteenth century, further advances on the basic cellular level had to wait for further technical know-how. Finally,
the mid-twentieth century brought the electron microscope, and,
quite literally, endless new vistas were opened up to curious,
probing scientific eyes. Now they could see what was going on
inside cells!

Meanwhile, the unraveling of the code of DNA—that microscopic programer in the nucleus of every living cell—was trigger-
ing molecular research on cancer in laboratories all over the
world. Perhaps DNA carried a gene for it, making the disease
hereditary?

Immunology was brought into the act, through organ transplants and the accompanying use of heavy quantities of certain
drugs. A disproportionate number of transplanted kidneys became malignant. Other kinds of cancers also appeared in these
patients. "Why?" scientists wondered. "Because of the drugs used
to prevent the body's rejection of the foreign organ," some an-

swered. "These immunosuppressant drugs are also lowering resistance to other things." Other experts said these cancers were
not due to the drugs at all, but to stimulation of the body's immune system by something in the alien kidney.

Using this bit of knowledge about immunology, some irradiation here, chemotheraphy there, doctors found they could cure
some skin cancers. Some of the leukemias (there are many types)
are now also long-term chronic diseases, instead of being immediate death sentences.

On another front, the American Cancer Society (founded in
1913) made public education a top priority. Massive publicity
about the seven danger signals began to bring cancer out of the
closet it had shared with syphilis and gonorrhea. With financial
support from the ACS, in the late 1950s Dr. George M. Papanicolaou developed the "Pap test" for detecting cervical cancer,
and this once lethal women's disease can now be entirely cured
if caught in time.

And breast-cancer progress? No change in the "end results"—
the mortality rate—since 1930. One reason more women are
living now in spite of having breast cancer is that surgical and
operating-room improvements have reduced the number of
deaths resulting from mastectomy itself. In addition, techniques
for earlier detection have prolonged the life span from the time
of diagnosis. Certainly much is known about the disease that was
not known in 1930. But all this has not decreased the absolute
number of tumors found. On the contrary, the incidence of breast
cancer has risen. Nor has the mortality rate dropped. In the
countries of the world from which data are available, half of the
women who develop breast cancer die of it sooner or later. The
number of deaths each year from breast cancers diagnosed in
previous years equals about one-third of that year's incidence rate
(the latter is estimated at about 90,000 cases in the United States
in 1975). There has been one ominous change in the statistics
since 1930. While the incidence rates (the number of cases per
100,000 of the population) have been rising, the average age of
onset is dropping—more and more women under thirty are becoming victims.

So those awful "end results" logged by the statisticians are no
better than they were fifty years ago.

And in the awful beginning, when a woman learns she has the disease and becomes a part of the incidence rate?

"Unfortunately," Dr. Paul Carbone, of the National Cancer Institute, told me, "the first course of action is still some kind of radical mastectomy. The best treatment to produce a cure first requires removal of the breast and the axillary nodes."

That is exactly what Mr. Charles Moore was saying in 1867. More than a century ago.

MYTHS

No history of any disease is complete without telling some of the myths about its causes and cures that have accumulated over the centuries. There are probably more myths about cancer than about any other disease except, perhaps, epilepsy or leprosy. Only these three have been so enshrouded in an aura of fear and mystery through the ages. Some of the most persistent—and most easily refuted—myths concern breast cancer.

To get right to one of the more prevalent of these, breast cancer is not contagious, and neither are any other carcinomas. Viruses are under investigation as a possible cause of cancer, and this viral research is described in a later chapter. But even if every laboratory in the world should prove beyond a shadow of a doubt that a virus is the cause, it would not be the kind that can pass along the flu, a cold, or any other contagious disease. As far back as Eve, there has been no indication—and certainly no hard evidence—that anyone ever caught breast cancer from someone else.

And no kind of cancer can be caught from a sick animal, either. I recently read of a woman who was convinced that her breast tumor was somehow caused by contamination from cleaning up after her cancerous dog. When I asked scientists about this, I was laughed at so many times that I finally stopped from embarrassment. It is nonsense.

The idea that germs can enter the breast either through the ducts of the nipple or through a cut or scratch is also without scientific foundation.

Many women say they were hit or bumped on the spot where

a tumor later grew. An ordinary injury will not develop into a malignancy. But it is true that a woman is more likely to develop a neoplasm if she has a prior history of breast disease—by which doctors generally mean benign growths, breast abscesses, mastitis, inflammations of the milk ducts when nursing, and the like. So it might be that certain kinds of breast injuries could be classified as prior diseases. This, then, may not be altogether a myth, after all.

It is also true that a trauma can call attention to an already existing cancer that had simply not been noticed before. In any case, soreness or a lump caused by a fall or blow should be reported to a doctor if it does not go away within a reasonable period of time.

I interviewed two patients, in two different countries, who blamed their breast cancers on their husbands' overeager manipulations while making love. A radiologist laughed when I told him this story. "It was probably the husbands' constant attention to their wives' breasts that led to the early discovery of cancers that were already there," he said. As a matter of fact, I had asked the women who first discovered the lumps, and both admitted it had been their husbands.

I also interviewed several women who blamed malignancies on their babies, for having sucked too hard and painfully during breast feeding. If the baby caused real damage to the breast, would this qualify as a prior breast disease? I asked, and was told, "Nature provides for the skin of the nipple to become very tough during breast-feeding days, making it unlikely for a child to inflict serious trauma." But if that does happen, a woman should follow the rule for any injury: report it to her doctor.

Pregnancy does not cause breast cancer, either. Unfortunately, the myth that it does has some factual underpinnings. If a woman has a cancer at the time she becomes pregnant and it remains undetected or untreated, her outlook is not good. The body sends a flood of estrogens, the female hormone, into the blood stream to prepare first for the nine months of creating the baby and then for feeding it. This hormonal overload is fine for the baby, but it also feeds the developing cancer, which spreads like weeds after rain.

One woman I interviewed thought her cancer came from

having had too many chest X-rays to detect tuberculosis. She was a restaurant cook, and the law required that she be X-rayed every six months. A radiologist told me that, while it was possible, he doubted her tumor was caused by the semiannual examination. "The average chest X-ray gives so very little irradiation," he explained, "that the chances of its happening are almost zero. A mammogram exposes a woman to about two rads of irradiation per breast, for example, and yet we recommend it annually for older women. The TB examination gives only a fraction of one rad."

Possibly one of the hardest myths to die—it isn't dead yet!—is the notion of "implantation by knife." The myth persists because often patients do die soon after a mastectomy or other cancer surgery. The reason, however, is not that the surgeon spread the cancer into the blood stream with his scalpel. While this may sound plausible, scientific evidence does not support it. For one thing, after a biopsy of a cancerous breast, malignant cells are frequently left at the site of the surgery, but they usually die or are killed by the body's defense system. It is also now known that all malignant tumors constantly shed living cells into the blood stream, in the same way that healthy tissues do. While these could travel on and start new cancer colonies somewhere else, most die. Random blood tests of cancer patients show that about 70 per cent of the test samples contain either living or dead cancer cells that did not metastasize. But they were not put there by the surgeon's knife; they were "sloughed off" by the tumor.

Then why do some cancer patients indeed seem to fade and slip away from life so quickly after surgery? Is it a false illusion? Is it a bizarre coincidence? One doctor told me his theory. "Some kinds of cancer cells are anaerobic, that is, they require very little oxygen. So long as they are tightly enclosed in the body, they grow slowly but steadily and could probably stay that way for a long time before causing death. Then surgery exposes the internal tissue to air, and that shot of fresh oxygen might make the cells grow faster." This is but one man's theory, however; nothing more. I could find no evidence to support it.

Originally, I had planned to put the statement that lactation —the production of milk for breast feeding—is a protection against breast cancer into the myth category, because some renowned epidemiologists in the United States had announced that nursing does not give a mother protection. However, I found that most European experts disagreed strongly with the new view. Further inquiry showed that many American authorities share the European opinion that woman *is* protected while she is breast-feeding. So I have moved lactation out of the myths and back where it had rested comfortably for decades—among the epidemiological aspects of breast cancer, which are discussed in the next chapter.

Does going bra-less cause breast cancer? Dr. Dao did not think there could be any connection, and everyone else I questioned agreed. "Too many cultures that have never seen a brassiere have very low incidences," he explained. Immediately, a mental picture of the legendary "topless" women of Bali came into my mind. "But no woman should think that, just because of these data, being bra-less gives any protection against breast cancer," an epidemiologist cautioned. "It's just one of those statistical coincidences."

Does being amply endowed make a woman a higher breast-cancer risk than one who cannot fill a size-32AA bra? No, but it makes lumps harder to find. For this reason, large-breasted women should be careful to examine their breasts every month and, after the age of forty, have an annual checkup that includes a mammogram. Mammograms are much more accurate in finding cancers in large, fatty breasts than in small, dense ones, by the way. Fat, the major component of a 40DDD cup, provides what the technicians call "good contrast material," and even small tumors are easily picked up.

What about silicone inserts used to enlarge the breasts? There has been no evidence that the added filler *causes* cancer. But any extra padding inside makes a tumor more difficult to find. Also, those under-the-skin stitches feel like tiny growths themselves, and can therefore lull a woman into neglecting a malignant growth. Women whose breasts have been enlarged by surgery should take the same precautions as their naturally large-breasted sisters.

The Pill? So far, all authorities say there is no definite proof that oral contraceptives cause breast cancer in humans. In fact, some scientists maintain that the Pill offers protection. Most doctors I talked to would not commit themselves to either side of the controversy, but only mumbled something about "it's too soon to know." Myth or fact, the whole subject is so important that I've given the Pill an entire chapter to itself.

QUACKERY

"Cures" for breast cancer over the ages have included exorcism, the laying on of hands, concoctions to drink or apply, and even fire. In the Middle Ages, when herbs were virtually the only medicines for any disease, a mixture of herbaproserpinaca (knotgrass) and butter was prescribed to make tumors disappear. Sweet butter was in almost all the medicinal ointments, mixed with other ingredients, such as milk or vinegar. Burning out a suspected cancer was another favorite treatment. This was done either with red-hot irons or with instruments called "fire drills."

In the Arab world, external applications of caustics were popular, because the Moslem religion forbade any kind of mutilating surgery. But Christian doctors also used caustics for chemical burning. French physicians of the thirteenth century applied arsenic and zinc-chloride pastes. In Germany, in the fourteenth century, the breasts were squeezed between heavy lead plates.

In England, Queen Elizabeth's personal physician, William Clowes, decided that the laying on of the royal hands was the perfect treatment, although there is no record of any cures being effected by Elizabeth's "divine, royal touch," or by the ring she wore between her breasts. If Elizabeth had her ring, the common people had amulets and talismans of their own—preventatives that are probably still worn in many places around the world today.

Lourdes and many other religious shrines have always had their share of breast-cancer patients seeking a miracle cure, and no doubt, in the United States today, faith healers like Oral Roberts have a good many visits from them.

Shortly after my own mastectomy, I began to receive in the mail literature about three substances—laetrile, hydrazine sulfate, and abscissic acid—that were described as being able to prevent a recurrence of cancer. Every authority I questioned, if he had heard of them at all, felt they were a waste of money, and a

biochemist who examined the formulas thought they might even
be dangerous.

Laetrile (amygdalin) is nothing more than ground-up apricot
pits—an ancient Chinese cancer remedy, according to a friend
from Shanghai—but even with my limited chemistry background I
could see that cyanide was somehow involved in its action, and
this persuaded me not to try it. Hydrazine sulfate and abscissic
acid were not so easy to reject out of hand. Apparently they have
some effect on the respiration of cancer cells (the words aerobic
and anaerobic were all through the booklets plugging them),
and many researchers mention respiration problems in discussing
the causes of cancer. But anything that interferes with a cancer
cell's respiration might do something to a good cell's respiration
as well, so I decided to wait for more solid evidence of their
promise and rejected the idea of being a guinea pig.

Krebiozen, a drug that caused a furor just a few years ago, has
apparently been dropped by the promoters of quack cures (or
else they have simply not found my name yet). The only mention of it I found concerned the dispute several years ago between
the "cancer establishment"—the American Cancer Society, the
Food and Drug Administration, the National Cancer Institute,
and the American Medical Association—and patients who were
clamoring to have this horse-serum derivative legalized. For some
reason, the issue has since disappeared from the news.

Let me define my notion of a quack cure and differentiate it
from one that simply has not yet been accepted by the medical
establishment. To me, a quack cure is something that does not
permit any conventional treatment during or after its use. For
example, a doctor in Switzerland advertises, via the grapevine,
that his special blend of an extract of mistletoe cures breast cancer. The vital—or should I say fatal?—"catch-22" is that no other
treatment can be administered until the six-to-eight-week course
of mistletoe injections is completed. The doctor's prime targets,
naturally, are desperate women who know that their mastectomies
did not stop the spread of the cancer. These unfortunate victims
do not have six to eight weeks to waste on something that is
utterly useless. If they go to the Swiss doctor, it may be too late
for proven treatments to do them any good. (As far as I have
learned, the promoters of laetrile, hydrazine sulfate, and abscissic

acid make no such demand, but leave the patient free to go ahead with alternative therapies. Nonetheless, these have been denied FDA authorization for use as cancer treatments, and the American Cancer Society lists laetrile as quackery.)

"Cures" come and go like long skirts. So-called "vaccines" turn up periodically on unauthorized markets. One, reported in 1968, was a liquid saturated with bacteria, which was to be inhaled by means of an aerosol spray. The unique feature of this treatment, so its promoters said, was that if the patient was too weak to get out of her car, it could be administered at the curb outside the doctor's office. There is a "cure" that stuffs the patient with grapes, and another of red cabbage, either eaten raw or applied as a poultice of some kind. Many similar "miracle" diets are based on the belief that eating an excess of a particular food, vitamin, or mineral will cure cancer.

Then there are the gadgets—panels of knobs, colored lights, and switches, with controls to measure whatever response the patient is supposed to be giving. A wooden box lined with zinc has been touted as a device to renew the body's store of a cosmic energy called orgone, which, the manufacturers claim, is a very beneficial treatment for cancer.

These examples do not come from medieval medical tracts; they are from advertisements in pamphlets and newspapers published in the last half of the twentieth century. There is an underground cancer press that has many subscribers. For when cancer strikes and all hope is gone, intelligent, normally well-balanced people grab at anything. What do they have to lose but money? And someone is always there to take it.

Another kind of quackery must be mentioned, along with the grapes, gadgets, and orgone: the kind perpetrated by the doctor who deceives a patient. Moreover, general practitioners and surgeons who know little or nothing about the management of cancer but who, nonetheless, insist on treating patients with the disease are, in my opinion, just as dangerous as real quacks. Although they are physicians and they "mean well," they, too, cause patients to lose valuable time by giving inadequate or inappropriate treatment.

Most cancer specialists probably agree, although it is unlikely that any would ever say so for the written record. General physicians and surgeons should not be angry or insulted, since no one can fairly expect them to be experts in cancer when they have to deal with almost every ailment that exists. Unfortunately, however, they do not know what they do not know.

In the first few months after my mastectomy, I had a personal experience with a woman whose doctor either deceived her, out of misguided kindness, or was unaware of his lack of knowledge. She was a friend of a friend, and not long after I came home from the hospital she called to wish me good luck. She had undergone a mastectomy the previous January and knew what I was going through. "My doctor said he got it all out," she said happily. "He said I didn't need radiation, chemotherapy—anything. All my nodes were clean as pins."

Two or three months later she called again. This time she was hoarse and coughed after every other word. "That son of a bitch!" she cried. "I went in to see him because I had a cold that just wouldn't go away. He did a chest X-ray, and my lungs are loaded with cancer. It must have been there all along—it couldn't have spread that fast. Why didn't he put me on some kind of treatment? Why didn't he tell me it was spreading, instead of saying I was clean as a pin?"

A month later, I heard that the cancer had metastasized to her brain. Less than a year after her mastectomy, she was dead.

Her doctor was a general surgeon, with no expertise in the management of cancer. He knew only how to amputate malignant organs. She did not have preoperative scans of her lungs, or X-rays during her postoperative checkups. Until that chest X-ray eight months after the mastectomy, she had nothing but general physical examinations.

Perhaps the surgeon did not lie to her. Maybe he really thought she was all clear. Only he and the pathologist, of course, know what was found when her breast and nodes were removed. But *she* knew what was done afterward: nothing. If he did not deceive her, he was at best incompetent to manage a breast-cancer patient. Either way, he deprived her of perhaps a year of treatment as surely as the Swiss doctor takes away six or eight weeks. That year might only have further postponed her death, but even so, the extra time would have been worth it to her.

"Most women can't take the truth" is what one general surgeon gave me as his reason for not telling his patients the whole truth after a mastectomy. "If I find eight or ten positive nodes, they're lost anyhow. Why tell them? Or even their families? There's nothing to be done."

For this Hippocratian healer, and for all others who think as he does, I have one answer: You tell her, so that she can find someone who *does* know what to do about the eight or ten positive nodes. She is *not* "lost anyhow." Unless the cancer is so far advanced that all a woman can look forward to is a great deal of pain, even an extra six months is worth aiming for.

Of course, this inexcusable fatalism of general doctors does not apply only to breast cancer; it is true for all cancers. Oncologists are not so quick to write their patients off. They know of many things that can now be done to prolong life and keep it pain-free.

So, dear general doctor, do your best to remove all physicians from inclusion in anyone's "quackery" chapter. Tell your patients the truth—they can take it, or their families can—and help them find good cancer specialists to continue their treatment. You will be surprised to see how long we women can live today—even with eight or ten positive nodes.

Everyone, apparently, wants to make money from our free-enterprise medical system; and some doctors, misled by delusions of omniscience, are not excluded.

In the autumn of 1974, when both Betty Ford and Happy Rockefeller were struck by breast cancer, panicky women began stampeding to doctors' offices and hospital radiology departments for breast examinations. Established and reputable X-ray clinics suddenly had waiting lists that were weeks—sometimes months—long. To accommodate those who would not wait, general practitioners and gynecologists around the country began buying thermographs, the only breast-cancer detection device a physician who is not a radiologist is permitted to use. Several established detection clinics, while others used the equipment as a supplement to their regular physical examinations—at an additional cost of $40 to $50.

Thermography, based on the principle that malignant tissue retains more heat than healthy tissue does, picks up and films heat patterns from the breast. No potentially harmful radiation is involved; it can be used every week, if indicated. It sounds like the miracle we have all been hoping for, doesn't it? But thermography has one very grave flaw: its diagnoses of women who were later found to have breast cancer have been wrong more than 60 per cent of the time. This was reported on September 30, 1974, two days after Betty Ford's operation.

At the end of the first year of a mass screening program, when diagnoses made by the heat-recording device were compared with those from physical examination by an expert and from conventional mammograms or xeromammograms, the thermograms had *not* found the hidden cancers in 97 of 160 women subsequently diagnosed as "positive" by surgical biopsies. Mammograms and xeromammograms had been wrong in only 8 per cent of the cases in these demonstration projects—12 of the 160. The physical examination had made a correct diagnosis of "suspicious" or "positive" 57 per cent of the time, and had missed 69 cases. (But these were found by X-ray.)

Thus, thermography gave a rather poor third-place showing. Even the local medical representative of the manufacturer of the leading United States machine—General Electric's Spectrotherm— told me it alone should not be relied upon to find a malignancy in a woman having symptoms of one. Certainly not, experts at the National Cancer Institute and at hospital breast-cancer clinics agreed.

In March 1975, updated information reported by the American Cancer Society, cosponsor with NCI of the screening programs, showed that thermography had improved somewhat; "false negatives" had run about 55 per cent over the preceding six months. But women continued to flock to physicians who advocated thermography as a reliable diagnostic tool, heeding its "false negatives" and too often refusing to believe the machine is not accurate.

Thermograms are helpful adjuncts to mammograms in diagnosing breast abnormalities and are not themselves "quackery." But thermography clinics that rely only on this heat device for detection are. Perhaps the technique will soon be perfected so that it is as reliable as the X-ray, if not more so. But that has not happened yet, and no woman with a symptom indicating possible breast cancer should rely solely on a thermogram for a definitive diagnosis.

As the General Electric spokesman said, "Someone will always come along to make a fast buck out of somebody else's troubles." This, unfortunately, has been the history of quackery in cancer. Its victims have always been perfect lures for fast-buck artists.

4

Who, When, Where?

"It looks as if breast cancer is a cold-weather disease, doesn't it?" the statistician said, pointing toward a world map with the high-incidence countries colored red. "Look at them. Except for Israel, where a large part of the population originated in Europe, breast cancer seems to be confined to the top and bottom of the globe."

I studied the red blotches. "What could cold weather have to do with it?" I asked.

"I'm just commenting on the geography, that's all." He smiled. "As far as we know, weather—cold or hot—doesn't have anything to do with breast cancer. But there is a strong geographical pattern world-wide. You shouldn't ignore the epidemiology of the disease. It could give a valuable clue toward finding a cause."

I stared at the map hanging on his office wall. The United States and the southern half of Canada were a solid red, and so was the northern part of Europe, including the British Isles and Scandinavia (except for Finland), from the top half of France across to the eastern border of European Russia. In the southern hemisphere, South Africa was red, as were sizable portions of Australia and New Zealand. Iceland was colored in, and there was a red spot for Israel and a dot for Bombay, India. There certainly did appear to be a pattern.

"Not only does it seem to be geographical," he continued. "There are other interesting epidemiological aspects as well."

First, he reminded me that the term epidemiology has nothing to do with whether or not a disease is contagious and thus can cause an epidemic. "Both words, epidemic and epidemiology, come from the same Greek root, meaning 'staying among the people.' But epidemiology is the science of studying the kinds of people who get a disease, at what ages, and where it is most prevalent. Obviously, mammary carcinoma is primarily a disease of women, but there the obvious ends. There are dozens of epidemiological mysteries—especially the concentration in the upper northern hemisphere."

The statistician went on to say that until recently his young science has been virtually ignored by cancer researchers. "Their ears perk up when we talk about medical factors. But nutrition, industrialization—nothing doing."

"I've never read anything about those . . ."

"And the incidence keeps nosing up every year," he continued, not even hearing me. "There doesn't seem to be any explanation."

I called Dr. Sidney Cutler, the associate chief of the Biometry Branch of the National Cancer Institute, keeper of the records of cancer-incidence rates and those dire statistics known as "end results." (Biometry is the investigation of biological phenomena by mathematical and statistical means.)

"In 1974," he said, "cancer of the breast achieved the dubious distinction of having become the number-one cancer in the United States. That is, if intestinal malignancies are separated into colon and rectum, as they should be. It outranks lung cancer of males and females together." Dr. Cutler added that these data had not yet been published, but would be in the next edition of the NCI epidemiological report. The 1972 edition still showed lung cancer in the top position.

"But be careful to distinguish between incidence and mortality," he warned. "Breast-cancer incidence is higher—more women are getting it. Lung and bronchus still have the greatest mortality, however; fewer people are getting this carcinoma than breast cancer, but fewer survive. That's important to remember. Caught early, mammary carcinoma is more easily cured."

"Of course, it's mostly women," I said, "so half the population is counted out right there."

"About 99 per cent female," he agreed. "When you take that

into account, the impact is enormous. It's not spread around the population."

For unknown reasons, Dr. Cutler said, the age of onset appears to be dropping, and the disease is attacking younger women now than it did in earlier decades. He credited the wide publicity given to early detection, breast self-examination, and mass screening programs like those of the American Cancer Society for some of the age drop. "More women are finding tumors earlier, while they are small. That could account for a discovery at age forty-two instead of forty-five."

"Early detection would have absolutely nothing to do with the increased incidence, though," he said flatly. "That has just been going on too long. If the reason were earlier detection, there would have been a hook in the graph, showing a sudden increase in the level, for maybe five years. Then you would have a shift back to the preceding levels." He predicted such a hook on graphs for the last three months of 1974, representing the thousands of tumors discovered after Betty Ford's mastectomy. "But the rise is temporary in such instances," he added. "The steady annual increase in breast-cancer incidence has got to be due to something other than earlier detection."

At a breast-cancer conference held at the National Cancer Institute two days after Mrs. Ford's surgery, I had overheard a visiting oncologist talking to a colleague at the coffee bar. "I've never seen anything like it," he said. "It's almost an epidemic in Connecticut. What's it like in Cleveland?"

If the doctor from Connecticut should ever look up Dr. Cutler's data, he would learn that there is not much difference between his state and Ohio. In both, about 14 per cent of all cancers found are located in a woman's breast. Around the country, one of every fifteen women will develop a breast cancer sometime in her life. Grimly, in spite of all the advances in treatment and in earlier detection, about one-half of all these women will eventually die of the disease.

Some women run a higher risk of getting breast cancer than others, however, and that is where epidemiology comes in. Someday, the statisticians hope, their science will yield clues that result in pinpointing the cause of breast cancer. It is already yielding clues that help to identify the high-risk groups.

The red-blotched map suddenly became more important. On a mortality-rate table titled "Cancer Around the World, 1968–69," issued by the World Health Organization, I discovered that the United States was not first in the breast-cancer column at all, but was twelfth. The Netherlands had the highest mortality rate of the countries listed. Second was Scotland, third was England and Wales combined, then Israel and Northern Ireland. Denmark, Ireland, Iceland, Canada, New Zealand, and Switzerland also came before the United States. All are "cold-weather countries" except for Israel, and, even there, most of the population is Caucasians who originated in cold-weather countries.

At the other end of the statistical pole, the Dominican Republic had the lowest death rate, according to the table. "But who knows what data are available there?" said the medical librarian who had found the chart for me. "There are a lot of countries where cancer is still unmentionable—even if it is diagnosed."

Now I noticed that Taiwan and Japan had the second and third lowest reported mortality rates. "How are their data?" I asked.

"Well," the librarian answered, "Japan is mentioned by statisticians quite a lot, so I suppose the figures from there must be fairly reliable. I don't know about Taiwan."

A word about statistical charts, graphs, and tables, and the various ways they are compiled. With respect to incidence data, some countries collect absolute figures—the actual totals of patients during a given year, based on doctors' reports and hospital admissions. In other countries, where years of record keeping have marked a specific region as being typical of the nation as a whole, biometricians often collect figures from that single region and use them as a model to project the nationwide average. This is faster, but not as accurate. Still others average the rates of selected areas in different regions.

Most incidence data (and survival-mortality rates, too) are expressed as the number of cases per 100,000 of the total population. With breast cancer, many countries more realistically base the rate on the female population only. However, this usually includes females below the age of twenty, not just those in the vulnerable age groups. Since children and teen-agers rarely get breast cancer, their inclusion in the base has the effect of lowering the incidence rate. Some tables "age-adjust" the data, to take this distortion into account.

Some countries collect no raw data at all; some perhaps collect data but do not report them to the World Health Organization or any other international agency. Within a country, the quality of data can vary from region to region, city to city, or even neighborhood to neighborhood within a city. Comparing statistics of one country with those from another can, therefore, result in considerable confusion. Throughout these pages, I give comparative figures only when they all come from the same table or graph.

Returning to the WHO table, I studied the numbers for Japan. More than the Pacific Ocean separated that country's 4.01 breast-cancer deaths per 100,000 from the United States's 22.18 per 100,000. Even a data-collection system that was full of errors could not alone account for the huge difference.

The librarian was watching me. "I don't think you should be looking at death rates at all if you want meaningful information," she remarked. "Diagnosis and treatment are so spotty in some countries that mortality rates aren't necessarily a reflection of anything. After all, if only two out of 100,000 women in a place develop breast cancer and both of them die from it, you have 100-per-cent mortality, but only a fraction of a per cent in incidence." As a case in point, she found a mention of a small town in Argentina that had a 50-per-cent-higher mortality rate one year than the United States had. "And yet the incidence rate is much lower in South America than it is here." She smiled. "So, you see, there's no real connection between incidence and mortality in some countries."

She was right, of course. Not only would her suggestion to look at incidence rates be more accurate; it would also be more cheerful.

I began with the "who." Who are the women most likely to develop breast cancer?

The highest-risk category of all is made up of women who, like me, have already had one cancerous breast removed. We are the most likely of all to develop a malignancy—another one, in the second breast.

This I had already been told. But nowhere could I find a comprehensive summing up of other high-risk or low-risk groups. I had to wade through isolated and scattered reports from all over the world to make some sense of all the statistics. It became a fascinating detective story.

An interesting discovery I made at the outset was that, where breast-cancer incidence rates are concerned, epidemiologists and biometricians distinguish between women of Latin or Mediterranean backgrounds and other white women—though all are Caucasians—because the Latin-Mediterranean groups' rates are considerably lower. Over all, however, in the United States, white women have a higher incidence than women of other races, a pattern that seems to prevail all over the world.

Several surveys I read stated outright that being black was in itself a protection, but Dr. Marvin Schneiderman, the associate director of field studies and statistics at the National Cancer Institute, told me this is not so and that there is no difference in incidence rates between the two races. The puzzle was cleared up for me by a report that linked affluence and breast cancer. "As black women climb socio-economically," it said, "their life styles change and their breast-cancer incidence by income and social status is the same as that of white women in the same group." The survey concludes that there simply are far fewer affluent black women in the United States than affluent white women and that this distorts the data.

"It's what we call a statistical artifact," I was told by one statistician. "You can't always go by absolute numbers. There are other factors." It will be interesting to see if the breast-cancer incidence rates of American black women continue to rise along with a better life style and higher incomes.

An international study done in 1970 compared the breast-cancer incidences of six countries. The United States and Wales were rated "high," Brazil and Greece "intermediate," Japan and Taiwan "low." Why? No one knows. But, again, the implication is clear: being white raises the risk.

So does being Jewish—sometimes. An American Jewish woman whose parents or grandparents came from Europe is in a higher-risk group than the rest of American white women. But if her family is from a North African or Asian Jewish background, her risk of developing a breast cancer is lower than the average for all other American women.

Being overweight is another factor that increases the risk of developing a malignant tumor. Not only that, but excess avoir-dupois also can make it more difficult to find one that is already there.

Cancer frequently "runs in the family." Whether this means that the disease is actually hereditary, the way brown hair or blue eyes are, is hotly debated by scientists, since familial diseases can be caused by other factors than genetics, such as having the same diet or environment. One cancer specialist told me he feels the most important factor is the age of a woman's mother or sister at the time either developed her breast cancer. "If they were seventy-five or so," he said, "there would be little risk. If they were premenopausal, a real risk; if in their thirties, a severe risk."

The heredity debate is immaterial so far as risk is concerned. If a woman's sister had breast cancer, her chances of getting the disease are higher than for someone without this factor. If her mother had the disease, the risk is somewhat lower than with a sister, but higher than for someone with no breast cancer in the family. Some specialists say that having a maternal aunt or maternal grandmother with the disease also qualifies a woman for the high-risk category.

Having a history of benign breast disease similarly increases a woman's risk. This includes fibrocystic disease, adenomas, chronic mastitis, a tendency to be "cysty" or "lumpy," infections and abscesses, and some kinds of accidental injuries to the breasts. Cysts, adenomas, and the like rarely become malignant, but any-one with a tendency to grow benign lumps may have a predisposi-tion to develop malignant ones as well. Also, being accustomed to having breast masses makes it easy to overlook or neglect a new one.

Women in all of these high-risk categories should give them-selves a breast self-examination—BSE—every month (the pro-cedure is described in detail later). They should also have mammograms at least once a year after the age of forty and be examined every six months by a physician trained in breast pal-pation. In addition, a woman with a family background of cancer

must be sure her doctor knows this history. Some oncologists think
high-risk women over age thirty-five should be X-rayed twice
each year.

A variety of factors involving reproductive life—the years from
the onset of menstruation through the menopause—affect a
woman's risk of getting breast cancer. No one knows exactly
why, except that the secretion of female hormones must somehow
be involved. But epidemiology, remember, is based on analyses
of statistical data collected from patients, doctors, and hospitals,
not on laboratory experimentation or clinical trials, and for the
moment we are concerned only with identifying the "who," not
the "why."

Women who begin menstruating at an early age (in the United
States, before twelve) are more likely to develop breast cancer.
Early menarche, the medical term for early menstruation, presup-
poses a long reproductive life.

On the other hand, if a woman has her ovaries removed before she is thirty-five, or has a natural menopause at an early
age, her chances of developing breast cancer drop considerably.

A woman whose first full-term child was born before she was
twenty (that particular age applies only in the United States)
has substantially reduced her risk of developing breast cancer.
At the other end of the age line, a woman who has her first child
after thirty-five has elevated her risk, as has someone who has no
children at all.

The significance of the number of children a woman has had—
her "parity"—is a subject of debate among breast-cancer experts
around the world. There seems to be little question that nulliparous women—those who have no children—are high-risk
candidates, and it has also been widely accepted that bearing the
first child at a very early age confers some protection, for reasons
as yet unknown. The dispute centers around whether having
many children is protective.

In Moscow, I was given a plausible explanation by Professor
O. V. Sviatukhina, a slim, graying woman of perhaps fifty-five,
who is both a surgeon and an endocrinologist, and heads the
all-female staff of the breast-cancer section at the Institute of
Experimental and Clinical Oncology. Professor Sviatukhina believes that a woman is less vulnerable to mammary carcinoma

while she is actually breast-feeding. Therefore, if she has four
or five children and nurses each for two years, she gains eight
or ten years of immunity that a non-breast-feeding mother does
not have. If Professor Sviatukhina is correct—and other experts
abroad agree with her—it is not the number of children but the
years of breast feeding that count.

And this brings us directly to the most controversial of the
reproductive-life factors in relation to breast cancer. *Does* breast
feeding protect a woman against the disease? For decades, it
was commonly accepted that it did, at least during the period
of actual breast feeding. Then Dr. Brian MacMahon, a Harvard
epidemiologist, said, "No, it does nothing one way or the other."

Suddenly all the authorities did an about-face. In his book
Early Detection, Dr. Philip Strax, a diagnostician-radiologist at
New York's Guttman Institute, agreed with Dr. MacMahon. "It
used to be thought that breast-feeding—especially prolonged
breast-feeding—was associated with a lower incidence of breast
cancer," he wrote. "The latest data on a world-wide basis refute
this concept. Apparently there is no relationship between nursing
and breast cancer." Since I had been weaned on the gospel according to La Leche League, to me this was heresy. But science
is science. That was when I moved "protection conferred by
lactation" firmly into the myth category.

But then I visited Russia and heard Professor Sviatukhina describe her theory. I asked her what evidence she had found in
her laboratories or clinics to support it.

She explained that the hormone prolactin, which triggers milk
production, but is always present in a woman's blood in smaller
quantities, contributes to the growth of mammary carcinoma during periods when she is not nursing. For reasons not yet known,
prolactin loses its ability to produce neoplasms when a woman
is breast-feeding; the professor believes it is because the brain
signals the production of some kind of inhibiting hormone
during this period. The more children a woman has and the
longer she breast-feeds them—three years or more is common in
the Soviet Union, Professor Sviatukhina said—the longer she has
this protection against the adverse effects of prolactin.

And the professor thinks the theory has been proven in her
clinics. Russian women who live in cities usually work; therefore,

few of them are able to breast-feed. They are also more likely
to take oral contraceptives, which could increase their prolactin
levels. In rural areas, most women breast-feed and few of them
take the Pill—and there is much less mammary carcinoma than
in the cities.

Professor Sviatukhina reconverted me. In spite of hard data
to the contrary from top epidemiologists, I have taken breast feeding out of myths and put it back into epidemiology—but with a
question mark. Every woman must decide her superstition for
herself.

One caution: Some evidence indicates that a woman who has
had one cancerous breast removed may transmit suspicious particles via the milk of the other breast. For this reason, most doctors
recommend *against* breast feeding by anyone who has had a
mastectomy.

Now, according to all this data, who in the United States is
most likely to develop breast cancer? Jewish white women of
northern European descent who are overweight, have cancer in
their families, began menstruating early, and had a first child
after they were thirty-five years old.

And who, so far, is least likely to develop it? Oriental or American Indian women with no history of breast disorders, no cancer
in the family, late beginning of menstruation, and motherhood
before age twenty. Orientals have less risk than any other women
in the world. A short reproductive life because of an early menopause—surgical or natural—helps lower the risk for everyone.

When is breast cancer most likely to appear?

The disease rarely develops in girls under twenty, and until
recently it was seldom found before thirty. Today more and
more women under thirty are becoming victims. For unknown
reasons, when it does occur under thirty it is more virulent than
is the case with older women.

As Dr. Cutler had told me, the incidence peaks between the
ages of forty-two and forty-seven. Then an eight-year plateau
appears on the graphs—the statistical phenomenon known as
"Clemmesen's hook."

The term describes a "bump" in graphs on which age and
frequency of occurrence are plotted together. The bump occurs

after about the age of forty-five. Until then, the graph shows a steadily climbing line, beginning at about age thirty and continuing until forty-five. Now comes the bump, and the line levels off into the eight-year plateau. Starting in the early fifties, the rate again climbs, though not as steeply, until very old age.

Many experts interpret this as statistical support for the belief that breast cancer in young women is a different disease from that in older women. The theory received support from American investigators in a study published in December 1974. Three Johns Hopkins researchers, Dr. Thomas J. Craig, Dr. George W. Comstock, and a nurse, Patricia B. Geiser (the study was done at the Johns Hopkins University, with funds from the National Cancer Institute), reported a distinct difference in the histories and risk factors of women who developed breast cancer before the age of forty-five and women who developed it later in life. According to their findings, a family history of breast cancer and a later age for the birth of the first child were more often associated with the younger women, while breast feeding was a factor mainly with the older ones.

Many women think the risk of getting breast cancer disappears after age seventy. That is not true. The total number of new cases does drop with age, because fewer women are still alive, but the incidence rate among women over seventy actually increases. Anyone lucky enough to have reached threescore and ten must not think she is home free. She should pick a set day every month for self-examination and never forget to do it, as well as have an annual physical examination by her doctor.

Here is a simple "scorecard" by which a woman can test herself and see roughly where she falls in the risk areas discussed so far.

Anyone scoring 225 or higher should practice monthly breast self-examination (BSE), and have a physical examination of the breasts by her doctor every six months and a mammogram annually. Between 100 and 220, she should examine her breasts monthly, have a physical exam as part of an annual checkup, and have periodic X-rays. Below 100, BSE remains a must, along with a physical exam as part of an annual checkup.

Where are the risks highest?

Self-test Scorecard

Age group   **Your risk**

20-34 10 points	35-49 40 points	50+ 90 points

Race group

Oriental 10 points	Black 20 points	Caucasian 30 points

Family history

None 10 points	Mother, sister, aunt, or grandmother with breast cancer 50 points	Mother and sister with breast cancer 100 points

Your history

No breast cancer 10 points	Previous breast cancer 100 points

Pregnancy

First pregnant before 25 10 points	First pregnant 25 or after 15 points	Never pregnant 20 points

Your total

Reprinted by permission of the *National Enquirer*

Only within the past few years has much attention been paid to the possible role of the environment in relation to breast cancer. But today, when we have more and more potentially harmful substances all around us, the "where" of breast-cancer incidence has become increasingly significant, and the epidemiologists are beginning to come into their own.

For example, they have found that the region around Birmingham, England, has more cases of breast cancer than the Liverpool area.

Why?

That women living in the European republics of the Soviet Union have more than five times the breast-cancer incidence rates of those in the Asian republics. Yet when Asian women move to the European sections their rates rise to match the existing ones.

Why?

That, in Israel, Jewish women from American or European families have at least three times the incidence of breast cancer as do Jewish women whose backgrounds are North African or Asian, while those from Yemen have less than the Africans and Asians.

Why?

That the Parsi women of Bombay have twice the breast-cancer incidence of Hindu, Christian, and Moslem women there.

Why?

That those red high-incidence blotches on the world map do seem to form a weird geographical cold-weather pattern.

Why?

What could possibly explain all these statistical oddities?

I looked again for clues in the World Health Organization's mortality-rate tables. The highs were primarily cold-weather countries; the lows were the Dominican Republic (whose data may not be the best), and Japan, Taiwan, and the Philippines— Oriental.* With a mental reservation about the reliability of data, I saw that Mexico, Colombia, and Mauritius, also toward the bottom of the list, had mortality rates so low that even bad reporting could probably not explain the gap between them and

---

* Data are not available from most Oriental countries.

the high-risk countries. Not quite so low, but far lower than the United States, were Bulgaria, Chile, Rumania, Venezuela, and Greece. Toward the middle were Finland and Italy.

Finland? Its relatively low incidence did not fit the northern-hemisphere, cold-weather geographical picture I was trying to paint. What was Finland doing so low? I called a cancer epidemiologist.

"Well, you know that genetics plays some role in breast cancer," he began.

I nodded, even though he could not see me. "Yes, I've read about the Parsi women, and about families with a lot of—"

"Centuries ago," he interrupted, "Asiatic tribesmen came westward on horseback to escape Genghis Khan. Some of them settled in the Danube basin and became Magyars—now Hungarians. Others kept going northward and became the ancestors of today's Finns and Estonians. I would guess that their Asiatic heritage may have given Finnish women some kind of built-in genetic protection, which has survived over the centuries of intermarriage and exposure to a different environment. Their incidence rates are higher than Japan's, aren't they?"

Genetic protection?

My thoughts turned to those Parsi women, who have twice as much breast cancer as the Hindu, Christian, and Moslem women of Bombay. The Parsis, some 100,000 strong, are descended from Zoroastrian refugees who escaped from Persia about 1,300 years ago. They live mainly in Bombay and have kept themselves very much segregated from their neighbors, so that they are perhaps the most inbred people in the world. And their women have so much breast cancer that it accounts for half of *all* Parsi cancers. No wonder breast-cancer researchers are interested in them. The value of having a naturally bred 1,300-year-old population like this cannot be measured. I couldn't help wondering if modern Persian women have high unreported incidences.

But what is the reason for all the Parsi breast cancer? No one knows, except that it must be something genetic—a predisposition of some kind for these women to develop the disease.

Then I stumbled onto another mystery, which made no apparent sense in relation to what I had learned about breast cancer —differences in diet. Dr. Frits deWaard, a professor at the University of Utrecht, in Holland (the country at the top of the mortality list), has spent years studying nutrition and the role it might play in mammary carcinoma. He has found a definite correlation between what he calls total body volume—a combination of weight and height—and the incidence of the disease, and he thinks that large women—those who are unusually tall or fat or both—are very high risks.

To support his argument, Dr. deWaard cited the differences in the diets of Yemeni women in Israel and of Israeli women who have a more European life style. "Yemeni food was very tasty," he told me, "but I would not like to eat it every day. There is very little meat, mainly vegetables and starches. They use primarily vegetable fats, no butter. In Holland, we are not accustomed to that kind of food."

"Did I understand you correctly?" I asked. "Height is a factor, as well as weight?" Most authorities, I knew, agree that obesity is a factor in computing risks, but until then I had heard nothing about height.

"Height as well," he insisted. "It is total body volume. Height and weight cannot be separated. You know that in your country children of immigrants are usually much bigger than their parents. Not only are the girls taller than their mothers, but also they are heavier in general. And they tend to begin their reproductive lives earlier. In the United States, the average age of menarche is twelve or thirteen. But elsewhere, in Finland, for example, it is not at all unusual for it to be sixteen or older."

He reminded me of studies of the Japanese in California and Hawaii, where Japanese-American women are being surveyed for just this kind of generation gap. Those who were born in Japan and who have maintained a basically Japanese diet and way of life in the United States have breast-cancer incidences as low as in Japan. However, their daughters, who have adopted more of the American dietary and other habits, have more breast cancer. Now the granddaughters are reaching the vulnerable age group, and they are developing even more breast cancers than their mothers did. While some kind of racial genetic protection may exist that will always keep their rates below average, the incidence has been increasing with each generation.

A similar survey was done of Jewish women in New York, I

learned. Being Jewish, and knowing that women with my background have a higher risk than others, I looked into this as soon
as I read of it. Between 1949 and 1951, American Cancer Society
analysts compared the breast-cancer incidence among immigrant
Jews with that of their American-born daughters. The older
women had about the same rate as did the control group of
non-Jewish New Yorkers. Their daughters' rate was much higher.
Diet and nutrition were not specifically mentioned, but the different environment was pinpointed as a possible contributing
factor, and diet is certainly a part of one's environment.

Herbert Seidman, the Cancer Society statistician who ran the
survey, said the explanation was really quite simple. "The daughters became more affluent and were able to afford things their
mothers could not." He agreed that one of the first things people
buy when they have more money is richer and more varied
foods. "Certainly they began eating better," he said. "But there
are other factors. A good many of them went to college, and
this meant marrying later and having their first children later.
That sort of reproductive change would also be significant, I
think."

I thought that Dr. deWaard had been more convincing, and
in Moscow, talking with Professor Aleksandr Chaklin, chief of
epidemiology at the oncology institute, I brought up the question
of diet. He, too, felt that Dr. deWaard's conclusions made sense.

Professor V. M. Dilman, an endocrinologist at the Petrov
Research Institute of Oncology, in Leningrad, was even more
emphatic. "Fat women have more mammary carcinomas than
skinny women," he said. "Of that, there is no question. There is
something found in some foods that contributes. There is also
a high correlation between women who developed both diabetes
and mammary carcinoma in later life—and, as you know, diabetes is a disease connected with foods."

He showed me some of his data. "I feel strongly," he said, in
his excellent English, "that a young woman who shows signs
that she may have diabetes should be doubly watched for signs
of mammary carcinoma as well." He explained that one early
diabetic symptom is giving birth to a baby that weighs ten
pounds or more. "Rich diet, obesity, and diabetes go together,"
he said. "And I believe mammary carcinoma goes along also."

My beautiful northern-hemisphere geographic picture was
being badly muddled by affluence, nutrition, and now diabetes.
Also, several references had been made to city women versus
rural women. And then those genetic factors could not be forgotten. What about those countries whose people were descended from Asiatics—Hungary, Finland, and Estonia?

"How are Estonian incidence rates?" I asked Professor Chaklin. "Pretty low, no?"

His eyebrows lifted to his hairline. "Oh, very high! All of the
Baltic republics have very high rates of mammary carcinoma.
See here." He showed me a chart. "Here we see Turkmen has
an incidence rate of 5.4." (He pronounced it as "five and four.")
"Now here we have Estonia." He pointed higher on the list.
"Estonia has 28.6. In Estonia, there is almost six times the mam-
mary carcinoma as in Turkmen."

"That doesn't make sense, Professor Chaklin," I said, surprised.
"Estonians and Finns are first cousins. Even their languages are
alike."

"You mean because they are both descended from the Mon-
gols?"

I nodded. "The Finnish incidence rates are much lower than
they are in other northern countries."

Professor Chaklin shrugged. "Estonia is higher than Finland,
and, as I told you, the republic of Turkmen is much, much
lower. By my data, it seems that Estonia is even higher than
Holland." He suggested I go to Tallinn, the capital of Estonia,
to talk to Professor Maret Purde, that republic's chief cancer
epidemiologist. But it was impossible to hop a plane for a fast
interview with her.

I recalled my conversation in Helsinki with Dr. Matti Hakama,
one of the chief epidemiologists in Finland. "Finnish women
have a lower incidence than other Scandinavian women because
our people still are more rural and have a lower standard of
living. The diet has far less protein and fats. Our women marry
earlier and have their children earlier, and—especially in the
rural areas—they have many children." He rejected the Mongol
theory sharply, and I dropped the subject. "It is simply not true,"
he said—sharply.

Dr. Hakama went on to say that breast-cancer incidence in

Finland had been climbing since the urban population began to grow. "In 1967, there were 550 city women and 354 rural women with the disease. In 1971, the totals were 704 for women living in cities and 452 in the country. I think there is a definite correlation between urbanization and the rising incidence in Finland."

His opinion about city living agreed with what I had been told by Dr. Helen Westerberg, at the Karolinska Institute, in Stockholm. "In Sweden, I suppose the incidence rate is about the same as in the United States," she said. "We have around 3,000 cases annually—somewhat more than Norway, but far fewer than Denmark."

"Why is Finland so much lower?" I asked.

"Well, because Finland is, I think, predominantly a more rural country than Sweden is," she replied. "There is some work showing a correlation between high blood pressure and breast cancer. That would be urbanization as well, don't you think?"

I remembered what Professor Sviatukhina had said about the differences in the city and country women who came to her Moscow clinics, and Professor Chaklin confirmed this with data from the rest of the Soviet Union. "In the cities and in the European republics, there are many more mammary carcinomas," he said. "Estonia is an excellent example." Again he urged me to visit Professor Purde in Tallinn.

"Next trip," I promised, thanking him for his help.

Help? Now I had the added puzzle of what had happened in Estonia to make it so different from Finland.

Back home, I found there was not much information available about breast cancer in Estonia. I wrote Professor Purde, but received no answer for several months. When she replied, she said that her statistics showed Estonia's breast-cancer incidence rates to be *lower* than those of Finland. However, Dr. Schneiderman, one of the top international epidemiologists at the National Cancer Institute, thought she must be using different statistical bases for her data, and he referred me to Professor Calum Muir, director of the International Agency for Research in Cancer, in Lyon, France. By telephone, Professor Muir confirmed that, according to his agency's data, Finland's breast-cancer incidence rate was lower than that of any of the Baltic Soviet republics or of the other Scandinavian countries.

But all this was three months after my return from Europe. Until Professor Purde's reply arrived, I had not been sure I would have an answer soon enough to include it here. What to do?

People who live in Washington have the habit of picking up the telephone and asking the federal bureaucracy for information on almost anything, and that was what I did. I called an agency that keeps track of current happenings in various parts of the world—only to learn that nobody in Washington collected statistics on breast cancer in Estonia. "However, we do have other recent information about Estonia," I was told. "If you have any nonmedical questions that we might be able to answer, please put them in writing. We'll do our best."

I struggled with all the factors I had collected. Race? ethnicity? being Jewish?—genetics. Diet and nutrition? affluence? urban versus rural?—environment. Oral contraceptives? breast feeding? age when first baby was born?—reproductive life. Finally I boiled it all down to this:

"Using World War II as a dividing line, is the over-all population [of Estonia] still as ethnically (genetically) related to the Finns? Has there been much migration between Estonia and other European republics of the USSR? What are the possible ethnic breakdowns, if available, between women with Asiatic heritages? Jewish women? Other non-European stock, such as Laplanders or Eskimos? Are more women working in factories than formerly? Do more women live in urbanized areas than on farms? Are they marrying later—or, more directly, are they giving birth to their first child at a later age? Are they having fewer children? Are they taking oral contraceptives? Are they breast-feeding their infants as they did before?"

In the middle of the composition of the letter came a report that Seventh-Day Adventists (who eat no meat at all) and Mormons (who eat much less meat than the general population) have much lower breast-cancer incidence rates than the rest of the United States population. Meat! Dr. Hakama had said that Finns ate little animal protein or fat; Professor Chaklin had said that Estonia was a big cattle-raising country.

"Have there been changes in diet?" my letter continued. "Is more animal fat used in cooking and baking, as opposed to vegetable oils? Is more meat being eaten? What kind? What is butter consumption?"

The letter was sent, and I really expected to hear from Tallinn first. In the meantime, I studied a risk chart I had put together and tried to guess from it what could have pushed the Estonians' breast-cancer incidence rates higher than those of their cousins in Finland. Estonia, I discovered from our tattered and worn *World Book Encyclopedia*, is a "granary" of northern Europe. Granaries mean cattle, and cattle mean a lot of relatively inexpensive beef. It might be a clue. Also, there were strong suggestions that the population of Estonia had changed after World War II, while Finland has remained quite homogeneous.

But who knew? The various military occupations during World War II, the deaths and immigrations and emigrations, might have left Estonia without many ethnic natives. Certainly the environment must have changed considerably since the country became part of the Soviet Union. Collectivization of farms usually means mechanization and fewer people needed in the countryside. If city women there are like the women in Moscow and Leningrad, they are working, not staying at home. This could mean later marriage, later first babies, and little or no breast feeding. More important, perhaps, it would mean two family incomes: affluence.

Now that my projections were made, based on what I had learned from other high-risk areas, I waited impatiently for a reply. Considering that Washington was still going through the post-Watergate upheaval, the answer came quickly. I had it in less than three weeks.

In 1970, only 68.2 per cent of the population of Estonia was ethnic Estonians. The rest were mainly Russians and Ukrainians. During and after World War II the native population apparently was reduced. So almost one-third of the people were *not* first cousins to the Finns.

"Prior to World War II," the letter said, "Estonia had been predominantly a rural nation. With war [came] a large-scale industrial build-up and urbanization, primarily in Tallinn and the surrounding areas. More people are living in urban areas now than earlier. There are many more women in factories now than prior to World War II." More women in factories meant more women in the cities, of course.

The report went on to say that since Estonians are among the more westernized of the Soviet peoples, the women might be taking oral contraceptives; there was no real knowledge, however, just an assumption. There were also no data about the average age of marriage or the average number of children. But the report said that the birth rate had been dropping and that the average woman in the Soviet Union married between the ages of twenty and twenty-five. As seems to be the case everywhere, rural women were having more children than city women.

"We have no statistics on whether Estonian women breast-feed infants as often as was done prior to World War II," my researcher wrote. But he guessed that, with more women working, there was an over-all decrease in the number of nursing mothers.

"There was a 14-per-cent increase in meat consumption between 1965 and 1971." My old *World Book Encyclopedia* had already confirmed what Professor Chaklin had said: that Estonia is a top cattle-raising region, known for beef, milk, butter, and other milk products, and that apparently it produces enough for export. If there was enough to sell abroad, I guessed, the local consumption had probably increased by more than 14 per cent since 1971.

Everything in the report fit the format.

Meanwhile, I had managed to obtain one report (in Russian) about breast cancer in Estonia, written by the same Professor Purde I was waiting to hear from. Translation showed that the paper concerned the role of several hormones in breast-cancer development. In addition, to my surprise, she gave some evidence that, in Estonia, there is a high correlation between breast-cancer incidence and a certain kind of goiter (not the one caused by an iodine deficiency) called thyrotoxicosis. Could that be another factor? Thyroid trouble?

Library research showed that scientists in the United States were also hot on this trail. Dr. Bernard Eskin, in Philadelphia, has been working for years on the relationship between thyroid disease and breast cancer, but he is certain there is a connection that involves iodine deficiency. His goal: to use possible thyroid problems as early indicators of potential breast-cancer victims.

Professor Purde made another point that did not fit my format. According to her data, a large number of breast-cancer patients began their reproductive lives *late*—at age seventeen or older. If she had not emphasized the age several times, I would have passed it off as a printer's error. But she did repeat it more than once, and data cannot be changed simply because they fit no format.

The Estonian reproductive clock must be set for a few years later than ours, by the way. In the United States, ages twelve to fourteen are the usual years for the beginning of menstruation; Finland's average age is sixteen. Also, the average first-child age here is twenty; Professor Purde's comparable age was twenty-six.

Since her report was primarily about hormonal aspects of breast cancer, the environment was not mentioned. But genetics was. In 1,802 families of breast-cancer patients, she reported finding twice the number of cancer victims she had expected from general-population statistics.

What to make of all this? Some of the new factors made sense; others were a puzzle. Elsewhere, I found still more new correlations—I should say "suspected correlations." For example, Dr. Nicholas I. Petrakis, of the University of California, has been comparing breast fluid extracted from Chinese women with fluid from Caucasian women, in an attempt to link the low Oriental breast-cancer incidence to the presence or absence of some substance in the body. In the course of these analyses, described in the chapter on early detection, he and his colleagues found an association between breast cancer and ear-wax secretion. Women with small amounts of dry wax, common among Orientals, have a much lower incidence than do those with wet, sticky ear wax, which is more prevalent in Caucasians. No one knows why.

Another correlation, reported in 1968, is that women having a certain kind of salivary-gland carcinoma have eight times the normal breast-cancer incidence. Again, no explanation.

There is even a funny side to breast-cancer epidemiology. A serious scientific study several years ago said that a woman is more likely to develop a first cancer in the breast opposite from her husband's handedness. In the fall of 1974, at the Royal Marsden Cancer Hospital, in London, one of the younger oncologists took me aside during a tea break. "Is your President Ford, by any chance, left-handed?" he asked.

"Yes," I told him. I explained that much had been made in the American press about the southpaw President.

"From newspaper pictures, he looks to be left-handed, but that, of course, could be a reversed negative as well."

"I am certain he is left-handed," I insisted. "There was a lot about it the first time he signed a batch of bills."

"That's all very interesting," the doctor commented, telling me about the study.

"What do you think of it?" I asked. "Mrs. Ford's cancer was in her right breast."

"A coincidence, I'm sure," he replied.

Or is this another mysterious factor?

"Oh, pay it no mind." He laughed. "It's probably just that most men are right-handed, and most women develop first tumors in the left breast. Correlation doesn't necessarily mean cause and effect, you know—just coincidence."

In epidemiology, this is an important difference to remember. All the risk factors may not be actual cause and effect; living in cities instead of rural areas, for example, may be coincidental, not contributory. Nonetheless, no one knows, and women must respect the high-risk factors epidemiologists have identified. On the chart here, possible risk factors whose effects are unknown are listed at the bottom.

The following chart has no point system. If a woman fits several of the categories at the high end, she should examine her breasts monthly and have a doctor's examination and a mammogram at least once a year. She should also be sure her doctor is aware of her risk status.

For the intermediate category, monthly BSE and annual mammograms after the age of forty should be enough. A woman blessed with being at the bottom of the page must remember that low risk does not mean no risk. Monthly breast self-examination and regular visits to a doctor experienced in palpation are essential after thirty-five. However, mammograms may not be indicated; it depends on the physician.

Epidemiology may ultimately provide clues about the causes and cure of breast cancer. The science has already produced

BREAST-CANCER RISKS FOR U.S. WOMEN

	WHO	WHEN	WHERE

HIGH	1. Family history of cancer
	    Self—breast or other cancer
	    Sister
	    Mother
	    Maternal grandmother or
	        aunts
	    Maternal first cousins
	
	2. Prior history of benign
	    breast disease
	
	3. Reproductive history
	    Early menstruation
	    No children
	    Late (or no) beginning of
	        sexual activity
	    First child born after age 35
	    Late menopause
	
	4. Race and ethnicity
	    Jews of European ancestry
	    Non-Jews of northern
	        European background
	        (including Iceland)
	    Affluent blacks
	
	5. Diet
	    Obesity due to high amounts
	        of animal proteins and
	        fats, including butter, lard,
	        cheese, whole milk
		Age 40 and
		up (includ-
		ing women
		over 70)
			Large in-
			dustrial
			cities,
			especially
			in the
			Northeast
			
			Also:
			San Fran-
			cisco-
			Oakland
			
			Minne-
			apolis-
			St. Paul
			
			Detroit
			
			Pittsburgh
			
			Iowa
			
			Colorado

INTERMEDIATE	1–3. Average rates in the above
	        categories
	
	4. Race and ethnicity
	    Middle-income blacks
	    Latin Americans
	    Southern European
	        ancestries
	
	5. Diet
	    Moderate amounts of animal
	        protein and fats
	        (e.g., Mormons)
		Ages
		25–39
			Medium-
			sized cities
			
			Also:
			Dallas-Fort
			Worth
			
			Atlanta

LOW	1. No family history of cancer 2. No history of prior breast disease	Under age 25	Small towns and rural areas

WHO	WHEN	WHERE

3. Reproductive history
   Late menstruation
   First child born before age 20
   Early beginning of sexual
      activity
   Early menopause (natural
      or artificial)
		Also:
		Birming-
		ham, Ala.

4. Race and ethnicity
   Jews of North African or
      Asian ancestries
   Non-Jews of Finnish ancestry
   Low-income whites
   Low-income blacks
   American Indians
   Oriental ancestries		

5. Diet
   Mainly nonmeat protein and
      vegetable fats (e.g., Sev-
      enth Day Adventists		

Other possible risk factors, effect unknown or subject to debate: Breast feeding, use of oral contraceptives, number of children, height, blood pressure, role of paternal ancestry, diabetes, enlarged thyroid gland, salivary-gland cancer, emotional stress, mental depression, quantity and quality of ear-wax secretion.

Data compiled by Rose Kushner; copyright © 1975 by Rose Kushner

LOW

enough information to help women pigeonhole themselves on the risk chart and, perhaps, find a breast cancer early enough to be cured.

If they will take advantage of it.

5

And Why?

It was a day to be marked in red on my calendar. The bandages were coming off, and I was told I could wear a loose bra and stuff absorbent cotton into the empty cup. I cannot explain why, but it made an enormous psychological difference to look down and see two elevations instead of one.

As if this were not enough, Dr. Dao suggested I get dressed that afternoon and come over to see what his Endocrine Research Laboratory was doing about finding a cure for breast cancer. "I am a biochemist as well as a surgeon, you know," he said. "Being able to do a good mastectomy is only part of dealing with this disease. We must find a cure, so that we won't need mastectomies at all. The really important work is going on in the laboratories. Why don't you come down after lunch? I'll be expecting you."

The invitation was exciting for two reasons. I did want to see what the lab looked like and what was going on. But, more important personally, it showed that Dr. Dao felt I was in the clear and rid of the cancer. He was treating me like a science reporter, not a patient.

Elated on all counts, I surveyed my wardrobe: a blue-and-white-striped cord pantsuit and a sleeveless blouse. They were what I had had on my back when I rushed to New York. After lunch, I dressed and scrutinized myself in the mirror. Nobody, but nobody, would be able to guess which one was real and which one was absorbent cotton.

Dr. Dao was wearing the white, stiffly starched laboratory over-coat researchers all over the world wear. It changed his person-ality completely. No longer was he my surgeon making daily rounds. He had become *Herr Direktor,* Chief of the Endocrine Research Laboratory. Even his floppy, brightly dotted bow tie did not detract from the picture of scientific endeavor.

I looked around at the banks of expensive electronic equip-ment, with names ending in -meter and tongues of computerized print-outs drooping from mouthlike slits, that could measure and analyze a minute fraction of a substance in a droplet of fluid. Although there were also traditional centrifuges, microscopes, and test tubes, the laboratory looked like a Mission Control Center. It was not what I had expected.

Dr. Dao walked over to greet me at the door. "First of all, you can see from the name of the lab that my research is concerned with the hormonal, or endocrine, aspects of breast cancer," he began. "We have known since 1896 that removing a woman's ovaries often caused her breast cancer to improve. But it took years to find out why."

"You mean estrogens?" I broke in.

He nodded. "Yes, the estrogens, the female hormones. These substances are produced by the ovaries, and removing them from the blood stream has a marked effect on slowing the growth of a breast cancer in many cases."

I was about to break in with another question, but Dr. Dao was not to be interrupted.

"Although the principle had been known since 1896," he re-peated, "the reason was not discovered until much later. Remov-ing the ovaries helped, and that was it. So oophorectomy, or ovariectomy—surgical removal of the ovaries—was done routinely after a mastectomy in a younger woman with metastatic disease."

"Did doctors think the female hormones caused the breast can-cer?" I managed to ask.

"Some did and some didn't," he replied. "But no one could disagree that oophorectomy improved the condition of many breast-cancer patients." Dr. Dao went on with his brief history of the rather confused estrogen picture.

First, while a good many women improved, some did not respond at all after their ovaries were taken out. Their tumors continued to flourish, unaffected. "In these cases," he said, "we had to assume the cancers were different—what we call hormone-independent, not influenced or controlled by estrogen secretion. Another inexplicable factor was the presence of estrogens in a patient's blood stream even after oophorectomy. This means that there must be other glands in the body that either take over estrogen production when the ovaries are removed or produce female hormones along with the ovaries. A third mystery was that many women—especially postmenopausal women—were considerably improved when given the very same estrogens that were causing so much trouble in younger patients."

After more research, Dr. Dao continued, scientists learned that the adrenal glands, near the kidneys, and the anterior pituitary gland, deep inside the brain, are also involved in estrogen production—the pituitary directing the ovarian hormone factories' production. To stop secretion of the female hormones altogether, it was necessary to get rid of all these glands.

"The anterior pituitary also secretes the hormone called prolactin," Dr. Dao went on. "This is the hormone that causes milk production to begin after childbirth, but it is also present in the body at other times, although its function aside from lactation is not clearly understood. However, it is known to contribute to the fast growth of a cancerous breast tumor when a woman is not breast-feeding."

"Why would the body do that to itself?" I asked.

He smiled. "The brain must intend for the body to have a correct balance of all the hormones, but the delicate balance somehow becomes altered. We don't know exactly what 'correct' is. We know only that when an imbalance exists, it creates a nourishing endocrine, or glandular, environment for the growth of breast cancers, as well as carcinomas of other reproductive organs."

"Then what about oral contraceptives? The Pill? They've got estrogens in them. And what about the female hormones given to cattle and sheep so they'll get fat faster? What about—"

"Wait a minute, now. You are getting ahead of the story. What I have been talking about are endogenous estrogens—hormones made by the woman's own body, to prepare her for menstruation, ovulation, possible pregnancy, and then lactation. These are all normal secretions, which are controlled by the brain, probably the hypothalamus."

The hypothalamus? That is the part of the brain involved with the emotions. Could cancer be psychosomatic? I tried to ask, but got no chance.

"For a long time, scientists thought it was the pituitary gland that regulated all other glands. It was called 'the conductor of the body's hormonal orchestra.' Now we know it is only the concert-master, not the boss."

He stopped. Here was my chance. The Pill or the hypothalamus? "What about the oral contraceptives?" I asked quickly. He probably was not much interested in the psychological side of cancer, anyhow.

He paused. "We have no proof that such exogenous hormones—those obtained from outside the body—cause breast cancer in humans." He seemed to be choosing his words very carefully. "However, three of them, estrone, estradiol, and diethylstilbestrol —as well as prolactin—do stimulate breast cancers in lower animals."

"What do you mean by stimulate?"

"Exactly what I said. Most estrogens enhance the growth of a mammary carcinoma. For example, in mice who have first been injected with a carcinogen—a substance we know causes cancer—tumors appear much earlier, their rates of growth are much faster, and the tumors are larger if they are also given female hormones, especially prolactin. But prolactin alone does not do this without estrogens. Remember, though, that in these experiments the initial cancers were not *induced* by hormones, but by a chemical we are certain is carcinogenic."

"Where does that leave the exogenous estrogens in oral contraceptives?"

"In the suspicious category." Dr. Dao smiled. "Anything that upsets the body's hormonal balance contributes to a favorable environment for cancer growth in the breast. We have evidence of this in several species of animals, but not in humans."

"What about heredity?" I asked, changing the subject. "Cancer seems to run in families, doesn't it?"

"There's no question that there seems to be some kind of in-born predisposition. In our own lab, for example, we use certain strains of mice that have been deliberately bred to develop mammary carcinomas quickly and with very little stimulation. The same principle could apply in human families. It could be a predisposition for the body's endocrine balance to be upset easily."

"Are there strains of mice that never develop breast cancer, no matter what you do?"

He nodded. "However, as these mice get older, they become more vulnerable, too."

I was the only breast-cancer patient in my family on both sides, as far as I knew. Was I starting a new, awful strain? But then, I had been given hundreds of hormone tablets. Could it be that?

"Where does a breast-cancer virus come into the picture?"

"It could be a trigger. Like the chemical we used in those mice to set off cancer growth."

"And X-ray?"

"Not the tiny quantities from dental examinations or tuberculosis checkups. But, in larger quantities, X-ray could also be a trigger. First, however, there must be that nourishing endocrine environment, before a cancer will grow at all. If the environment is hostile, the original microscopic tumor will die and disappear."

"And the hypothalamus helps to create a good environment?"

"Yes."

"Do you think there is a psychological cause of breast cancer, then? After all, that's the part of the brain that controls things like sex drive, fear, and anger." Good grief! Too much sex? Too little sex? Too many arguments?

"Not sex drive." Dr. Dao laughed. "But some investigators have mentioned stress as a factor, and it might be. Plenty of hormones are secreted during stressful times. One hormone could stimulate another. A stress hormone that stimulated estrogen secretion could help to create the nourishing endocrine environment the cancer needs."

Looking for the cause of breast cancer was like wandering in a labyrinth. One path that seemed clear ran into another that was blocked.

"Breast cancer is a multifactorial disease," Dr. Dao concluded. "There just is no one, single cause that works alone."

Later, while trying to digest all I had learned, I realized Dr. Dao had not said anything about why postmenopausal women respond to treatment with estrogens, but younger women have to have their ovaries removed. This mystery was finally cleared up for me months later, in Finland, when I first heard the theory that breast cancers in the two age groups are two completely different diseases.

Dr. Dao had given me some reports published by his laboratory, and, from them, one problem in studying breast cancer in humans was apparent immediately. His mice developed tumors within weeks of being injected, and the entire life span of a mouse is only a few months. In humans, the trigger setting off the first malignant cell could be separated from the appearance of a tumor by as long as twenty years. I tried to recall some events of the last twenty years of my life.

I had never taken birth-control pills, but now that I was thinking of the Pill as a female hormone, an estrogen, rather than as a contraceptive, I realized how many times I had been given prescriptions for one estrogen or another: to regulate menstrual periods, to prevent miscarriages, or to "dry up" after weaning my children from the breast. And who knew how much diethylstilbestrol (DES)—the hormone used to fatten livestock—I had eaten in chopped liver and chicken soup? Even without the Pill, I must have taken in plenty of exogenous estrogens.

Dr. Dao had very cautiously shied away from discussing oral contraceptives. However, I was left with the strong impression that he frowns on their widespread, indiscriminate use, and he is not alone among the experts. But there is no proof of any connection between use of the Pill and human breast cancer. Of course, there has not been enough time yet; oral contraceptives have been best sellers only a few years.

What Dr. Dao had said about the significance of endocrine environment for breast-cancer growth meant more to me after I learned about the epidemiological aspects of a woman's reproductive life. The start and the finish of reproductive life are especially dependent on the proper balance of female hormones, and now

I understood why early or late beginning of menstruation and early menopause affected the risk category.

While the significance of the mother's age when her first child is born remains a mystery, it also must have something to do with her hormonal balance.

Understanding that breast cancer can be stimulated by excess hormones also made it easier for me to see why diet might be a major factor. A 1953 experiment restricting the caloric intake of cancer-prone mice, for example, showed that a one-third reduction in calories virtually wiped out their breast cancers. In the German concentration camps during World War II, cessation of a woman's regular menstrual periods was one of the first signs she was suffering from food deprivation, and the same symptom was found in Japanese internment camps. A shortage of food must lead to a shortage of estrogens and thus to an imbalance in the endocrine system regulating the monthly cycle. And there was that link between diet and breast cancer in countries where, like the Netherlands, the consumption of animal fats is very high, while in Japan and other countries that use few animal fats the breast-cancer incidence rates are very low.

Dr. Philip Cole, of the Harvard Medical School, has suggested that the cholesterol in the animal fats is somehow converted inside the body into estrogenlike substances, thus upsetting the hormonal balance. Although animal fats were the suspects in a survey Dr. Cole made, many scientists think meat proteins as well as fats are responsible.

Several researchers have pointed out that most of the meat we eat comes either from female animals—hens and ewes, which are loaded with natural estrogens—or from castrated males—steers and capons, whose androgen-producing testicles have been removed. (Lambs, calves, and piglets have not yet developed their hormone-producing equipment.) Since even male animals secrete some estrogens, most people get only female hormones in their meat from these eunuchs. Although no study has been done to ascertain what this means in relation to breast cancer, it must be remembered that Seventh-Day Adventists (who eat no meat at all) and Mormons (moderate meat eaters) have far fewer cases of all kinds of cancer, including breast cancer.

Some such diet factors probably explain why obese women

are in the high-risk category. They may also explain why the daughters of low-incidence immigrants to the United States develop more breast cancers than their mothers—too many hamburgers and creamy milk shakes. And the quantity of animal fats or meat in their diets might account for the difference in the incidence rates of Israeli Jewish women with Yemeni and with European backgrounds.

With regard to the high risk of obesity, Dr. Frits deWaard, the Dutch epidemiologist who has developed the total-body-volume theory, believes that each cell in the body is a microscopic factory that produces estrogens independently of the ovaries, the adrenals, or the pituitary. This extraglandular phenomenon, as Dr. deWaard calls it, would give large women extra estrogen-producing equipment, and therefore more hormones in their bodies.

Whatever the cellular biochemistry, though, an excess of female hormones floating in the blood stream helps cancers find a nourishing home in the breasts.

But what triggers that first cell and causes it to transform from normal to malignant?

Scientists have decided there are four basic causes of all cancers: genetic mutations, chemical carcinogens, irradiation, and oncoviruses (*onco-* is a medical prefix meaning "cancer"). In one way or another, any of the four can do the malignant evil of wrecking a cell's control over its growth and reproduction.

To find out about genetics, I went to see an epidemiologist at the National Cancer Institute. "Is breast cancer hereditary or isn't it?" I asked. "On the one hand, I have read that Dr. Brian MacMahon thinks genetics plays a minor role in breast cancer, and on the other there are Jewish women, and the Parsi women in India. And what about the Japanese and Yemeni women?" I fished a paper from my briefcase and put it on his desk. "Now I have just found this study, done at the M. D. Anderson Hospital and Tumor Institute, in Houston, saying that women have forty-seven times the risk of getting breast cancer before the age of thirty-nine if both their mother and a sister had it. It doesn't make sense to insist it isn't a genetic disease."

He shook his head and laughed. "I can see why it's so confusing. You get the epidemiologists and the statisticians on one side, and the doctors in the clinics on the other side. They seem to conflict, don't they?"

"They certainly do." I sighed. "I hope you can straighten it out."

"Well, I'll try," he began. "But first, MacMahon used the term 'genetic role,' not hereditary. What do you mean by hereditary?"

"Running in a family," I replied.

"There are many ways a disease can run in a family and yet not be hereditary in the same way as hair and eye color are," he said. "Traits like coloring are passed along physically, by the genes in the sperm and egg of the parents, and these are genetic. But a characteristic can be transmitted to the next generation in other ways."

In 1936, he went on, Dr. Joseph J. Bittner, a scientist at the University of Minnesota, did a series of now classical experiments that proved there is a mammary-tumor virus in mice—the scientific shorthand for it is MuMTV, for murine (mouse) mammary tumor virus—and that the virus can be passed along to their young via their milk. Baby mice fed by mothers with breast cancer subsequently developed breast tumors, too. Then Dr. Bittner took a group of baby mice away from their cancerous mothers immediately after birth and had them suckled by healthy mothers. None of these babies developed breast cancers. Nor did the offspring of healthy mice who were fed by their own mothers; but they did if nursed by the cancerous mothers.

"Do you think something like this happens with humans?" I asked.

He shook his head. "Nobody knows. Particles similar to the MuMTV have been found in human milk, and some women swear that their infants refused to take milk from a breast that later became malignant. But the only way to prove anything would be by a Bittner-type experiment, and scientists can't ethically mix and match people the way they can mice."

I persisted. "There must be a reason for the high risk of a woman who has a sister or mother with cancer, compared with the risk of a woman who has no cancer in her family. Not everyone is breast-fed. I'm sure thousands of women with breast cancer were fed by bottle."

"It could be a statistical artifact." He smiled. "Don't forget, 6 per cent of all American women get breast cancer. This means there is one chance in fifteen for any woman in the United States to get it. Now, in a family with three sisters, two grand-mothers, possibly a few aunts, and lots of female cousins, there's a good chance that some of them will develop breast cancer just because of its national incidence, not because it runs in the family."

Statistical artifact? That is probably what is meant by "doing anything you want with statistics." But here it made no sense. "That wouldn't explain the Finnish, Japanese, Jewish, and Parsi women," I said. "What about the Jewish women from Yemen compared with—"

He laughed. "I'm just putting you on. Of course there must be a genetic factor somewhere. All cancers have a genetic compo-nent, to a greater or lesser degree. For example, there's an eye cancer, retinoblastoma, that is caused by a mutant gene. We don't know why the gene changes, but we know what happens afterward if the children's lives are saved by removing their eyes, and they grow to adulthood and marry someone else with the same problem. Half of *their* children will also get retinoblastomas, but half won't. The risks of passing this mutant gene on are so well established that patients are usually advised not to have children."

He also explained how hereditary factors can influence the development of a cancer even if they do not actually cause the disease. For instance, blond, light-skinned people are more vul-nerable to skin cancers that come from long exposure to the sun than are dark people, whose skin pigmentation and thickness—both hereditary qualities—protect them from the ultraviolet rays of the sun. "But," he stressed, "both light- and dark-skinned peo-ple would have far less skin cancer if all of them stayed out of the sun."

"There are no hard-and-fast rules about genetics and breast cancer," he said. "If all the risk factors were based on heredity, Japanese women, for example, would have a low incidence rate no matter where they lived. But they don't. Low-risk women develop more breast cancer when they move from their native countries to high-risk areas."

A few months later, in Moscow, I asked Professor Sviatukhina what she thought. "The evidence is there for all to see," she said, adding that she had known of too many families spotted with breast cancer from one generation to another to say that heredity is not a factor. But not the only factor.

In other countries I visited, in different accents, the same opinion was given again and again—whatever the cause may be, there is no doubt that breast cancer does run in families. But why? Another mutant gene, like the one that causes retinoblastoma?

In studying the possible role of genetics in diseases, scientists try to find sets of identical twins who grew up in different environments. If the twins have been separated throughout their lifetimes and yet have had illnesses in common, those diseases could be genetic. But apparently no such twins with breast cancer have been found, for I discovered nothing of this nature in the medical literature.

A second-best approach is a computerized study of family incidence now in progress in Iceland. That northern island has a high incidence of breast cancer. It also has a relatively closed society: there has been little migration in or out for decades. Because of this, most Icelandic family trees can be traced back to 1910, many back as far as 1842.

It has not always been so. Professor Calum Muir, of the International Agency for Research in Cancer, in France, told me of a historical study of breast-cancer incidence in Iceland showing that ethnic Icelandic women (not Danish or other European immigrants) once had incidence rates as low as those of Japanese women. Then the population began to change and become more European. The incidence rates rose, and have remained at the same high level since. All this, Professor Muir said, seems to be evidence of a strong genetic component, introduced by the European immigrants, in the "why" of breast cancer in Iceland— although he, too, agreed that family history is just one factor, not the only answer.

The historical data are now being entered into the computer for the new study, however, beginning with the year 1910, after Iceland had already become Europeanized. Since 1911, the island has had 1,600 cases of breast cancer. Of these, ninety have been chosen at random for analysis. Each woman's family has been traced back as far as its records go and the data put into the computer in the form of a "linkage file" by which various family relationships can be studied.

The project will be a lengthy one, and not even preliminary results have been announced yet. But the scientists in charge warn that high family correlations do not necessarily establish a definite genetic link. The same environment, the same foods, or other characteristics of Icelandic life—such as marrying late and having a first child late—could also be factors in the correlations, they caution. However, the computer is expected to calculate the relative breast-cancer risks for daughter, sister, first cousin, and niece more accurately than they have been known. In addition, the results should show if running in the family is confined to the maternal side, or if the father's family is also involved.

Chemical carcinogens in tobacco have been tagged as the cause of lung cancer; vinyl chloride, of a rare cancer of the liver; and various pesticides as possible causes of other cancers. Only two chemicals (female hormones are not considered chemicals) have been proven to be linked with breast cancer: urethanes (no relative to all those foam-rubber products) and anthracines. Neither group of chemicals is found in the air or in any food, household product, cosmetic, or medicine. I have been assured that both are laboratory chemicals, not used for any purposes other than scientific experiments. Moreover, the only mammary carcinomas these have induced have been in mice.

So they say. The truth is that no one really knows whether these chemicals pose a risk of human breast cancer, or if there are any other chemicals that do.

Dr. David Rall, the director of the National Institute of Environmental Health Sciences, admitted this ignorance at a national conference of scientists in late 1974. "The chemical industry has really only grown up in the last twenty or thirty years," he said. "We have an enormous number of new, unique synthetic chemicals, and with a latency period of twenty or thirty years [before the appearance of malignancies] there is little reason to be confident that the dimensions of the problem have been revealed. Society has largely ignored the problem of delayed, irreversible effects of chemicals, swept it under the rug. We are so terribly uncertain about the risk these chemicals entail for the population in general and for individual members of the population. There is still no way of determining this risk."

An important function of the National Institute of Environmental Health Sciences (NIEHS), a branch of the National Institutes of Health, is to correlate known epidemiological statistics with data from the few animal experiments involving chemical carcinogenicity.

To take just two examples: large numbers of people in certain industries develop certain kinds of cancers. Why?

Mountainous parts of the country have higher incidences of some cancers than coastal areas do. Why?

Could chemical factors be the explanation in either case?

A 1974 article entitled "Cancer and the Environment," in *Science* magazine, said, "Between 60 and 90 per cent of all human malignancies are believed to be caused by environmental factors ranging from ultraviolet light to synthetic chemicals." The statement is widely accepted as true, and yet little or no scientific evidence exists to implicate most carcinogenic substances. The reason for the lack of proof, according to the *Science* article, is the problem of extrapolation—that business of applying to men what has been learned from mice. The results of cancer experiments with rats, mice, and other animals are almost impossible to apply to humans with any certainty.

For one thing, the animals are usually given enormous doses of suspect chemicals, so that they will show cause-and-effect results more quickly. Second, the species-specificity of cancer—the fact that most kinds will grow only in a certain species of animal and not in any others—gives chemical manufacturers a perfect loophole in defending their products. It is easy (and scientifically accurate) for them to argue that traces of a certain substance in a detergent, say, would not necessarily cause breast cancer in humans just because larger quantities of it induced mammary carcinomas in a thousand mice. And the chemical industry uses that loophole all the time!

After three days of talk, the NIEHS conference reached no decisions on how to estimate the risks to humans of getting cancer from exposure to low doses of known chemical carcinogens. But it did agree on these points:

1. The effects of most such substances are cumulative; they collect in certain organs of the body and are not usually excreted. Therefore, no matter how low the dosage, if a large population is exposed to carcinogenic substances over a long period of time, a risk of cancer exists for some of those people.

2. The production and use of carcinogenic substances that our society can get along without—chlorinated pesticides, for example—should be stopped.

3. Carcinogens that cannot be removed entirely from the environment should be subject to legal limits on the amounts that can be released, just as emissions from automobiles are being limited.

However, the first and most vital problem—identifying all the chemical carcinogens—is far from solved. Nonetheless, enough chemicals are already known to be carcinogenic that these three suggestions, if carried out, could be helpful.

But having an official government agency make suggestions and seeing them implemented by law are two different ball games. As I discovered in my prowling into the Pill, both chemical and drug manufacturers have extremely powerful and well-financed lobbies on Capitol Hill. "Look at the benefit-risk ratio" is their favorite line. And much of the time—*not* all, by any means—it is a valid argument.

Is the risk of famine if insecticides are banned greater than the risk of cancer if they are not? If chlorine were not put into our drinking water, how many more people would die of typhoid fever than are possibly dying now of cancer? In the case of synthetic hormones, what are the medical, social, and economic risks of unwanted pregnancies if oral contraceptives are outlawed?

Obviously, not every chemical that might cause cancer can or should be banned. But more must be known about all chemicals, so that the more dangerous, less essential carcinogens can at least be regulated.

We have almost no control over one well-established and dangerous carcinogen, ionizing irradiation, which sends electrically charged particles into the atmosphere.

I don't mean the ultraviolet rays of the sun; these are nonionizing and, as far as anyone knows, have no effect on breast or most other cancers. Too much exposure to sunlight can cause cancer of the skin, especially in people with light complexions, but the rays do not penetrate to the inner tissues. Nor am I referring to the kind of ionizing irradiation given off by the diagnostic X-rays ordered by a physician or dentist. This we can limit, or can avoid entirely if we choose.

The virtually uncontrolled irradiation I am talking about is the invisible fallout that may be bombarding us every minute of every day from nuclear equipment and some other devices.

Several government agencies, including the Atomic Energy Commission and the Nuclear Regulatory Commission, have been responsible for setting what they call "acceptable" levels of radiation emission. According to current standards, half a millirem of emission is acceptable. (A millirem is one-thousandth of a rem; the standard unit of radiation measurement.) However, when a nuclear power plant being built about 150 miles from my home, in Maryland, was found to be leaking as much as twenty times this level, Marylanders were assured that the leakage was not enough to be hazardous to employees in the plant or to people living nearby. Then what is an "acceptable" level? No one knows what it should be.

Randolph S. Rae, a physicist and a government consultant, explained to me how the maximum acceptable levels are computed. "We know how much exposure is dangerous," he said. "So we go down and say, 'Well, a thousandth would certainly be safe, and a millionth even safer.'" That, according to Rae, is why no one need worry about "small multiples" of the so-called maximum acceptable levels.

"Usually," he continued, "these levels are even less than what we are exposed to all the time from irradiation in the atmosphere. There is no way—it's absolutely impossible—for anyone to be protected from what is in the air around us all the time."

Scientists do know more about the cancerous effects of irradiation than of chemicals, however. Results of the atomic blasts in

Hiroshima and Nagasaki, which are still showing up in Japanese incidence rates, have taught them much. The many experimental explosions on the ground, underground, and in the air have also yielded a great deal of information. It is known, for example, that ionizing irradiation is, paradoxically, both a cancer cure and a cancer cause, and for the same reason: it does something to the gene on the DNA molecule that controls the cell's growth and reproduction. In the massive doses given to cancer patients, irradiation destroys a malignant cell by preventing it from reproducing. In lesser doses, irradiation damages the chromosomes of a normal cell, without killing it; if the damage takes place in the growth-and-reproduction gene, the mutation can create cancerous daughter cells.

While it had been known since Marie Curie's day that ionizing irradiation causes cancer, for many years mammary carcinomas were thought to be an exception. The reason the danger to breasts was not recognized is logical: it takes a long time for a breast tumor (as well as other slow-growing cancers) to become apparent, and the X-rays that might have caused it are usually long forgotten by the time the cancer is discovered. So, until four years after World War II, X-ray was used to treat anything from bleeding nipples to tuberculosis to eczema. By then, bits and pieces of evidence appearing occasionally in the medical literature were telling of women who had developed cancer in the affected breast as long as twenty-five years after X-ray therapy for a benign disease. Indiscriminate use of X-ray declined— though doctors believed it aggravated a cancer already in existence, but did not cause one to develop.

Not until six Japanese survivors of Hiroshima and Nagasaki developed breast cancer in 1965, twenty years after the blasts, was the cause and effect of X-ray considered proven. Six cases are not many here, but in Japan they are a large number, and the fact that all had been A-bombed was too much to be a coincidence. As a result, scatter-shot use of X-ray stopped, and it is rarely a cause of primary breast cancers today.

Many physicians are reluctant to expose their patients too frequently to even the small quantity of irradiation from a mammogram or chest X-ray. But this is one of the times when possible risk must be weighed against possible benefit. I believe that the choice a high-risk woman over thirty-five *must* make is at least an annual mammogram, no matter what her family doctor says. More about this later.

But *take special note:* I am talking about diagnostic X-ray, not radiotherapy. A doctor occasionally wants a patient to have "prophylactic X-ray treatment" in the area of the surgery or the axilla after a radical mastectomy. As will be detailed in another chapter, such postoperative irradiation is dangerous.

Two avoidable sources of irradiation, aside from sunlight and X-rays, should be mentioned briefly—microwave ovens and color television sets.

"Is there anything to the scares we've had about them?" I asked Dr. Joseph Sharp, formerly a radiation specialist at the Walter Reed Army Institute of Research, in Washington.

"As far as we know," he said, "they're as safe as they can be—by current standards, whatever the standards are right now. No one has really gotten any evidence to show that either machine, in good working order, can cause cancer." He smiled. "For that matter, there is no evidence that either machine in bad working order can cause cancer. I would say that the best thing to do, based on the information we have now, is just to turn the contraptions on and keep your distance. We might as well play it safe with the few things we can do something about."

That is a fair summary of irradiation and cancer: play it safe wherever you can.

If extrapolating results from mouse to man is a problem in studying hormones, genetics, chemicals, or radiation as causes of cancer, it is an almost total road block in virus research.

Scientists have known about that MuMTV—the virus that causes breast cancer in mice—for four decades, but they have found no way to investigate whether a similar virus causes breast cancer in humans. The reason is obvious. Scientists can't duplicate the crucial animal experiments in humans without running the risk of causing cancer in their subjects.

The usual procedure for proving that a particular "thing" causes an illness is to inject tissue suspected of harboring it into an animal, thus causing the disease to develop. After that "guinea pig" becomes ill, some of its diseased tissue—in the case of cancer, the tumor—is injected into a second animal. If the same illness appears again, the process is repeated several more times. Then, and only then, will it be stated without doubt or qualification that this disease was caused by that "thing." The procedure is known as Koch's postulates, and it has been success- fully applied in finding the causes of a great many diseases. With the common cold and other minor diseases that simply don't "take" in experimental animals, scientists have used paid human guinea pigs or have gotten volunteers for their Koch's procedures. Prisoners have occasionally been recruited, in ex- change for early release. But to do this with cancer? Impossible.

"How was it done with polio?" I asked Dr. Ernest Plata, a virologist at the National Cancer Institute. "They certainly didn't go around inoculating human beings with polio to find that virus, did they?"

"This is the cause of a lot of confusion," Dr. Plata said. "The 'thing' we suspect of causing some breast cancers—*some*, not all, by any means—is totally unlike the polio virus or the viruses that cause the cold, measles, mumps, and so on. First of all, no one has been able to transmit this suspected virus from humans to lower animals, as was the case with polio.

"In the second place, it is *not*—repeat, *not*—contagious. With contagious viral diseases, the virus invades a cell and reproduces, using the machinery of the cell to make new viruses. In the end, the cell may be killed and will expel through its membrane dozens of newly made viruses into the surrounding tissue. To study these simpler diseases, all the scientist must do to get a sample of the virus is to break up a piece of diseased tissue and extract it."

Dr. Plata went on with his viral explanation. "In cancer, the process is different. As soon as the virus invades a cell, its genes —because viruses have them, too—hide in some way among the genes of the cell itself. The body of the virus disappears. All that is left is an extra, infinitesimal piece of genetic material— a dot."

Dr. Plata added that these small pieces of gene, these dots, were only recently found in cancer cells. The sophisticated tech- nical know-how was not available earlier, he explained. Again, progress in cancer research was directly related to the higher lens power of the latest microscope and to the development of other technologies.

He gave a thus-far-imaginary scenario of how an HuMTV—human mammary tumor virus—might work. The "thing," or virus, would enter a healthy cell and be incorporated so that nothing remained of it but the dot of gene among the host cell's chromosomes. The dot would somehow change the growth genes of the cell—and, by doing so, create a malignant mutation. During the S period, when the cell's DNA molecules were twinning, the mutation would be duplicated in both sets of new chromosomes. In the succeeding D period, the daughter cells would be born transformed into cancer cells.

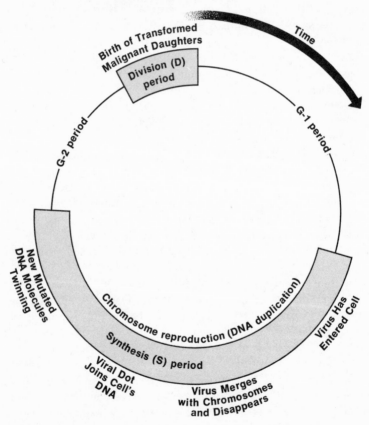

The HuMTV Scenario

Dr. Plata said that this viral theory does not conflict with any known facts about breast cancer. In addition to the transforming mutation, he explained, it is likely that genetic predisposition makes the body's defense mechanism vulnerable; otherwise, the transformed cells would simply be killed.

The idea is based on a concept, supported by many immunologists, that every "immunocompetent" body has an elaborate immune surveillance system to kill off invaders when they appear. The system includes the lymph nodes, bone marrow, the thymus gland, and the spleen, as well as individual cells, which, according to this concept, are constantly roaming through the lymphatics and the blood stream searching for and destroying foreign invaders.

Studies have shown that patients with malignancies have large numbers of living cancer cells just floating around, and not establishing new cancer colonies. Dead cancer cells have been found, as well. Immunologists who support the surveillance-system concept suggest that only about 1 per cent of the stray malignant cells manage to live long enough to become metastases; the dead cells were killed by the various components of the immune system. If this were not so, they argue, few cancer patients with metastatic disease would live very long, because every live cell that was shed into the blood stream or into a lymph vessel would grow into a new tumor.

Sometimes, however, even in immunocompetent bodies, this front-line militia is overcome. Some immunologists blame it on a "sneaking-through" phenomenon, by which malignant cells somehow manage to evade their killers. Of course, if the patient is immunodeficient, for one reason or another, the surveillance system is already weak, and it is much easier for the cancer cells to sneak through. As we know, breast cancer, in sneaking through, usually spreads first to the axillary lymph nodes, by way of the lymphatic vessels, and then, if the nodes themselves become cancerous, to other parts of the body.

In addition to a genetically deficient immune system, a hospitable endocrine environment—natural or artificial—would aid and abet the viral breast cancer's growth. As Dr. Dao had told me, the cancerous cells could not multiply without lots of nourishing hormones.

Like irradiation, chemical carcinogens, and genetic mutations, the oncovirus is one more instrument that could foul up a cell's control of its own destiny.

"How can you ever prove this theory if the virus disappears?" I asked Dr. Plata. "Have you been able to take cells from a human breast cancer and grow a tumor in a laboratory animal?"

"In reality, no. With extracts from tumors, no." Dr. Plata shook his head regretfully. "But we learned a trick from the heart transplants of a while back, when doctors discovered how to prevent the body from rejecting foreign tissues. By knocking out an animal's ability to reject foreign tissue, we can grow human tumor cells in its body. In other words, the animal acts as an incubator."

"Can you grow healthy human breast tissue in a test tube or Petri dish?"

"Only for about twenty or thirty generations," he replied. "That generally means from one month to, at most, three months. Healthy cells eventually stop living and growing *in vitro*—in glass. Only cancer cells keep on growing indefinitely. That is one way we have of knowing when cells have been transformed—when the tissue in the dish never stops growing. We don't even need a microscope."

"Then you have grown human cancer in a dish?"

Dr. Plata nodded. "Human cancer cells are now grown routinely in most laboratories. But, as yet, a confirmed human cancer virus has not been detected or produced in any cultured human tumor." On the other hand, he added, several researchers have obtained suspicious particles "somewhat resembling" viruses from human milk. Attempts are being made, without success so far, to have the particles invade and transform healthy human breast tissue growing *in vitro*. "These human particles have some of the characteristics of the MuMTV—the mouse virus," Dr. Plata said. "Some even look a little like it. But that is as far as we have come."

Before going to see Dr. Plata, I had made up a list of questions to ask him based on the polio-virus kind of invasion. I had planned to ask why scientists were diddling around trying to decide whether a virus did or did not exist. Why not simply assume there was a HuMTV, develop a poliolike vaccine, and forget the whole Koch's-postulates business? Now that I knew the suspected cancer virus is completely different from the polio virus, the fancy argument I had concocted evaporated. I must have looked quite disappointed.

"It's not so very hopeless." Dr. Plata smiled. "There are some really promising human-breast-tumor cell cultures, in several laboratories around the country, that, with a little work, may yield viruses worthy of study."

He told me about a two-and-a-half-year-old "particle-producing" culture of cancer cells taken from the chest fluid of a woman with breast cancer. Particles from the culture—named MCF-7, for the Michigan Cancer Foundation, where it was first grown—are being intensively studied in several laboratories, including those at the National Cancer Institute. "There isn't yet a large enough quantity of the particles to do much experimentation—only a few micrograms. If a thimble holds about two grams, can you imagine what a few micrograms are?" Dr. Plata was certain, however, that when more is available scientists will be able to study the suspicious MCF-7 particle as a purified virus—if it is a virus.

In anticipation of that, he has no fewer than fifteen normal and malignant human-breast-cell lines already growing *in vitro* in his laboratory. "If I could infect"—in cancer jargon, to infect means to cause an invasion; no contagion involved!—"any of my well-defined cultures of normal breast cells with a purified virus, and if those cells transformed to resemble the cultured breast-tumor cells, there would be little doubt that the MCF-7 was the breast-cancer virus we are looking for."

"And then what?" I asked hopefully. "Will you be able to develop a vaccine?"

He shook his head. "Oh, perhaps yes, but that is not the immediate answer. Let me explain. Take measles as an example." Doodling on a pad of paper, he pointed out that, before the measles vaccine was developed, the disease was very widespread —much more so than breast cancer is. But, he reminded me, as prevalent as it was, it was not generally a serious or fatal disease.

Breast cancer is another story. "We must look at the fatality rate of the disease before we begin to think of giving every woman a vaccine against it. Even a vaccine that is 99.999999-

per-cent perfect is potentially too risky. Suppose there is a bad
batch. It happened with polio, if you recall. The catastrophic
results of having a bad batch of a breast-cancer vaccine are too
enormous even to consider."

I leaned back in my chair, very discouraged. "Then are you
playing scientific games here just to prove that breast cancer
is caused by a virus? What's the point? Why spend all this time,
talent, effort, and money to find something that won't do any
good even if it is found?"

"It would do a lot of good." Dr. Plata smiled. "Once we find
the virus, we will be able to look for a part of it—an antigen on
its surface, a completely harmless substance—that we can use for
a vaccination. If necessary, once that antigen is recognized,
it could then be synthesized. By copying it chemically," Dr.
Plata continued, "we would totally avoid the possibility of virus
contamination. The antigen—the small part of the virus—would
resemble the oncovirus closely enough to trigger the body into
producing antibodies against just that antigen. Then, by attacking
the antigen wherever in the body it would be found, the antibodies would kill the entire virus or the tumor cell of which that
antigen formed a part."

"Is that what's meant by immunotherapy?" I asked.

"Yes," he replied. "This would be especially effective if a
particular breast cancer were found to be caused by an exogenous
—external—oncovirus."

"What other kind of virus is there?" I asked. "Don't all viruses
come into the body from outside?"

Dr. Plata shook his head. "That is true for most viruses. But
unfortunately, in cancer, according to new evidence, and the
oncogene theory of Dr. Robert Huebner and Dr. George Todaro
of NCI, at least some oncoviruses may be an integral part of the
animal host to begin with. There may well be an oncogene built
into every cell." He told me of experiments by many investigators
showing that these oncogenic viruses can be "demonstrated"—
shown to be present—in nearly all animal species tested so far,
by manipulating healthy, normal cells with certain sophisticated
chemical and irradiation procedures.

"In almost every case," Dr. Plata told me, "the oncovirus 'pops
out' of the cell when these manipulations are done."

"What does that mean?" I asked.

"It may mean that every cell in the body has an endogenous, or internal, gene that could trigger a cancer if all the other circumstances were suitable for its growth."

I was startled into silence.

"A built-in cancer gene," he repeated.

"That would mean everybody has a genetic predisposition to get cancer, wouldn't it?" I finally gasped.

"Perhaps." He nodded. "This is being carefully studied. What are the different mechanisms that activate the oncogene? Why is it expressed differently in various hosts? How is it naturally controlled? This would also mean that, at least in some instances," he continued, "the immunological system of the body would naturally do little to attack and kill such a virus. Endogenous oncoviruses would not be recognized as foreign bodies, for the simple reason that they aren't. They are part of the body that made them."

"It sounds as if you were telling me that all animals may be born with built-in 'cyanide pellets,' which will kill them by cancer if something else doesn't kill them first. Is that right?" I asked.

Dr. Plata nodded again, this time gravely. "If the theory turns out to be reality, it may be one way by which most animals are preprogramed to die." *

I had gone to the virology department of the National Cancer Institute with high hopes of hearing that a vaccination against breast cancer was imminent. Or, at the least, that a major breakthrough was expected any day—dawn, at last, at the end of the black night.

Instead, I had learned that cancer may be nature's own solution to the population explosion.

An inborn, suicidal oncogene!

---

* Since this was written, three other laboratories in the United States and one in Germany have discovered the presence of a cancer-causing gene in the cells of several lower animals.

6

The Problem of the Pill

I was talking to Frank Korn, a public-information officer for the Food and Drug Administration, about the rumored relationship between the Pill and our rising breast-cancer rates.

He recited the standard litany: "At this time, there is no proof that oral contraceptives cause breast cancer." Then he added, "When Betty Ford and Happy Rockefeller both got it, the first thing that popped into somebody's mind here in FDA was 'I wonder if they were taking OCs.'"

OCs, I quickly learned, is medical jargon for the Pill. "Why would anyone at FDA say that if there wasn't some risk you know about?"

"Don't misunderstand me," he snapped. "We have no evidence at all of a cancer risk with OCs. It was just something someone said."

When I was in the fifth grade, thirty-five years ago, the Johns Hopkins Hospital and the Baltimore and Maryland departments of health decided to screen elementary-school children for hearing defects. I was found to have a deficiency in my right ear. The hospital and the two government departments generously decided to do something about the hard-of-hearing children, which included me. Every Thursday, a bus took me to Hopkins for an afternoon of radium treatments. I was the envy of all my "hearing" friends.

"I forgot all about the radium," I told an otorhinolaryngologist (ear, nose, and throat specialist) twenty-five years later. "Then a friend of mine told me her daughter had a thickened eardrum like mine. So I suggested radium treatments. 'Good Lord!' she yelled to me. 'Thousands of people who got radium treatments are getting cancer of the thyroid and larynx.' That's why I'm here to see you," I explained to the doctor. "Is my throat okay?"

He examined me carefully. "Everything seems to be all right." He smiled. "I doubt that, after twenty-five years, anything would happen now. But let's keep checking. You may be walking around with a time bomb inside you."

For the next five years he examined me frequently. Finally, thirty years post-radium, he cut me down to annual checkups. "I think you can breathe a bit easier now," he assured me in 1970.

But who really knows?

Now here was Frank Korn insisting that oral contraceptives—after less than fifteen years on the market—had no cancer risk.

"You mean there is no risk that you know of *so far*. Isn't that more accurate?" I questioned.

"There is absolutely no proof."

I told him about my radium treatments. "That was thirty-five years ago, and I'm still being watched. It took twenty-five years for most of those radium cancers to show up."

He was silent for a moment. "There is no proof OCs cause cancer," he repeated. "The FDA is monitoring all the time."

That was at the end of 1974, before Drs. Huebner and Todaro announced their oncogene theory. If they are right, if everyone is born with that built-in "cyanide pellet"—and it looks as if they may be—what a wonderfully nourishing endocrine environment the oncogenes have to thrive in, from all those estrogens in the Pill!

The tour through Dr. Dao's lab had made me suspect the Pill immediately. How could it not be dangerous?

"So is smoking," one of the doctors at Roswell Park said. "But people don't read that 'Warning: The Surgeon General Has De-

termined That Cigarette Smoking Is Dangerous to Your Health'
on every pack. As far as the Pill is concerned, there are a lot
of women who would rather risk cancer instead of a pregnancy."

"But do they know there's a risk? Is there a surgeon general's
warning on the Pill package?"

"I'm sure there is," he insisted. "The risk is too obvious. The
government must have made the drug companies put a warning
on."

"Don't be so sure. The government can be very strange," I
told him.

"Well, get some and see. There must be contraindications where
cancer is concerned. There is a Food and Drug Administration,
you know."

I followed his advice. No, there is no warning of possible cancer risk on the label attached to the package, which is known,
in FDA jargon, as the "patient package insert." It carries the
manufacturer's instructions for use of the product, prefaced by
this warning, printed in boldface type:

ORAL CONTRACEPTIVES (Birth Control Pills)
Do Not Take This Drug Without Your
Doctor's Continued Supervision

The oral contraceptives are powerful and effective drugs which can
cause side effects in some users and should not be used at all by some
women. The most serious known side effect is abnormal blood clotting
which can be fatal.

Safe use of this drug requires a careful discussion with your doctor.
To assist him in providing you with the necessary information, [the
manufacturer's name is inserted here] has prepared a booklet written
in a style understandable to you as the drug user. This provides information on the effectiveness and known hazards of the drug including
warnings, side effects and who should not use it. Your doctor will give
you this booklet if you ask for it and he can answer any questions you
may have about the use of this drug.

Notify your doctor if you notice any unusual physical disturbance
or discomfort.

Caution: Oral contraceptives are of no value in the prevention or
treatment of venereal disease.

I asked a pharmacist for the booklet mentioned in the label,
but he had none. They are available only from obstetricians and

gynecologists, or from drug-company "detail men." Other physicians do not receive copies. Finally my husband's secretary got one for me from her obstetrician.

"You aren't given one of these automatically," she explained. "My doctor only gives it to patients who ask for it." She had been taking OCs for several years, and the booklet she had, *What You Should Know About the Pill,* pertained to her prescription. She decided to stop using it as soon as she finished the last page.

"Oral contraceptives, like all potent drugs," this booklet said blithely, "have some side effects. Fortunately, serious side effects are relatively rare."

Among the nonserious side effects it mentioned were: tenderness of the breasts, nausea and vomiting, gain or loss of weight, spotty darkening of the skin, vaginal bleeding, elevated levels of sugar or fat in the blood, nervousness, dizziness, some loss of scalp hair, increase in body hair, an increase or decrease in sex drive, and appetite changes. Also, a nursing mother was warned that she may find a decrease in her supply of milk.

There were also light references to migraine headaches, mental depression, fibroids of the uterus, heart or kidney disease, asthma, high blood pressure, diabetes, and epilepsy. These were all listed under "Special Needs."

The *serious* side effects? Statistical evidence about thrombophlebitis—a potentially fatal circulatory disorder—did force the FDA to order drug firms to give women some information about a risk of blood-clotting problems resulting from use of the Pill. One of about every 2,000 women on OCs, the booklet said, is hospitalized every year because of blood-clotting trouble; also, one in 66,000 pill-taking women under thirty-five dies each year from thromboembolic disorders. But only *one in 500,000 women not taking OCs* dies annually from clotting disorders.

Although cancer was omitted from the patient package insert, it *was* mentioned in this booklet. "There is no proof at the present time that oral contraceptives can cause cancer in humans," it said. "However, the possibility that they may continues to be studied, based on observations that large doses of female sex hormones have produced cancer in some experimental animals."

And, buried deep in "Special Needs": "There are some

women . . . who should not use oral contraceptives. These include women who have cancer of the breast or womb." This
booklet did not say that the Pill is contraindicated where there
is a family history of cancer, although I was told by Dr. Louis
Hellman, chairman of the FDA advisory committee that approved
the Pill for sale in November 1959, that his copy of the *Physicians' Desk Reference*—a drug guide for doctors—did have the
warning. The 1975 edition does not, however.

Dr. Hellman, now the deputy secretary for population of the
Department of Health, Education, and Welfare, was not aware
that breast-cancer incidence rates have been climbing steadily
upward. He also did not know that the package insert carries
no warning aimed at women who have had cancer, in spite of
having helped write the first label. "The original insert specifically mentioned cancer . . . as a contraindication," he told me.
"Certainly whatever is in the booklet and the physicians' instructions about cancer should also be on the patients' label."

Oral contraceptives, by the way, are the *only* drugs on the
market in the United States that carry a warning label about
any contraindications that is addressed to patients. Although
there are many medications that should not be taken by certain
people, only their doctors are told.

A former obstetrician-gynecologist and a professor of both,
Dr. Hellman had testified before Wisconsin Senator Gaylord
Nelson's Select Subcommittee on Monopoly in January 1970—
shortly after the Pill's tenth birthday. He had told the senators
then that he was "uneasy" about possible carcinogenic effects on
the breast, that the fear "is always at the back of my mind." But,
he said, there was no evidence that a cause-and-effect relationship existed, and so he had advised the FDA to approve the Pill
for marketing. Women were to be warned, however, about the
possibility that estrogens should be avoided if they or close relatives had cancer.

He stressed to me that correlation must not be confused with
cause and effect. "Just because the breast-cancer rate is going up
at the same time as use of OCs is going up, that doesn't necessarily mean the drug is causing the increased incidence."

Another witness at the 1970 Senate hearings was Dr. Roy Hertz,
then an associate medical director of the Rockefeller University.

He had also been a member of the FDA committee that evaluated the Pill. During his career, Dr. Hertz has been a professor of obstetrics and gynecology, and has taken part in research programs at the National Institutes of Health. At the time of my telephone interview, in late 1974, he was a research professor in obstetrical pharmacology at the George Washington University Medical School, in Washington.

He told me that he still stands by his 1970 testimony. "I don't think that between then and now we have obtained the definitive information we need to know whether the estrogens in the Pill are carcinogenic or not. The same possibility of risk is still there."

In 1970, he had testified that "it was clear from the outset such an innovation, like all new medications, [carries] with it certain inherent risks." Increased cancer of the breast and uterus, Dr. Hertz had said, were his prime concerns. Asked by one senator if he thought estrogens were the whole cause of breast cancer, he replied, "I think they are to breast cancer what fertilizer is to the crop. They are not the seed."

Dr. Hertz had helped to write the physicians' instructions, which warn that women who have had cancer should not be given OCs. He had assumed the patient package insert repeated the warning.

The 1970 Nelson hearings brought together an impressive array of medical experts on all the diseases that might be affected by the Pill, not just cancer experts. As far as mammary carcinoma was concerned, the consensus was that it was too soon to know. Even one of the FDA's own witnesses, Dr. Robert Kistner, of Harvard Medical School (also, at the time, a grantee and part-time consultant to Searle Pharmaceuticals), admitted that ten years were not enough time to judge.

Dr. Hugh Davis, a Johns Hopkins professor of obstetrics and gynecology, was vehement in his objections. "Shall we have millions of women on the Pill for twenty years and then discover it was all a great mistake? Breast cancers have been induced on at least five different species of animals by treatment with the same synthetic hormones being marketed in the oral contraceptives."

Dr. Marvin Legator, then the chief of the Cell Biology Branch of the FDA's Division of Pharmacology, a defender of the Pill, nonetheless agreed that its effects had to be carefully watched. "The earliest period for detecting an increase in genital or mammary tumors . . . would be the mid-'70s," he told the subcommittee.

We have arrived. It is now the mid-1970s, and there has been a definite increase in mammary-tumor incidences. But oral contraceptives still carry no warning of cancer on the patient's label.

Paradoxically, in 1959—the year before OCs went on the market—the Food and Drug Administration banned the use of diethylstilbestrol (DES) in poultry feed, because tests had proved this synthetic female hormone caused breast cancers in mice. Edible tissues of poultry getting the feed, the FDA ruled, retained traces of DES that were too high to be safe, under the food section of the 1938 law that authorized creation of a supervisory agency. DES was also banned in feed for cattle and sheep in August 1972. However, in January 1973, the District of Columbia Court of Appeals reversed the latter ruling on a legal technicality.

Edward Nida, an information officer at FDA, explained why estrogens are FDA-OK for women but prohibited for chickens. "Oral contraceptives are voluntary and available only by prescription," he said. "Drugs put into animal feed are what we call 'surreptitious,' and consumers may not be aware they're getting them."

Nida, like Korn, reiterated the line about there being no proof that estrogens cause cancer in humans. "The pharmaceutical firms are required by law to report any adverse effects immediately," he declared. "If they don't somebody goes to jail. We don't play around with them."

The FDA is depending on the proverbial fox to guard our chicken coop.

"We have medical officers who follow all drugs," Nida added. "We also have literature searches and automated medical libraries." He said the FDA continues monitoring all drugs even after approval is granted.

The questionable efficiency of the FDA's estrogen monitors was demonstrated on October 9, 1974, when the approval of an injectible contraceptive—Depo-Provera—was delayed just three days before it was to go on drugstore shelves. The delay was at the direct order of Secretary Caspar W. Weinberger, the head of the Department of Health, Education, and Welfare, of which FDA is a member agency.

Congressman L. H. Fountain, of North Carolina, had told Weinberger that his Intergovernmental Relations subcommittee—the House's biting watchdog over FDA—had evidence showing Depo-Provera to be the possible cause of cervical cancer in twenty-two of 1,000 women involved in clinical trials of the drug. In the course of his eleven-page, single-spaced letter, Congressman Fountain said the relevant data had been published by the National Cancer Institute *in 1971.*

There are other examples of FDA's failure to exert tight surveillance over the Pill. For example, its Metabolic and Endocrine Section did not know that breast-cancer incidence had increased since OCs were approved, as Frank Korn admitted. "But let's thank God it's easily cured," he said.

Korn apparently did not know that the "cure" is to have the breast amputated and then to be given a fifty-fifty chance of living longer than ten years.

Korn said he knew of no work in progress to study a possible relationship between the Pill and breast cancer. Again FDA monitoring had failed. Several investigations were under way.

Two contracts to study the problem were then being funded by the Center of Population Research (CPR) of the National Institute of Child Health and Human Development. Dr. Philip A. Corfman—whose name was mentioned by several FDA officials as that agency's unofficial monitor on OCs—is the director of that institute. The chief of CPR's Contraceptive Evaluation Branch, Dr. Heinz Berendes, was tracking the results. He told me one investigation involved 200 women in Connecticut and the other about 450 women in California. Both were "retrospective studies": women with recent diagnoses of breast cancer were compared with a closely matched control group.

"We ask the cancer patients, 'Did you take the Pill?' " Dr. Berendes explained. "Then we analyze to see if there is an association." After two years, he said, no cause-and-effect relationship had been found. However, he admitted that 650 is a small sample and "it is too soon to know with certainty."

I did not try to track down the Connecticut scientists. However, I did call Dr. Ralph Paffenbarger, in Berkeley, California, and was referred to Dr. Elfriede Fasal, who directed the California investigation Dr. Berendes had cited.

"I did not say there was no relationship," she told me. "I simply gave some preliminary findings at a national public-health meeting. At that time, I merely gave these findings with no conclusions, except that some of the comparative data were not statistically significant. The actual report has not even been published yet." (This was in April 1975.)

As an example of the study's statistical insignificance vis-à-vis breast cancer, Dr. Fasal told me she found that all the women over the age of thirty took the Pill less frequently than did those under thirty—regardless of their illness. (The control group, by the way, was hospitalized patients who had medical or surgical problems other than breast disease, not healthy women chosen at random.) The thirty-to-thirty-nine age group averaged 65.6 per cent Pill users; the forty-to-forty-nine group, 38.6 per cent. She said the differences in usage between breast-cancer patients and others in the older age groups were not "statistically significant"—only a few percentage points.

However, Dr. Fasal said that of the fifteen women between the ages of fifteen and twenty-nine who had breast cancer, *100 per cent* were on the Pill at the time their tumors were found. Only 81 per cent of the younger women in the control group, on the other hand, used OCs. This difference, according to Dr. Fasal, is also not statistically significant, because the sample was so small. But, since breast-cancer risks are normally low in this age bracket, she thought the 100-per-cent use of the Pill by the young cancer patients "warranted further investigation."

I found no mention anywhere of this aspect of the Berkeley study, and when I called Dr. Corfman for more information, he told me he was not aware of the data. He had not heard the oral report given by Dr. Fasal and was waiting for the final results to be published in an NIH journal. Dr. Berendes was not available.

Then I called Dr. Herschel Jicks, at Boston University. His Boston Collaborative Drug Surveillance Program had been so widely referred to that I was certain he must have found something important. Also, it involved 25,000 women—an enormous sample.

"We were not primarily concerned with breast cancer," he told me, "but with all diseases—short- and long-term—that could be related to oral contraceptives." He said that only twenty-three of the 25,000 women studied had breast cancer, and the major pharmaceutical suspect was reserpine, not the Pill. However, he agreed that reserpine along with estrogens could have a relationship to breast cancer, because reserpine increases prolactin secretion and because prolactin must have estrogens to interact with in order to be carcinogenic. Logically, more estrogens in the blood, from oral contraceptives, would give the higher prolactin levels a more favorable environment to do their cancerous work. This, Dr. Jicks told me in a telephone interview in April 1975, is the suspected link between breast cancer and the various Rauwolfia drugs—reserpine is just one. From another doctor, however, I learned that this connection is to be studied in greater depth by other scientists before it will be accepted as fact.

As far as I could see, the widely touted Boston Collaborative and Berkeley studies incriminated oral contraceptives even more deeply than I had suspected.

"I just don't understand how anyone could interpret their results as proving no relationship between breast cancer and the Pill," I told Harvey during dinner that night.

"In my business, we're working with statistics all the time." He laughed. "You can always find some number to support what you want to prove."

One problem seems to be that all the Pill studies have been retrospective. As Dr. Berendes said, women with breast cancer are asked if they have ever taken the Pill, and if they have not they are listed in the "no-oral-contraceptive" column of the chart.

When I entered Roswell Park, I was also asked if I had ever taken oral contraceptives. I said that I had not. "But," I told the young physician who interviewed me, "I've taken lots of estrogens."

Without even trying to add up the gallons of chicken soup, DES-impregnated until 1959, and the DES-impregnated chopped liver I have eaten in my life, I told him about the hormones prescribed for me as a teen-ager to regulate my menstrual periods and to clear up my skin. I added that I had been given estrogens to prevent miscarriages and to "dry up my milk" after breast feeding.

"Estrogens are estrogens," he said laconically.

"Prospective studies" are analyses of women who are followed "ahead of time." In such controlled surveys, a random group would be chosen and studied for years—some taking the Pill, others not—to see what diseases they developed over as long as twenty years. Estrogens taken for any other reason would be included. A prospective study, it is agreed, is a far more reliable technique, but it takes a very long time to get adequate data.

So, as of early 1975, all the evidence against the Pill as a carcino*trophic* factor in breast cancer—cancer-nourishing, not cancer-causing—is based on retrospective studies, simply because it has not been around long enough.

Another statistical problem is that postmenopausal women with breast cancer are combined in the same data base with younger victims, considerably diluting the impact of the actual number having the disease. Since so much evidence now indicates that there are two different, age-related kinds of breast cancer, it would seem to be more accurate to base studies of the effects of Pill use on only the younger population.

In contrast to the Food and Drug Administration, Dr. Corfman does not depend on drug firms to report adverse effects of the Pill.

"I don't think the industry has hardly any good data." He laughed. "That's the reason we're doing the studies here." He also places little reliance on National Cancer Institute research, but for different reasons. "We keep in touch," he said, "but we don't find we get much from their work. The only way to study pills is to study pills and not try to piggyback on bigger studies."

Because of the lack of close communication with NCI, neither Dr. Corfman nor Dr. Berendes was aware that today's breast-cancer incidence rate is much higher than it was in 1960. Even without knowing this, however, Dr. Berendes admitted he would be "reluctant" to have his wife take OCs for ten years or longer.

After I told him what the current incidence rates are, Dr. Berendes recalled that during the 1970 Senate hearings there had been unanimous agreement that, unlike cervical cancers (also linked with OCs), breast tumors could take as long as twenty years to develop. The witnesses—including Dr. Corfman—had testified on the need for periodic re-evaluations of oral contraceptives. "We knew there would have to be continuing surveillance . . . at least for maybe ten years," Dr. Berendes said. "We simply don't know how long someone would have to be exposed . . . and what the interval would have to be."

In a report published in the medical journal *Contraception,* in late 1974, Dr. Corfman wrote a résumé of current methods of birth control. Using as evidence the Berkeley and Boston studies, as well as work done in Britain, he said, "At least to date, there is no relationship between the use of OC's and breast cancer."

However, the editor of the journal followed Dr. Corfman's report with this statement: "I find myself again in the position of calling for moderation and against over-enthusiasm in accepting and interpreting data in regard to oral contraception. . . . Subjecting well young women over long periods of time to potent drugs with widespread generalized reactions is certainly not good medicine."

Now we are told that all of us probably have an oncogene— a hidden trigger in every cell in our bodies—which might produce a cancer virus under the right circumstances. What might be the consequences of disturbing the delicate hormonal balance of a young woman by adding unnecessary estrogens?

Married women, who usually get their prescriptions for the Pill from family doctors or obstetrician-gynecologists, are presumably under their constant care. Presumably, these physicians know their patients' family backgrounds and personal medical histories. But what about the thousands of teen-agers and young women who get their pills through friends or from various birth-control clinics, mostly after one-shot visits and with no continuing care? No one is keeping a watchful eye over them.

In Europe, no one I interviewed hesitated to say that oral contraceptives are carcinogenic. This seems to be the "catch-22" of OCs—the three-letter syllable *gen,* Greek for "produced by." There is indeed no proof that the Pill produces breast cancer in humans. There is, however, a great deal of proof that, whatever the seed might be, the estrogens in these drugs are fertilizers that stimulate and speed the growth of mammary carcinomas. Research literature shows evidence that, while OCs may not be carcino*genic* in humans, they are certainly carcino*trophic*—cancer-nourishing.

With regard to animal studies, the FDA's spokesman, Frank Korn, told me the law specifies "toxicity" in three species of animals as being enough to rule a drug unsafe for human use. Five species of animals have developed mammary carcinomas after being given the same hormones that are in the Pill. Here is some of the additional evidence.

- Scientists needing cancerous tumors for experimentation routinely grow them quickly by giving estrogens to specially bred vulnerable strains of mice.
- Two compounds, Ethynerone and Neonovum (trade names for estrogenic OCs), were not even submitted for FDA approval, because they had caused breast cancers in dogs and monkeys over a seven-year period.
- Clinical data show that both the withdrawal and the administration of estrogens affect the rate of growth of breast cancers in women.
- Premenopausal women with the disease whose ovaries—a natural source of estrogens—are removed usually improve.
- Women who have had their ovaries surgically excised before the age of forty have a lower risk of developing breast cancer; the same is true of women with natural early menopause.
- Most breast cancers that develop in pregnant women are particularly virulent and fast-growing; the accepted reason for this phenomenon is the high estrogen level in the blood during pregnancy.
- From the late 1940s through the 1960s, millions of American women were given diethylstilbestrol routinely to prevent miscarriages early in pregnancy. Now their "DES daughters"—most of them teen-agers—are developing rare forms of vaginal and cervical cancers. Scientists suspect that the prebirth doses of DES somehow activated a "time bomb" in the affected girls. Estimates of the number of DES-linked cancer cases vary from 3,000 to 27,000.
- Giving estrogen to men with prostatic cancer has led to the

development of cancer of the breast—a very rare disease in males.

- Breast-cancer specialists know that some tumors are hormone-dependent and some hormone-independent, and that knowing the type helps determine the best postoperative treatment.

What is the Food and Drug Administration doing about warning women of the risks of the Pill? The same thing it is doing about reinstituting the 1973 ban on feeding DES to cattle and sheep. Nothing.

Ed Nida told me the FDA admits there are many unanswered questions about cancer and the Pill. "No drug, including aspirin," he insisted, "is absolutely safe. What we look at is the benefit-risk of a drug. Do the benefits of preventing pregnancy outweigh the risks in having a baby?" He admitted, however, that the Supreme Court decision of January 22, 1973, liberalizing abortion laws has virtually eliminated one of those risks—the danger of botched abortions. In using the mortality rates of childbirth as a risk factor, it would seem that FDA is equating pregnancy with a serious disease, like meningitis. By FDA criteria, to be pregnant is a pathological illness, where the benefit of a potentially dangerous drug that can prevent or cure—like chloromycetin, which can also cause the destruction of white blood cells vital in fighting disease —is weighed against the risk of possible death. But the dangers of giving chloromycetin are usually spelled out clearly to the patient or the patient's family.

Nida contended that the FDA is doing all it can about the Pill, under the circumstances. "When you have drug companies chewing on us for not approving drugs and creating a drug lag, and the Ralph Naders and the rest of the world chewing on us for putting risky things on the market, questions are not easily answered."

Gilbert S. Goldhammer, a consultant to Congressman Fountain's oversight subcommittee, said that one of the FDA's major problems in dealing with the Pill is simply that the agency is too "business oriented," and OCs are big money-makers. "There's no real chicanery," he told me. "No bribery or things like that.

It's just that the people at the top of FDA are not really scientists. They are medical people, but they're more management types. They have a business outlook on salvaging a product and making it work out." He chuckled. "And if they're wined and dined by the pharmaceutical people, that makes them all pals. You can't turn around and hurt pals."

Goldhammer added that Richard Nixon's longtime friendship with the founder of the giant Warner-Lambert firm, Elmer H. Bobst, undoubtedly had had an effect on the FDA's attitude toward all drug companies. "Bobst is godfather to one of the Nixon girls," he laughed, "and close to Nixon. By taking over Parke-Davis, he got one of the OCs—Norlestrin. Now, you know that kind of relationship had to affect the bosses at FDA. Nixon never needed much encouragement to be on the side of any business, and everybody knew what direction to go in." In early 1975, most of the top FDA officials were still Nixon appointees.

Goldhammer said that the Fountain subcommittee had held hearings on DES in animal feed, but, except for the Depo-Provera matter, it had not devoted much time to oral contraceptives. "I certainly think that all cancer risks should be put where the woman can see them," he said. "That means on the patient-package-insert label." They have not been added.

Paradoxically, in early March 1975, the FDA withheld authorization of an estrogen compound containing large quantities of DES that had been developed as a "morning-after" contraceptive, citing fears that it could cause cancer. Why bar a morning-after drug but not the standard OC? Who knows? The ways of FDA are strange and uninterpretable. Less than a month later, the potent compound was approved, because, according to Nida, doctors were simply prescribing multiple doses of ordinary DES to be taken for five consecutive days after the "accident."

"We are just recognizing current medical practice," he explained. "This way, the morning-after DES will have a warning on it that it is for emergency use only—rape or incest—and can be taken only once in a lifetime."

Approve a drug so dangerous it can be taken only once in a lifetime? As I said, who can understand the FDA?

Why is DES not permitted in chicken feed when it is all right in the feed of steers, sheep, and other animals?

Why were cyclamates banned as carcinogens on the basis of far less evidence?

Why is high blood pressure going to be mentioned on the Pill label as a contraindication—at least, newspaper reports say it will be—and not cancer? *

And it doesn't look like the cancer risk will be added. Spokesman Frank Korn told me in late 1974 that the patient package insert was then in the process of being reviewed, "but there are no great alarming facts that are going to be included. There are no plans to mention anything about cancer on the label."

There is still no proof positive that estrogens cause breast cancer in women. Probably there never will be; the hormones are carcinotrophic—fertilizers, not seeds. And even if they were the cause, a woman who would rather risk cancer than risk becoming pregnant should have the right—in the spirit of the basic individual freedom invoked by cigarette smokers—to make that choice.

I am not suggesting that oral contraceptives be summarily wiped from the shelves, as the "carcinogenic" cyclamates were. But Pill users should be warned, as smokers are. I see no excuse for keeping the possible consequences from them—especially those in the high-risk breast-cancer categories.

In January 1975, five years had passed since the Pill was last discussed in open hearings on Capitol Hill. Five years and about half a million breast cancers later, it was time for another congressional look. There was none.

Benjamin Gordon and Dr. Frederick Glaser, Senator Gaylord Nelson's top aides on drug matters, told me that no new hearings had been scheduled because of all the recent evidence that OCs were not related to breast cancer and might even be protective. What evidence? The Boston Collaborative and Berkeley studies. "We've also been told that breast-cancer incidence has not been soaring upward, as we and you thought," Gordon said.

"I can't believe that at all," I said. "One of the top statisticians

---

* As of January 1975, this warning was still not on the patient's label. According to FDA rules, drug manufacturers can use up existing supplies of labels before printing new ones—a situation that could create a lag of several years.

at NCI told me just a couple of months ago that it's been going up about 1 per cent every year since 1960."

"Well," he said, "that's all I can tell you. That's what they say."

I called Dr. Sidney Cutler, the NCI biometrician I had been quoting. He was on leave, but Susan Devesa, I was told, would have such incidence information. Immediately, she assured me that I had not been misquoting Dr. Cutler or giving out misinformation. NCI's statistical method had simply been changed.

"What he told you was based on information from Connecticut," she explained, "and we are not using that as our base now." Ms. Devesa went on to say that Connecticut—where the breast-cancer incidence had been going steadily upward, from 65 cases per 100,000 women in 1960 to 74 per 100,000 in 1969—had been the data base because it had a reliable state tumor registry, which had been in existence for many years. However, NCI had come to feel that Connecticut was not truly representative of the country as a whole. For example, few blacks, Orientals, Latin Americans, or American Indians were included.

Therefore, in the mid-1960s, money was granted to seven cities and metropolitan areas to establish tumor registries—Birmingham, San Francisco-Oakland, Atlanta, Dallas-Fort Worth, Detroit, Minneapolis-St. Paul, and Pittsburgh—as well as to two entire states, Iowa and Colorado. The registries began collecting and analyzing incidence data in 1969, and their figures for the years 1969–1971 were published, as the Third National Cancer Survey. Since most of the areas had no earlier statistics, there were no precedents against which to measure changes.

"But San Francisco has had a registry since 1960," Ms. Devesa told me, "and the breast-cancer incidence in that area has been rising. The age-adjusted rates for 1969–1971 were 84.1 per 100,000—even higher than Connecticut's." Sure enough, telephoned data from Alameda County (Oakland) showed a rate of 66.1 per 100,000 women—including Orientals, who have little breast cancer—for the 1960–1962 period, with a subsequent steady upward climb to 84.1 (which also includes San Francisco) for 1969–1971. I studied the table of statistics Ms. Devesa referred me to. Birmingham had only 58.8 per 100,000 for 1969–1971. But a phone call to its registry gave no further information; there were no earlier incidence data.

"Maybe I can find out how many women are taking the Pill in the two areas," I suggested to Harvey during my daily dinnertime report. "The difference of incidence around Oakland is enormous. I bet it's even 'statistically significant.'"

After hours on the telephone, I discovered it is impossible to learn any details about sales of oral contraceptives. The American Pharmaceutical Association, the Center for Health Statistics, Planned Parenthood, the Population Institute, and even Ralph Nader were no help. Finally I turned to Benjamin Gordon, in Senator Nelson's office.

"That breakdown is kept by a marketing research firm named IMS, in Pennsylvania," he told me. "I've never been able to get the information out of them." Sure enough, the appropriate persons at IMS said this was privileged information.

The Census Bureau told me that women in the San Francisco–Oakland area are generally more affluent, well educated, and sophisticated—all factors that might contribute to an increased use of OCs—but these same factors could contribute to the rising breast-cancer incidence without the Pill, as well.

"Another piece in the jigsaw puzzle," I lamented to myself.

But I did learn a great deal about statistics and their significance—and insignificance—to cancer in the course of my study of oral contraceptives. For example, I could not find a single scientist involved in breast-cancer research who believes OCs are safe where this disease is concerned. Everyone I queried was positive that adding large quantities of female hormones to a woman's body—especially a young woman's—is somehow dangerous, statistical evidence notwithstanding.

The arguments supporting the Pill are coming from doctors in clinical practice and from those scientists who play various numbers games. These are the people who constantly say, "That is not proof," "There is no evidence," and even "OCs are protective." Laboratory scientists like Dr. Dao pay little attention to numbers. When mice consistently develop mammary carcinomas after treatment with estrogens, this is proof enough to them that the female hormones are not safe. As for humans, Dr. Dao has often told me, "I don't need large samples. For me, ten out of ten are enough to prove anything."

But even the numbers players agree that a cancer warning should be on the patient package insert.

"Certainly," statistician-biometrician Susan Devesa said, "if the contraindication is in the physicians' instructions and in the booklet or other literature, it should be on the label the patient sees."

So why isn't it there? The reason can be found in the *Federal Register*, Volume 35, Number 113, dated June 11, 1970.

Organized medicine, speaking through the American Medical Association, the Association of American Physicians and Surgeons, the American College of Obstetrics and Gynecology, the American Society of Internal Medicine, the AMA Interspecialty Committee, the South Georgia Medical Society, the California Medical Association, the Rhode Island Medical Society, the Texas Medical Association and the Medical Society of Delaware, generally opposed [a label with assurances and warnings] on the grounds that (1) it would interfere with the physician-patient relationship . . . (2) that it would confuse and alarm the patient . . . (3) that the package insert cannot provide all the needed information . . . (4) that the physician is the proper person to provide the kind of information to his own patient . . . on a need-to-know basis; and (5) that the regulations should not control what information the prescriber gives to the patient.

Some physicians also felt that label warnings were an "unnecessary government intrusion into medical practice," and they said "the doctor's judgment as to what the patient should be told should prevail."

The Food and Drug Administration, created to protect and defend the people of the United States against impure, unsafe, and ineffective drugs, has bowed to pressure from pharmaceutical companies and "organized medicine."

"Why should we taxpayers be stuck with FDA salaries?" I complained to Harvey. "The FDA is looking after the drug companies and the doctors—not us."

Then I found an article written by Senator Vance Hartke, of Indiana, headlined "FDA Is a Sham That Looks After Its Cronies Instead of the Public." "An inescapable conclusion," he wrote, "is that industry will pay many FDA members' salaries when they leave government. The implication is obvious: Don't bite the hand that will be feeding you."

After weeks of reading, telephoning, and interviewing to find out why we were not being warned about the dangers of the Pill, I found the answer in one short article—an "economic incentive."

Early Detection

The telephone should ring at any moment to give me news about a friend who was scheduled for a biopsy this morning. Although she had found the tumor five months ago, it was "being watched."

After my mastectomy, it seemed as if every one of my female friends and relatives made a mad dash to her doctor for a breast checkup. In July 1974 there were no long lines or waiting lists, and all of them were examined quickly. Jerry was the only one to have a "suspicious" growth—and she had found it herself.

"It's in the left breast," she told me, after seeing her gynecologist. "He ordered a mammogram, and it was benign. So he said to forget about it for the time being. He just wants to keep an eye on it."

"How big is it?"

"About the size of a pea."

"Does it slide around and move, or does it seem to be stuck in one place?"

"It doesn't move a bit," she answered. "As a matter of fact, that's why he wanted a mammogram. He tried his best to move it, but it wouldn't budge, no matter how hard he squeezed and pushed—"

"Squeezed and pushed?" I cried. "What did you let him do that

146

for? You've read the instructions for self-examination. You're supposed to press and massage it with your fingers together, not—"

"I wasn't going to tell him what to do," she interrupted angrily. "He's a gynecologist, after all. He knows what he's doing."

I said nothing. What was there to say? My nephew had just passed his Obstetrics-Gynecology Boards examination with flying colors; his "cram book" had a total of two paragraphs about examining breasts.

"The mammogram did say it was benign, anyhow," Jerry continued. "Pushing and squeezing wouldn't bother it."

"Maybe you should get another opinion," I suggested. "Even a benign tumor should come out."

"As soon as I get enough sick leave, I will," she promised. "I'll wait till next year. The doctor said there was no rush."

To make a five-month story very short, Jerry's "benign" lump grew considerably after the examination. Two days ago, she abandoned her gynecologist and visited an oncologist. He did not like the way the tumor felt and scheduled the surgery for this morning.

Having breast cancer is bad enough. To know the cancer grew because of the arrogance, ignorance, or inexperience of a doctor must be unbearable. In the many lists of danger signals and instructions we are given, no one warns us about this obstacle to early detection of breast cancer: the inexperienced or incompetent physician who is confident a lump "is nothing" and "let's just watch it a couple of months."

Although patients are not told about them, the medical profession is very aware of such doctors. "Keeping an eye on it" is such a common habit it even has a name—"professional laxity." Physicians' delay and procrastination are so widespread and the consequences are so grave that *doctors themselves* have done surveys to discover the reasons. The results show that most general practitioners do not know enough about breast cancer to do a proper examination. Their breast checkups are perfunctory and inadequate—quick pats here and there—if the patient does not have a lump or other specific symptom. And if she does, they will too often poke and push it, unaware that harsh handling of a cancerous tumor could be dangerous.

After breast cancer reached the front pages in the fall of 1974, more doctors began to order mammograms, but a negative diagnosis usually reassured them into "keeping an eye on it." Yet months of "watching it" can turn a small, early cancer into a large, late one that could be lethal. Too few ordinary doctors have ever heard of doubling time.

Jerry's sister has just called. "They're cutting off her left breast right now," she sobbed. "It is cancer."

In every country I visited in Europe—England, Scotland, Sweden, Finland, and the Soviet Union—the practice is that all suspected cancer patients be referred to an oncologist immediately. "As soon as a woman shows up at a clinic with a suspicious symptom," I was told everywhere, "she is sent to a cancer specialist." But not in the United States.

It looks as if we women will have to depend on ourselves if we want to be sure we get every chance to survive. Vaccines and antibodies are still hopes for the future; fighting heredity and trying to avoid suspected carcinogens in foods or the environment are impossible. There is *nothing* we can do to prevent a breast cancer from developing.

But we can do a great deal to stop the disease from growing and spreading through our bodies. Any woman might easily save her own life by finding a tumor early, and this is possible if she faithfully practices breast self-examination—BSE. It is safe; it can be done as often as she likes; and she needs no appointment. About 95 per cent of all early breast cancers are discovered by the patients themselves, not by their doctors.

The basic technique for BSE is probably familiar by now to every woman who can read. Here are the instructions as given in an American Cancer Society pamphlet, available free from local ACS chapters.

This examination should be done every month. In premenopausal women, the breasts are most normal and free of cyclical bulges about ten days after menstruation begins, and that is when BSE should be done. Women who have already gone through the menopause might choose some date they will not forget and use it as the day for an examination every month. At first, the BSE may take several minutes, but after two or three times it will take no time at all.

Breast Self-examination (BSE)

1 1. Lie down. Put one hand behind your head. With the other hand, fingers flattened, gently feel your breast. Press ever so lightly. *Now examine the other breast.*

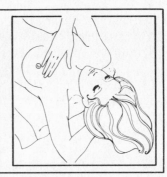

2 2. This illustration shows you how to check each breast. Begin where you see the *A* and follow the arrows, feeling gently for a lump or thickening. *Remember to feel all parts of each breast.*

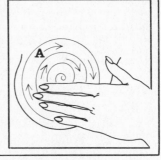

3 3. Now repeat the same procedure sitting up, with the hand still behind your head.

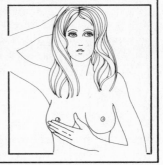

Reprinted by permission of the American Cancer Society

As all the standard instructions state, the first step in the BSE is done lying down, each arm alternately resting under the head while that breast is palpated with a gentle rotating motion, never a squeezing or pushing one.

A woman with large or pendulous breasts will need to alter this technique slightly. The side of the breast must be held steady, either with the hand or by resting it against something solid. Otherwise it would be like examining a plastic bag full of gelatin and a marble (the tumor, if one is present). Unless the bag is held steady, palpation will simply keep pushing the marble out of the way, and it will probably never be felt.

The axillas must also be palpated for growths, and this, too, is best done while lying down with the arm behind the head. For some reason, few instruction guides mention this important part of the examination.

For more sensitivity, the BSE should be done when the body is slippery from soap or oil. Or the hands can be coated lightly with powder. Even invisible bumps and dips feel like mountains and craters under slick fingertips. Lumps and thickenings are the most frequent first symptoms of breast cancer, but anything new or unusual should be noted.

If this part of the self-check does reveal a lump or thickening, the woman should call her doctor for an appointment immediately. In the meantime, she should ask herself these questions:

Does it hurt? If it does, this is a good omen. Early cancer, unfortunately, seldom hurts.

Does it seem to float freely inside? This is also a good sign. Most cancers are not movable, but fixed. Nor are they usually symmetrical; they can be irregular and fibrous.

Is she often "lumpy" and "cysty"? Has her doctor said she is prone to have chronic mastitis? If so, the lump is more likely to be benign. But the doctor must make the final diagnosis, not the patient.

Most instructions for BSE, excellent as they are, omit the less common symptoms of breast cancer, simply for lack of space in a small leaflet. Also, many symptoms are so infrequent that they are listed nowhere but in medical textbooks. To look for these, I recommend a second part of the self-check, which is done standing before a mirror.

First, the breasts should be scrutinized for any asymmetry. It is normal for one breast to be somewhat larger or to vary slightly in shape. But if such a change is recent it should be reported, even if there is no other symptom. Now for the skin: Is there a difference in the appearance of the skin of each breast? Any flaking or scaling? A variation in texture anywhere, giving an "orange skin" or "pigskin" appearance? Then the nipples: Are they cracked? Is any fluid coming from them? (Nothing should ever be flowing from the nipples except after childbirth.) The next step is to perform some gymnastics and contortions. Do the nipples react differently to the same movements? Does one seem to be forced into a different tilt? Any puckering or dimpling of the skin anywhere? Strange bumps or creases in the armpits? Yes answers to any of these questions call for a visit to the doctor.

Remember that signs of the two very rare carcinomas described earlier—the inflammatory and the generalized (the one with only pain as a symptom)—must be watched for, too. It is improbable that a hot, red, swollen, and sore breast would go unnoticed, but an odd, persistent ache or pain might. Doctors are just as likely as the woman herself to shrug off a simple pain as nothing but cyclical tenderness. If she knows the pain is not associated with her menstrual period, however, she should insist on a mammogram. With this generalized cancer, usually nothing is evident from a manual breast examination.

Here, then—in addition to the lump or thickening—is a list of less common warning signals:

1. Asymmetry in either appearance or movement of the breast.
2. Scaling skin around the nipple, changes in skin texture, cracked nipples, or any secretion from the nipples.
3. Puckering or dimpling of the breast skin.
4. Hot, swollen, and sore breast.
5. An unusual ache or pain that is persistent and not associated with cyclical changes and tenderness.

In his book *Early Detection,* Dr. Philip Strax, a veteran breast-cancer diagnostician, makes the excellent suggestion that every woman have one professional breast examination, including a mammogram and perhaps a thermogram, whether she needs it or not, in order to have a normal "map" for future comparison.

Before going on, I want to repeat the portion of the BSE instructions telling how the hands should be held, because it is so important that this be done properly. Use the flat of the hand, keeping the fingertips lightly together. The palpation should be gentle pressure and massage in a circular motion. Do *not* squeeze, push, pump, or pull.

And no doctor should squeeze, push, pump, or pull, either. If he does not know how to examine the breasts properly, the patient should put her clothes back on and find one who does.

Dr. Dao asked me how I thought the average woman could "really tell whether the doctor is doing a correct examination." My answer is along the lines of Dr. Strax's suggestion: go at least one time to a breast-cancer specialist—even if it means a trip to another city or state—and be examined by an expert. To judge by my experience, any woman who has paid close attention will easily be able to recognize a "correct" breast examination afterward. The difference is so dramatic that it could never be missed.

Now, suppose a BSE seems suspicious. An imaginary friend finds a tiny bump that was not there a month ago, or something else strange or unusual is present. She should never be bashful or shy about reporting anything, even a "nonsymptom" like a bruise that refuses to fade. What if her doctor does think she is a hypochondriac? If she wants to be examined and have a mammogram, and is willing to pay for both, why should he object? It's her life, after all.

In choosing a doctor, incidentally, she should never forget: the best BSE does no good if the doctor is one of those who want just to "keep an eye on it." Unless he or she is an expert whose hands have palpated hundreds of breast tumors, both benign and malignant, no faith can be put in fingers alone. Diagnosis by manual palpation has been proven wrong almost half the time. In hospital surveys comparing doctors' preoperative diagnoses with the postoperative pathology reports, manual examinations were inaccurate in 45 per cent of the cases. Nonetheless, having an examination by a doctor is the first step after finding a symptom.

Panicked, our friend has telephoned for an immediate appointment. "Don't delay!" the instructions insist. Unfortunately, she is just another in a long succession of women with like symptoms who began to arrive in doctors' offices after Betty Ford's mastectomy on September 28, 1974. There is no chance of her being examined for two weeks. Just as the tip of the tongue always finds the gap left by a lost filling, her fingers will automatically wander to the spot. She must do her best to avoid this reflex. When bathing or showering, only gentle patting and pressing are allowed—no squeezing.

Finally, though, the day of her appointment arrives, and she is in the examining room. (This doctor knows how to do a breast check, and she does not have to put her clothes on and storm out.) He finds the growth, but cannot tell what it is.

"Maybe it's a water-filled cyst," he mumbles, turning out the room light and flashing a powerful beam to see if the growth is hollow (this is the procedure called transillumination). "No." He shakes his head. "It's solid as a rock." Using a hypodermic needle, he tries to aspirate it, in the hope that something that can be examined will come out. "Nope," he repeats. "You'll have to have a mammogram." He writes the request on a prescription blank and gives her the name of the radiology clinic he deals with. "Maybe something will show up on the X-ray," he says.

Mammography has been with us since 1913, but not until 1960, when Dr. Robert Egan, a Houston physician, demonstrated its value, was its effectiveness in diagnosing early breast cancers widely accepted. Since then—a short fifteen years ago—the breast X-ray has become routine. Now its younger sister, xeromammography (that photocopy process for reproducing the X-ray film), is replacing the older technique as quickly as clinics can install the new equipment. The superiority of conventional mammography vis-à-vis xeromammography is being evaluated by the National Cancer Institute. So far, results show accuracy is dependent on which method the physician doing the reading was trained in or has had the most experience with.

Mammograms, with or without the xero-, are taken by a standard X-ray machine. The patient strips to the waist, and a technician bends her into strange positions while a cone-shaped device is focused on each breast and photographs it from various angles. The films are then developed and given to a trained radiologist for diagnosis.

As I said earlier, mammography is especially reliable for the woman with large breasts. The fatty tissue that makes her well endowed also gives the contrast needed for clearer and more accurate X-ray films.

A word of caution is needed about mammography. In my earlier discussion of the high-risk categories, and elsewhere in this book, I suggest that a high-risk woman should have a mammogram twice every year after the age of thirty-five. Many oncologists disagree. In spite of stringent inspection laws, apparently not all diagnostic X-ray machines expose patients to only the specified four rads (two per breast) of irradiation. Dr. Marvin Schneiderman, of the National Cancer Institute, told me that some equipment gives as many as fifteen illegal rads during mammography. "Exposing even high-risk women to that kind of irradiation twice every year might be more dangerous than not," he insisted. "I think saying all women over thirty-five should have mammograms two times a years isn't a good idea."

With Dr. Schneiderman's warning in mind, I must qualify my suggestion. The high-risk woman should find herself an oncologist, or an internist with a lot of cancer experience, who has access to good, nonleaking mammography equipment. Oncologists usually deal with radiologists they know and whose equipment they have learned they can trust. Then let the doctor decide how often X-rays are needed. The most important factor in breast-cancer (all cancer) treatment is, after all, the physician.

The doctor may suggest to our hypothetical patient that she have a thermogram, as well as the mammogram, to determine a baseline picture of the heat patterns of her breasts.

Like so many advances, thermography came to medicine from war. Scientists had long known that some materials collect and hold more heat than others. Using this principle, weapons designers invented rockets that home in on an enemy plane by following its engine heat. These are the "smart bombs" that simply track their quarries by the heat they give off. Knowing that malignant tissue and normal tissue have different heat-retaining qualities, medical scientists were able to adapt the principle for cancer detection. They have devised an infrared scanner that picks up heat patterns from the breast and records them on film. Although far from perfected, thermography is a useful "third opinion" in combination with the manual examination and the mammogram. It must *not* be relied upon alone, however.

Unlike mammography, thermography involves no irradiation at all, and thus can be used as often as necessary, even with very high-risk women. After undressing, the patient holds her arms up in the air or stretched out from her body for a few minutes, to give her skin a chance to cool. Then, using a specially treated paper, the scanner takes Polaroid color photos of the breasts. If the thermogram is to be done on the same day as the manual examination or the mammogram, it should be taken first. Even the small amount of friction involved in either of those could be enough to distort the heat pattern.

Initially, most of the thermographs in use were involved in twenty-seven demonstration projects funded jointly by the American Cancer Society and the National Cancer Institute. The projects were mass screenings of randomly chosen women with no breast-cancer symptoms, using the three basic examination techniques—manual examination, mammography, and thermography. The long-term goal was to find invisible malignancies during their first twenty generations of doubling—long before they could be palpated. There is good reason to believe the results will be well worth the cost.

Several years ago, the National Cancer Institute supported a screening of 31,000 women members of the Health Insurance Plan (HIP) of New York. Out of 132 breast cancers found, one-third were discovered by mammography alone; the malignant spots were too small to show up by manual examination. The most important finding of the HIP project, however, was that when radical mastectomies were performed on the women with these very early cancers, 75 per cent had no malignant lymph nodes at all, while normally about half of all patients have nodal invasion at the time of their mastectomies. In other words, a higher percentage of the screened patients were cured because their cancers had been discovered so early, before any cells had spread beyond the breast.

The success of the HIP project convinced the experts that more such mass screenings should be done. In 1972 and 1973, the NCI and ACS chose twenty-nine institutions (two cities have two projects), each to screen 10,000 asymptomatic women—those having no obvious signs of cancer—between the ages of thirty-five and seventy-five. During the first year each project examined 5,000; the second year, 5,000 were added for a first screening, and the original 5,000 were checked again. Then all 10,000 are to be followed annually until every woman has been checked for a total of five years. The hope is to repeat or improve on the results of the HIP screening, and so far the projects are succeeding. After only one and a half years and 125,000 screenings, more than three-fourths of the women in whom breast cancers were found had no invasion of the lymph nodes.

The procedure for the screening participants is not too different from that for an individual patient. After they have had all three of the tests—clinical examination, mammogram, and thermogram —radiologists and experts who have learned how to read thermograms study the pictures and make their diagnoses. Then the results of the three tests are evaluated and a consensus is reached. If the tests are all negative, no abnormal condition is present, and the woman is told to do a BSE every month and return in a year. If the three tests are positive, a biopsy is ordered. A "suspicious" or "indeterminate" diagnosis might require a second set of films for confirmation. If these are also suspicious, a biopsy would be recommended.

While the thermogram trails the mammogram in reliability, experts are working hard to perfect the new technique—not just because of the American love of gadgetry, but because no irradiation is involved. As we have seen, however, thermograms remain educated guesswork for the time being.

No matter what the three tests show, if there is a lump, thickening, or any of the other symptoms listed as warning signals, the only safe course is to have the growth removed and studied under the microscope by a pathologist. Biopsies are the only way to be sure today—although a lot of research is going on to find better and earlier methods of detecting breast cancer.

A reliable detection device that uses no irradiation is so desperately needed that even lingerie manufacturers are looking for one. An ingenious brassiere, wired to absorb heat, is being tested on thousands of women around the country. The principle is the same as that of thermography: cancerous tissue retains more heat than benign tissue does. By wearing the bra before any symptoms developed, a woman's normal pattern would be established, and white "hot spots" (malignant tissue shows up white under the bra's infrared heat sensors) that appeared later would indicate possible serious changes in her breasts. Inventors of the several variations being tested—most of them physicians —hope that wearing the bra only a few days every month would be enough to show whether changes of heat patterns had occurred.

Another technique being investigated uses ultrasonic waves. Also a by-product of war and weapons research, it is based on the knowledge that different materials give off different sounds, and that these can be converted electronically to pictures, as in the case of sonar. An acoustic beam is flashed through the breast and focused on a screen. But, instead of a submarine, the "sonogram" that appears is a cross-section of the mammary gland in great detail. A trained sonogram reader can distinguish between benign and malignant tumors, and all of the several variations of sonography being tried seem fairly accurate when the reading is done by an expert.

But a mass-screening device cannot be dependent on such a special skill; it must be simple enough to be operated by someone with only a little training. Another problem with breast sonograms is possible sound distortion. "Between the beat of the heart and the bellowing of the lungs," a National Cancer Institute expert told me, "the echoes bounce all over the place. There's just too much racket in the chest to get a breast picture that won't be affected by the noise."

One detection technique that will probably never be widely used is Dr. Nicholas I. Petrakis' method of analyzing breast fluid. Few women are aware that a constant supply of fluid is manufactured in the breast; it rarely drips out of the nipples, because their openings become plugged, and usually is reabsorbed unnoticed. This nonmilk is made by the acini, the tiny milk-producing glands in the lobules. To remove it from the breasts, scientists aspirate the liquid by suction or, sometimes, by putting fine pipettes into the nipple openings. According to the doctor reporting the research, "It is uncomfortable."

Breast-fluid analysis is not considered a diagnostic tool now, although it may be someday. The technique is being used experimentally in San Francisco to see what differences there are in the fluid composition of Caucasian and Chinese women. There is a difference, by the way, the scientists say. Chinese women have much less breast fluid than do Caucasians, and it contains fewer "atypical cells." Should the latter turn out to be precursors of cancer, breast-fluid analysis might well become a valuable early-detection technique.

Scientists have several detection dreams. One is a simple blood or urine test that would indicate the presence of breast cancer as readily as a Wassermann reveals syphilis. Another is a harmless substance that would collect only in malignant breast and nodal tissue. With a dab of radioactivity attached to it, such a chemical could be injected into a vein and followed through the body by a scanner camera. Any cancerous spot in the breast or armpit would light up on the film like a neon sign.

But so far these are still in the realm of "possible dreams." Neither can yet be included on today's list of early-detection techniques. To sum up, these are:

1. Breast self-examination monthly.
2. Manual examination by an experienced physician at least once every year.
3. Mammography or xeromammography.
4. Thermography.
5. Experiments (as yet unperfected) with bras, ultrasonics, and breast fluid.

Meantime, our friend with the breast lump is still waiting for the results of her X-rays and thermography. They finally arrive and are the same as mine were: X-ray—"benign fibrocystic disease"; thermogram—"suspicious, recommend a mammogram."

"Where does all this leave me?" she asks her doctor.

"Waiting for a slot on the operating-room schedule," he tells her honestly. "A biopsy is the only way to find out what's in there."

The day for the biopsy comes, and she is wheeled into the operating room. Even while the anesthetic is numbing her mind, the worry is still there—"How will I wake up, with one breast or two?"

Luckily, her tumor is benign fibrocystic disease. The mammogram was right! She and her husband go out to celebrate.

But now the watching game starts all over. Her risk of growing another tumor has risen. She must be even more careful to examine her breasts every month, and to have checkups by her doctor and a mammogram once or twice a year. There's no other way.

Shortly after Christmas 1974, on a Washington TV talk show, I saw an interview with Ann London Scott, a once dynamic feminist leader and one of the founders of NOW—the National Organization for Women. Ms. Scott, only forty-five, had advanced metastatic disease in her liver and did not expect to live much longer. Her cancer had begun little more than a year earlier as a breast tumor.

"Are you bitter about the prospect of dying?" the interviewer asked sympathetically.

The fiery organizer, her eyes flashing, stared into the camera. She was emaciated and clearly very ill, but her spirit was far from beaten. "Not about dying itself," she hissed, "but because it might have been postponed if I had had follow-up care. I thought the mastectomy would be the end of it, that I had to wear a stupid prosthesis and that was all. Finished."

Ms. Scott's luxurious black hair glowed with highlights under the television lights, and her fierce, expressive eyes blazed with anger. The rest of her slumped weakly in her chair.

"What I'm bitter about is the total lack of anything after the surgery—the X-rays, scans, and tests that could have spotted the cancer when it first began to spread. I never had any of them. If I had been put on chemotherapy immediately, it might have been stopped." She continued, her fury carrying across the airwaves onto my screen. "Okay, so I did all the right things. I found the lump and had the mastectomy. That was all I was told *I* had to do. For the rest, a woman depends on her doctor, and there is a lot of work that still needs to be done about that."

It was obvious that Ann Scott wanted to be around to do it. Unfortunately, she died not long afterward, on February 17, 1975.

There is no shortage of publicity about early detection of a first cancer. When the first and second ladies had their mastectomies, it was hard to find a newspaper or magazine, a radio or television program, that had missed giving instructions in BSE and the seven danger signals of cancer. For the general education of women, this is a marvelous contribution. But women like me, who have already had one cancer, have a very high risk of developing another one, and *nowhere* have I seen an article printed or a discussion aired on how to detect early signs of a recurrence or a metastasis.

In the reams of expensive brochures, pamphlets, leaflets, and booklets published by the American Cancer Society, there is not a single line addressed to patients to warn them about a second cancer. Ann Scott was right. All a woman hears about are BSE, biopsy, and the different kinds of mastectomy, as if these were the end of breast-cancer troubles. In fact, mastectomy is only the beginning of a lifetime of watching, examination, and testing —if the patient is lucky enough to have a doctor who knows what should be done.

An American Cancer Society spokesman told me the ACS has many and frequent meetings and conferences to "educate the profession." It is assumed, he said, that "once the cancer is discovered, the patients are under the care of physicians, and we direct our follow-up information to them." Having attended many a medical conference and meeting, I know how many doctors consider them nothing but tax-deductible vacations for brushing up on their golf, tennis, or fly casting. Science reporters covering such conventions usually return home knowing more about the subject of the meeting than the doctors do. Are the ACS-sponsored meetings any different?

"I think our professional-education programs are taken very seriously," the spokesman insisted. "The problem may be that general practitioners and general surgeons don't usually attend. Cancer specialists are our main participants."

Yet, according to statistics, about 90 per cent of cancer victims in the United States are being "cared for" and "followed" by general surgeons or by their family doctors, not by cancer specialists. Breast-cancer mortality rates have not dropped in forty years, in spite of all the advances in detection and treatment. Why not?

Ann Scott was not alone in her bitter anger at facing death sooner than she need have. In my more than 130 interviews with and letters from fellow victims of breast cancer, the lack of proper follow-up care was the one thing that prompted the most vehement attacks on physicians. Greater than their resentment at waking up "with one instead of two" without any advance warning, greater than their rage over unnecessary mutilation, the wrath of women with metastatic cancers detected too late was unmeasurable.

One woman in her mid-sixties called me from Florida. Her husband, on an extension phone, was even more passionately outspoken than his wife.

"I found my lump back in 1963," she recalled, "and I had a mastectomy. After that, I went to see the doctor about every three months. He'd feel around my other breast, check my pulse and blood pressure, and do sort of a quick physical. He never took X-rays or anything like that."

"And we were dumb enough to think he knew what to do," her husband broke in. "After all, what else can people do?" He continued, "Even that was only for the first two years. After that, he told her to come every six months. When the sixth year was over, he discharged her as cured. He never gave us any reason to think that the cancer hadn't been caught in time."

"Then, about three years later"—his wife picking up the story—"I had a very slight fall. It wasn't much of a fall, but I broke my hip. The orthopedist, in the same hospital, must not even have looked up the records to see what had happened to me before. He just operated, put in a pin, and never did any kind of an examination for bone cancer."

"I thought it was strange to break a leg from a little bump like that," her husband interrupted. "But she was getting older, having a lot of aches and pains, and bones break easier than they do when we're young. So we didn't think anything of it."

They learned later that her bone had broken so easily because it had been widely invaded and weakened by metastatic bone

cancer. But it took several months longer for her doctor to discover that, even after the break. Only when the upper part of
her spine—the cervical vertebrae—began to hurt were X-rays
finally taken, and then the spread of the malignancy showed up
plain and clear.

By the time I spoke with the woman, her skull was dotted
with tumors. She was then in the care of an oncologist, who had
prescribed drugs and X-ray treatments to lessen the pain. He
had told the couple this was all that could be done, barring a
medical break-through or a miracle.

"I can't help but think, knowing what I know now," the woman
told me, "that if the first doctor had taken X-rays or given me
more thorough examinations during those first six years, he
would have seen the spread to the bones. It must have started
back then."

Of course, medicine "back then," in the mid-1960s, did not
have all the treatments available now. Possibly nothing could
have been done for her even if the metastasis had been discovered. On the other hand, who can say? Even then, enough
was known to have perhaps slowed down the growth and given
her some added years.

Breast cancer—all cancer—is a chronic disease, like diabetes.
The first two postoperative years are the most critical, because
most metastases show up during this period. But five disease-free
years do not mean the cancer is cured. All they mean is that,
as far as any doctor or any test can tell, the cancer in the local
area of the surgery has been stopped.

Women who have just had mastectomies are at square one:
BSE every month, an examination by a doctor every three months
for two years, and twice a year for the following three. But now
the stakes are much higher. We are the most likely of all women
to develop cancer somewhere else. To protect ourselves against
careless and/or ignorant doctors, we ought to know what the
best procedures are. I am using as my model here the follow-up
examinations I am having at Roswell Park Memorial Institute,
in Buffalo, which, as I have said, is one of the best cancer hospitals in the world.

A second tumor most frequently appears in the remaining

breast. So, in between visits to the doctor—every three months during the first two years after surgery—BSE is imperative. The same technique of self-examination applies now, but more urgently.

The patient should be especially alert for any of the seven danger signals of cancer.

C hange in bowel or bladder habits.
A sore that does not heal.
U nusual bleeding or discharge.
T hickening or lump in the breast or elsewhere.
I ndigestion or difficulty in swallowing.
O bvious change in a wart or mole.
N agging cough or hoarseness.

Breast cancer has two usual routes for spreading: invasion of the bone of the rib cage and backbone, or metastasis to the lungs, liver, or brain via the blood stream or lymphatics. Any bone pain whatsoever, anywhere, should be reported to the doctor immediately, without waiting for the appointed checkup. So should a lingering cough or hoarseness, yellowing of the complexion, abdominal swelling, frequent and severe headaches, an unexplained loss of weight or appetite.

These are the specific warning signals we mastectomees can all watch for ourselves. But secondary malignancies, like primary tumors, are insidious. They often have no symptoms a patient can recognize until it is too late, and so she has no choice but to rely on her doctor's being alert for them.

During my first postoperative examination at Roswell Park, three months after my mastectomy, I had a thorough manual examination of the area around the incision and the affected armpit. Rarely, a stray cancer cell left behind after surgery will start a new malignancy in the surgical site itself. The remaining breast and the other armpit were carefully examined, of course, and my liver was palpated for tenderness or enlargement. If I had complained of a lingering cough or hoarseness, I would also have had chest X-rays. Any suspicious results would have called for more extensive tests and X-rays. However, everything seemed fine and nothing further was needed.

Six months after surgery, I went back to Buffalo for the second follow-up examination. This time, in addition to manual examination of the chest, armpits, and liver, blood tests were done to analyze how well my liver was functioning. Also, X-rays of my chest, pelvis, and spine were taken, from various angles, even though I had reported no symptoms of pain.

If all the results of the six-month follow-up are negative, as mine were, the next examination, three months later, will be a repeat of the first one, except that mammograms will also be taken, and the checkup at the end of the first year will be a duplicate of the one after six months, provided no symptoms have shown up in the meantime. Dr. Dao adds that he often has skull X-rays taken at this time, along with those of the chest, pelvis, and spine.

Besides having my checkups religiously, I am contributing some of my blood and urine every three months to the National Cancer Institute as part of a study to find "markers"—substances that may one day prove to be advance indicators of a cancer growing somewhere in the body. This is a search for one of those "possible dreams," a simple blood or urine test—about which, more shortly.

But suppose the results of my early tests had been suspicious. Suppose I had reported having pain. What would Dr. Dao have done? He told me that if a malignant tumor had been discovered in the second breast, I would have had another modified radical mastectomy, with a new beginning of the five years of follow-up examinations. Any sign of a recurrence in the operative site would indicate either surgery or some kind of chemotherapy, but not X-ray treatments. Strange spots on the chest or bone X-rays or abnormalities in the liver-function studies would call for scans.

Scanning is done in that hospital department menacingly named nuclear medicine. Scans are expensive and time-consuming, but, in spite of the skull and crossbones required by law to be plastered everywhere, they are nothing to be afraid of, and they do not hurt. The foundation of scanning is the simple principle that certain chemicals tend to be attracted to specific organs (iodine, for example, collects in the thyroid gland, leaving only traces elsewhere in the body) and that, once in the organ, the chemicals behave differently in normal tissues than in cancerous tumors. Thus, a radioactive "tracer" is put on one of these harmless chemicals, and the "tagged" substance is injected into a vein. For liver scans, gallium is the current favorite; for bone, a new element, technetium. The chemical eventually settles at its destination and shines brightly there for the scanner; films show whether the chemical has been "taken up" by malignant tissue.

Scans are more accurate and definitive than X-rays, but they should not be used routinely as a follow-up technique. They are indicated only when tests that use less irradiation are suspicious. Certainly, however, if there are symptoms of a possible metastasis, the danger of radioactivity from a scan is a fraction of the risk of having the cancer metastasize. Again, the question must be asked: Does the benefit outweigh the risk?

If a recurrence or metastasis is discovered, by a scan or some other means, appropriate chemotherapy must be started immediately. The drugs most effective against breast cancer are discussed in a later chapter.

Most general practitioners use X-ray to treat various kinds of bone tumors metastasizing from breast cancer. Also, if several positive lymph nodes are found after mastectomy, some doctors will irradiate the internal mammary chain of nodes, which runs along the breastbone under the ribs. However, there is evidence that X-ray should not be used at all on widespread metastases, for the same reason that prophylactic (preventative) irradiation has been dropped: it may do more harm than good. At Roswell Park and other cancer clinics and hospitals, therapeutic irradiation is used on bone metastases, but only when the X-ray can be sharply focused on isolated spots. Lower doses are also used for palliation—alleviating pain—when hope of destroying the cancer itself is gone.

Whether to irradiate recurrences or metastases that can be pinpointed, rather than treat them surgically or with drugs, is a matter of the attending physician's personal preference. It is one of those gray areas, with no solid proof of superiority one way or the other. For the patient, it becomes a matter of faith in her doctor's point of view. Inevitably, somewhere along the line, she has no choice but to cross her fingers and hope her doctor is right and his opponents wrong. There are a good many such gray areas in the treatment of breast cancer.

To review the basic elements of postoperative care during the first two years, here is what the doctor should be responsible for:

1. A thorough examination of the operative site, both axillas, and the remaining breast every three months.
2. A mammogram of the remaining breast every six months, unless the physician is very experienced in managing breast cancer. In that case, an annual mammogram should suffice.
3. A thorough manual examination of the liver every three months.
4. A liver-function blood study every six months.
5. Chest, spine, and pelvic X-rays every six months.
6. Skull X-rays if indicated.
7. Scans if indicated.

That is the pattern for the first two years after a mastectomy, the period when most recurrences and metastases appear. For the following three years, all these examinations should be done twice a year, although scans are only "if indicated" by symptoms or abnormalities. If a recurrence is discovered in the second breast, the nodes will usually be negative, since the cancer would have been caught very early. Nevertheless, the five-year follow-up would have to begin all over again.

Does it sound like an endless, hopeless treadmill? Thanks to early detection and good postoperative care, for more and more women it is not endless. And it is certainly not hopeless. I have now met many women who—with proper follow-up after mastectomy—have lived for years even with recurrences and metastases.

Through postoperative studies of thousands of women, scientists have discovered important clues left in the blood and urine by their breast cancers. These are the "markers" I mentioned earlier. Research on them is going on all over the world, and, at the National Cancer Institute, Dr. Douglass Tormey gave a progress report on his work to an international conference of breast-cancer specialists.

He told his colleagues that eight substances in the blood and urine of women with diagnosed metastatic breast disease are present in different quantities than are found in women with no signs of spread. While all are normal components of the blood and urine, the amounts vary with the stage of the disease. "Perhaps the most important potential use for markers such as these," Dr. Tormey explained, "is in the preoperative and postoperative settings. Measuring such markers . . . is an easy and efficient way of adding another screening variable."

Dr. Tormey said that, while some other illnesses can also cause abnormalities in the quantities of some of the substances, one in particular—carcinoembryonic antigen (CEA)—shows a far higher level in the urine of women with breast cancer than in patients having any other disease.

In London, a few months later, I met Professor Thomas Symington, chief of the Chester Beatty Research Institute, who is highly optimistic about CEA as a breast-cancer marker. He would like to computerize all the available marker information, especially that on CEA, so that the marker data of a given patient could be compared with that in the electronic brain. Instantly her doctor would know whether her levels were higher, equal to, or lower than the quantities found in known breast-cancer victims.

Professor Symington, who holds degrees in both medicine and biochemistry, bases his hopes for breast-cancer progress on molecular biology. He believes that when benign cells become malignant, chemical changes occur that cause some change in the wastes the tissue discards—wastes that, of course, eventually appear in the blood and urine. More important, the wastes would appear very early in the cancer's life—certainly during those first twenty generations of preclinical life, before a tumor is palpable.

Although markers are now only "a rough screening device" to detect recurrences, in Dr. Tormey's words, he feels that the technique "does show promise" as an early-detection method. Cautiously, not wanting to see bold black headlines reporting a miraculous breast-cancer test, Dr. Tormey would go no further than to tell the conferees that the quantities of the substances found in the blood or urine of breast-cancer patients did rise or fall according to the severity of their disease. And, as of the day of the conference (September 30, 1974), almost all the women in his test groups who developed metastatic disease (sixty-three of sixty-five) had abnormal levels of at least one of the markers. On the other hand, *no* woman showing normal levels had had a recurrence.

Dozens of labs around the world are, with Dr. Tormey and Professor Symington, chasing the "possible dream" of a simple, inexpensive, early test for breast cancer. Someone, somewhere, is bound to catch it. But it is not caught yet.

Any breast-cancer patient who lives near a hospital or medical school that is doing a marker study should try to take part in it. It means nothing more than giving a little blood and collecting a twenty-four-hour urine sample every three months. But this may be the test that will find a breast cancer before anything else can. As for metastases, it won't tell where they are, but it will tell a woman and her doctor that he has to look for them.

What does a patient do if her doctor laughs and tells her all those examinations and tests are a waste of time and money? Either she believes him, or she finds another doctor.

8

The Real Controversy: Surgical Biopsy, Staging, and the "Economic Incentive"

Everyone, by now, must know that a breast-cancer controversy is raging in the land. Are too many mastectomies being performed? Too many radical mastectomies? Why are most surgeons in the United States still doing the disfiguring and disabling Halsted radical, when the modified radical is just as good?

This is the "blazing" controversy we have been hearing so much about. But I think the real breast-cancer scandal has nothing to do with the kind of mastectomy at all. Other things are done that are not just mutilating, but actually murderous.

The single underlying basis for these practices is the penchant in the United States for performing the biopsy on the operating table and combining it with an immediate mastectomy if the frozen-section pathological diagnosis is cancer. Aside from the psychological trauma to the patient of going into the operating room without knowing whether she will awaken "with one or two," there are good medical reasons for separating the two procedures.

First, any chance of an error in the quick-freeze method of diagnosis would disappear immediately. Surgeons insist that in doubtful cases they "err" on the side of the patient—but what puts the doubt in their minds? Frozen-section diagnoses, admittedly, rarely differ from those of the more reliable permanent section, which takes several days. But mistakes have been made, and even one mistake is too many if it means someone's breast has been amputated for nothing.

A second medical reason is to guard against anesthetic traumas. Biopsies are usually performed under light anesthesia—an injection of a narcotic drug—which does not require a preliminary chest X-ray. All good hospitals insist that patients who are to be given inhalation anesthesia—gases—be X-rayed first, to be sure their lungs are free of infection and disease, which of course is not necessarily done with a biopsy patient. If the frozen-section diagnosis is "benign," all is well. However, the injected narcotic is not a deep enough anesthetic for a mastectomy. Gases of some kind must be used, and these should *never* be given unless the lungs have been examined and pronounced clear. But there is no time for chest X-rays when a mastectomy of any kind immediately follows the biopsy. I know of one young woman who died during a mastectomy—done under endotracheal anesthesia—because no films had been taken of her lungs. She had undetected "walking pneumonia."

In addition to these known and accepted contraindications for the one-stage procedure, evidence is coming from immunology laboratories that delaying the mastectomy for a few weeks, or even a month, after an excisional biopsy—removal of the entire tumor—gives the patient's defense system the time and strength to attack and destroy any residual cancer cells in the area of the tumor. While this hypothesis has not yet been proven, clinical data so far seem to support it.

Even without these considerations, however, there is ample reason for surgeons in the United States to stop combining biopsy with mastectomy. For in combining them, a vital medical step is skipped. It is far more critical than psychological anxiety and fear, the chance of frozen-section error, or a possible adverse reaction to anesthesia. The combined procedure means that the all-important "staging" of the disease cannot be done before the breast is removed.

Staging is the term used by cancer experts to describe the process of diagnosing the level of malignancy by X-rays, scans, and various blood tests. All cancers can be staged, although the parameters vary with the organ involved. With breast cancer, Stage I indicates that it is confined to the breast, as far as any test can predict. Stage II means some nodal involvement. Stages III and IV show that clear and definite signs of advanced metastasis are present and mastectomy would therefore be useless.

It must always be remembered that the only reason for ever performing a mastectomy is to stop the spread of the cancer beyond the breast. If preoperative tests show that it has already traveled beyond the axillary lymph nodes, there is absolutely *no* purpose in removing the breast. Such a patient will not benefit from mastectomy, and vital drug treatment will be delayed while she recuperates from the unnecessary surgery.

When the breast is routinely removed within minutes of a positive diagnosis, there is no time for staging. The usual practice in this country, if the pathology report shows that several axillary nodes are cancerous, is for the staging to be done afterward, to see whether chemotherapy is indicated.

Within recent years, a T-N-M code has been adopted internationally to define the stages of breast cancer more precisely, and this code was used for diagnostic examinations in all the countries I visited. The T stands for the tumor, N for the nodes, and M for metastasis. Ideally, a woman is $T_0N_0M_0$—no cancer at all. A small tumor would be T_1, a larger one or a second one T_2, and so on. The subscript numeral after the N tells how many nodes seem to be invaded, as far as the doctor can determine preoperatively by manual examination; if the nodes are removed and examined microscopically, this may change. The M refers to metastases, or the amount of spread, and the extent of metastatic invasion is also described by a subscript numeral. If the cancer is very advanced when a woman is first examined, the M may be obvious just from a manual examination. Usually, early metastases cannot be determined before surgery without X-rays, scans, and blood studies—staging.

The best way to explain the importance of staging is to recount a conversation I had with Dr. Maureen Roberts, at the Royal Infirmary in Edinburgh, Scotland. We went to her tiny cubicle of an office for a few minutes of talk between conferences. Over coffee, Dr. Roberts, a young and very pretty woman, shook her head, puzzled.

"In all of those newspaper and magazine stories about Mrs. Ford and Mrs. Rockefeller, it seems as if the mastectomies were done so very quickly," she commented. Her voice had a faint Scottish burr. "When could they have had time to do all the preoperative work-ups properly, if the mastectomy followed the diagnosis so quickly?"

"How do you do it in Edinburgh?"

"When a woman presents us with a suspicious symptom in the clinic," she explained, "we of course do mammograms or xero-mammograms immediately. If these are inconclusive, we biopsy the tumor."

"In the operating room?" I interrupted.

"Oh, that is only a last resort," she said. "Surgery for a biopsy is usually not necessary, because there are several other ways of finding out, in the clinic. First we try a fine-needle biopsy." *

That was what my first surgeon must have tried to do when he aspirated my tumor with a hypodermic needle. I nodded. "That's what was done with me," I told her. "But nothing came out."

"Of course, that does sometimes happen if the tumor is very solid. However, if it is filled with fluid that can be aspirated, the cyst simply collapses. Then we analyze the fluid, to be certain it was benign and not malignant."

"But what would you do if nothing came out? Wouldn't you have to do a surgical biopsy then?"

"Not straightaway," she said quickly, surprised. "We then use what we call a Tru-cut needle. It's a bit larger, and needs just a dab of anesthetic on the breast, but it invariably gets some tissue out, without requiring surgery. We rarely have to use surgical biopsies for the preliminary diagnosis here at the Royal Infirmary."

I remembered having heard a doctor at the National Cancer Institute say something about clinical trials of wide-bore needles for nonsurgical biopsies. As far as I know, the program is still in the talking stage in this country. In Edinburgh, it was already

* In the United States, where good pathology (cytology) is available, as at Roswell Park, the Cleveland Clinic, in Cleveland, Ohio, and at Memorial Sloan-Kettering, in New York, fine-needle aspiration biopsy in the doctor's office is routine. The experience of the Cleveland Clinic over the past twenty years, for example, is that if cancer is present, it will show up 85 per cent of the time.

routine, and the needle even had a trade name! The Royal Infirmary was only the second stop on my European tour. I learned afterward that, under one name or another, wide-bore-needle biopsies are also routine in Sweden, Finland, and the Soviet Union.

Dr. Roberts was still talking. "So, you see, before anything at all is done about removing a breast, every patient is staged, so that we know exactly what her over-all disease involves. If neither of the needles extracts enough tissue for a definite diagnosis to be made," she continued, "then and only then will we excise the tumor. As I said before, this is rarely necessary, but sometimes—yes, it must be done. If the lesion is not too large or deeply embedded, this procedure, also, might be done on an outpatient basis, without hospital admission.

"But there would be *no* frozen-section histological"—pathological—"examination. The tumor would be studied in paraffin, a permanent section. While waiting for the diagnosis, the patient is at home."

"Do you remove the lump if the needle biopsy says it is benign?"

"As a rule, yes. If the patient has objections, no. However, we do instruct her to come to the clinic frequently to be watched."

"And if the pathological examination shows it's malignant?"

Dr. Roberts smiled and took a big gulp of coffee. "That's what I simply cannot understand about your American way. Before we do a mastectomy here at the Royal Infirmary, we first scan the brain, bones, liver, and lungs, to see whether the disease has spread beyond the breast. If it already has, there's really no reason to do a mastectomy at all, is there?"

When I returned to the United States and asked Dr. Dao if such premastectomy scanning is his usual routine, he told me it isn't. "The public-education programs in this country have made women so aware of the early symptoms," he said, "that there are not as many patients being admitted to hospitals with advanced cases of mammary carcinoma." He credited education, early detection, and screening programs for the fact that in this country breast cancers are usually found in earlier stages than is the case in countries without such programs.

"Scans use radioactivity," he continued, "and I do not use these routinely for premastectomy or even postmastectomy diagnosis, unless other tests indicate something may be wrong or if the patient reports pain." He also told me that he and other experts feel scans may be useless in finding a hidden metastasis of Stage I breast cancer. "X-rays are enough, as a rule," he said.

Dr. Roberts went on with her explanation of the Royal Infirmary's practice with cases of advanced disease. The primary tumor in the breast is removed and other kinds of therapy are immediately begun. The breast itself is not amputated. "No major surgical procedure is ever justified if there is already evidence of metastases to other organs," she told me crisply.

"Then you never have women who don't know in advance that they will have a mastectomy?"

"No, never," she replied. "By the time the woman has come to the day of her operation, we know quite a bit about her. We have scanned her body and know the extent of the disease in terms of the rest of her organs, and we know the diagnosis absolutely. Of course, we have also done the other preoperative examinations—electrocardiograms, blood studies, urinalyses, and so on. The only thing we do not know with certainty is the status of her nodes. We cannot know about that until the mastectomy itself."

Dr. Roberts also pointed out that cancerous tissue removed during a mastectomy is immediately sent to the hospital's biochemistry section to be tested for hormone dependency. "By knowing the hormonal nature of the tumor," she explained, "we gain a good clue for future therapy, should it be needed. For example, if it's clearly hormone-independent, there would be no point in removing a patient's ovaries if a recurrence should appear later." A hormone-dependent cancer, on the other hand, would be helped by ovariectomy.

"But that"—the hormone-dependency test—"is done at the time of mastectomy. Staging takes place before surgery. So you see, we have been very puzzled here about the speed we read about in your country." She smiled. "That is, of course, if the newspapers were accurate."

She glanced at her watch. "Goodness!" She jumped from her chair. "It's time to hear about gynecomastia. Would you like to come along?" We left her office, and I dutifully listened to the lecture.

I listened, but did not hear much. My mind was absorbed in what Dr. Roberts had told me. Before my mastectomy at Roswell Park, I recalled, I had been X-rayed from stem to stern, in every conceivable position. Gallons of my blood had been taken for various tests before any surgery was scheduled. Obviously I had been staged without knowing it.

When I returned to London, I called Guy's Hospital and the Royal Marsden, and learned that staging and testing are standard preoperative procedures there, too.

In Stockholm, Dr. Helen Westerberg, in the Breast Section of the Karolinska Institute, was as adamant as Dr. Roberts. "Our policy is first to find out exactly how extensive the disease is," she told me. "You can't plan rational treatment unless you know the extent of the disease. It's not very sensible to talk about any kind of surgery without first doing the staging. Any kind of mastectomy is pointless if a patient's cancer is already far advanced."

Oncologists in the Soviet Union also have various techniques for diagnosing a tumor on an outpatient basis. In addition to the fine-needle biopsy, doctors in Moscow and Leningrad have a curettelike gadget that extracts a small specimen of the tumor, using a local anesthetic. "It is most important to know as much as possible before a mastectomy is performed," declared Professor Riurik Melnikov, the chief of surgery at Leningrad's institute of oncology. "This is the reason a woman knows she will lose a breast in almost all cases. We know the diagnosis in advance and warn her."

In Moscow, Professor Sviatukhina uses radioactive gold in an attempt to learn in advance of surgery how many nodes, if any, have been invaded. In a technique called lymphangiography, radioactive isotopes of gold are injected into the lymphatic channels that lie between the fingers. The isotopes ultimately settle in healthy lymph nodes but not in cancerous ones, and the nodes are then photographed. The professor told me that she had found this lymphangiography technique very reliable when compared with the results of pathological examination of the nodes after surgery.

Could lymphangiography eliminate the need to remove the axillary lymph nodes by radical mastectomy? When I returned from Russia, I asked Dr. Gerald Johnston, chief of the National

Cancer Institute's Nuclear Medicine Section, why radioactive
gold is not used here for evaluating the lymph nodes.

"Every woman has a different number of nodes, and they are
all in different places," he explained. "If I inject gold, and it
settles in the healthy nodes, that doesn't tell me a damn thing. A
place where a node might be in one woman may not show up
in another woman because the node is just not there. So a missing
node on the film would not necessarily mean it's cancerous. It
could just mean no node is in that spot in that patient."

He leaned back in his chair and shook his head. "Unless a
woman has so many malignant nodes that you only see four or
five healthy ones, instead of twenty or twenty-five, radioactive-
gold lymphangiography wouldn't be a bit of help. And," he
warned, "if a woman has that many nodes involved, I could
probably feel some of them by manual examination. So what's
the point of loading her with all that irradiation?"

Although lymphangiography may not be the advance I at
first thought it was, its use in the Soviet Union does show that
preoperative staging is a regular practice there. Why is it not
here?

The first answer I got was that—as Dr. Dao had told me—the
European approach is not applicable in the United States. "In
Europe," a general surgeon told me, "when a patient comes in
with her symptoms, she is usually more advanced than American
women are, because we have so much more emphasis on early
detection. We seldom have tumors, for example, that are three
or more inches in diameter when they are first found. Even a
one-inch tumor is large by our standards. So the chances of a
patient's having a metastasis when she first sees her doctor are
just not as likely here."

That argument does not tally with the facts. There is no question that tumors are caught earlier in the United States, because
of greater public awareness and massive early-detection programs. But, in spite of this, about half of all the radical mastectomies performed here show nodal invasion. In addition, a small—
even microscopic—breast tumor can already have metastasized to
another organ by the time it is discovered.

The notion that a tumor must reach a certain size before the
cancer spreads is a medical anachronism. National Cancer Insti-

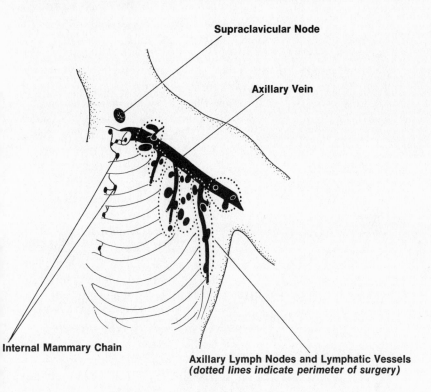

Supraclavicular Node

Axillary Vein

Internal Mammary Chain

Axillary Lymph Nodes and Lymphatic Vessels
(dotted lines indicate perimeter of surgery)

Approximate Location of the Nodes

tute studies of thousands of patients have shown that even a tiny lump, if strategically located, can disseminate malignant cells to other organs, sometimes by-passing the axillary nodes entirely and traveling via the blood stream. Thus a "small" or "early" breast cancer can spread "large" and "late" metastases. All of the experts I asked agreed—not for attribution—that most women who die within the first year after a mastectomy probably had metastatic invasion to a vital organ the day the operation was done. The metastases were not found then because the doctor had not staged to look for them.

Of course, even the most sophisticated preoperative diagnostic techniques and the most expert oncologists can sometimes miss a metastasis. Staging is no ironclad guarantee that undetected microscopic cancer colonies have not sprouted somewhere in the body. The fact remains, however, that the customary practice here, of surgical biopsy followed immediately by mastectomy, does not allow time for the search for those secondary cancers which, if detected, might make the mastectomy pointless.

A second argument used in support of the combined surgeries is that most women in the United States are well aware that a simple biopsy of a breast tumor could mean mastectomy, because of all the publicity and education regarding breast cancer. "Every American woman knows there are two chances in every ten a breast growth could be cancer," one surgeon said blithely. "Why should any patient wake up surprised or shocked?"

As someone who did know in advance I would have to have a mastectomy, and who has interviewed about 130 women who have had the operation, my only reply is "Baloney!" I had more than a week to adjust to the idea of losing my breast. Moreover, there were those two days of X-rays and tests while Dr. Dao looked for a possible metastasis, days that had left me hoping a mastectomy would be possible. Yet I had been stunned and pained when it was over and I looked down to see a level place where a gentle curve had been.

No, the few short hours separating two breasts from one—as it is in our system—are not enough time for any woman to absorb the staggering blow of losing a breast. While this may make no sense at all to the average, ordinary, commonsensical male surgeon, there it is. One woman in her seventies, who admitted she "really didn't give a hoot about losing the tired old thing," remembered her first reaction when she woke up in the recovery room: "I felt mutilated." Julia Child told Dick Cavett, in a television interview, that she had felt "mangled."

The third argument I heard against separating biopsy from mastectomy is that one operation under general anesthesia is safer than two. (This would not be an argument at all if the diagnosis were made by other techniques than surgical biopsy.)

As I said earlier, this does have some validity in certain cases. If the patient has a medical problem that would make it dangerous for her to undergo anesthesia a second time, she should have the single procedure. And if—like one unfortunate patient in London I was told about—she has a carcinoma that cannot be left, there is no alternative but to remove the breast immediately. However, such instances are rare.

Apparently, some surgeons think there is never such an instance. After reading the preceding paragraph in manuscript, Dr. Dao circled the words "cannot be left" and wrote a red "Why?" in the margin next to them. This must be another of those controversial gray areas. Most of the surgeons I interviewed feel that, indeed, some tumors cannot be left and that, in such cases, immediate mastectomy is imperative.

The fourth argument is that, by cutting into a cancerous breast during a biopsy and then closing the incision, the surgeon might "seed the cancer by scalpel" and cause it to spread. The surgeon I interviewed called it "implantation by knife," and I have referred to it elsewhere.

"There are no data whatsoever to support that point of view," Dr. Roberts told me, in Edinburgh. At the Karolinska Institute, Dr. Westerberg was just as firm. "Of course," she added, "the surgeon must know what he is doing. But, properly done, there is no danger whatsoever of seeding."

Dr. Westerberg's point of view, supported by Dr. Roberts in Edinburgh, as well as by other oncologists I have read or interviewed, is nonetheless controversial. This is another gray area. Many experts do worry about the dangers of seeding and "implantation by knife." But, as I have also said, surgical and immunological evidence does not support such a fear. As far as breast cancer is concerned, the seeding argument is based on myth, not fact.

One special situation should be mentioned in which a two-stage procedure does not make sense. This is when the mammogram is definitely positive or when there are other signs that a tumor is certainly malignant. Naturally, in such cases it is the diagnostic biopsy that is unnecessary. If the patient is then staged, by the time those tests are finished she—like me—will probably welcome a mastectomy.

In spite of current practice in the United States, it is rarely, if ever, necessary for a woman to be wheeled into an operating room and have a mastectomy without knowing in advance that this will be done. And she should never have a mastectomy without preoperative staging for metastases.

Of course, if this were done here, the lucrative business of doing surgical biopsies in hospital operating rooms would disappear. But there would be many beneficial by-products to patients. Even when all the other diagnostic tests fail to show a definite positive or negative and surgical biopsy is required, inpatient hospitalization for the operation could be reduced considerably, if not abolished altogether. Surgical and hospitalization costs would decrease; insurance premiums would drop.

Yes, getting rid of such biopsies would solve many problems (except for the one of the surgeon's decreased income). Of the ten women with breast growths, only the two whose tumors are cancer would need hospital beds. Only those two would have to take the surgeon's valuable time for comforting, condolences, and counseling about the various surgical alternatives. And they would have time for the premastectomy staging.

In criticizing surgical biopsies done under general anesthesia, I am *not* advocating that they be done in the doctor's office. I simply mean that there is little reason for hospitalization as an inpatient. A careful surgical biopsy—even under a general anesthetic, if necessary—can be done on an outpatient basis in most hospitals. Recently a friend had her Fallopian tubes tied, under general anesthesia, as an outpatient. Afterward she slept off the drug for a few hours and went home. Another young woman I know had a breast growth biopsied, under a local anesthetic, in the emergency room of a local hospital. She rested there for an hour and then returned to work while she waited for the pathologist's report.

It seems so simple and right. Yet no one is making any public outcry about this most basic aspect of breast-cancer mistreatment. Why? I don't know. I must admit it had never occurred to me that anything was wrong with this American custom before I went to Europe. My own reasons for demanding the two-stage procedure had been my distrust of frozen sections and my insistence that I be treated by a specialist. I had not heard of staging then.

———————

Abroad, a surprising—perhaps unfair—mercenary motive was often cited as the possible reason for our standard practice—an "economic incentive." Over and over, in England, Scotland, Sweden, Finland, and the Soviet Union, I heard the terms "economic motive" and "economic incentive."

The words reminded me of a conversation I had had at the National Institutes of Health library one evening with a young foreign doctor I had often seen there. Slender, dark, and curly-haired, he spoke in heavily accented English. "Is it true that in America your surgeons are paid for the number of inches they cut out?"

Instantly I was catapulted out of a grisly description I was reading of the controversial extended, or supraradical, mastectomy. "What did you say?"

He looked embarrassed. "I have been in this country only a few months," he explained. "Before, I trained in Scotland and Denmark. In neither country was there as much radical breast surgery carried out as in the United States." He looked around furtively, as if he wanted to negotiate the sale of some "grass." No one was within listening distance. "When the wife of President Ford was given a mastectomy which removed the pectoral muscles as well as the nodes, I was amazed to read that this procedure is accepted by almost all American surgeons."

I nodded. "Unfortunately, that's true. About 95 per cent—but it's dropping, because of all the publicity Mrs. Ford and Mrs. Rockefeller got after their mastectomies."

"That may be, but the only conclusion I could reach at the time is simply that the surgeons receive more money if more tissue is excised. I am familiar only with government-sponsored medicine, where wages are not dependent on the quantity of surgery. I have seen you always surrounded here by works on breast cancer, and I thought you would perhaps know the answer. There is so much evidence everywhere in American medicine of an economic incentive."

An economic incentive. A forgotten bell began to ring. When Dr. George Crile, Jr., had so vehemently condemned the Halsted radical mastectomy, he had written: "Partial mastectomies that remove the affected part of the breast and reconstruct the rest are not only more time-consuming and more difficult to perform but medical insurance plans pay surgeons less for doing them than for removing the breast. In short, the surgeon is paid 2 to 3 times as much for performing a mutilating operation than for performing one that leaves the woman relatively intact."

Now, in Europe, I was learning that high fees were laughingly blamed for the overuse in the United States of the Halsted operation. Yes, Dr. Foreign Exchange, wherever you are working now, it does look suspiciously as if our surgeons were paid by the number of inches they cut out.

Dr. Roberts, for example, told me that the top salary paid to a full-time doctor, under Britain's National Health Service, is £10,000 annually, *after* he or she has reached the status of "consultant." At the current rate of exchange, this is about $23,500. "But the average salary of a physician like me is far less," she added. "Most of us earn considerably less than £10,000 every year, but we are paid the same sum regardless of the number of patients we treat." She smiled. "So, you see, doctors in the United Kingdom have no economic incentive to treat women with mammary carcinomas. They are happy to refer them to oncologists."

In his book, Dr. Crile goes to great lengths to blame the continued use of the Halsted radical in the United States on the higher fees collected for it than for the modified radical or the lesser surgeries. To a degree, Dr. Crile is correct. Insurance companies do feel the Halsted radical is worth more money.

Surgical fees vary considerably around the country, depending on the local cost of living and other factors. Most insurance companies, however, base their rates on one national measure, called the California Relative Value Scale (CRVS). It tells just what the name implies, the relative values of different medical and surgical treatments, so that insurance-company clerks and bookkeepers will have some idea of what each procedure ought to cost. The CRVS uses proportions, not dollars, which allows the scale to be applied to any geographical area. (Manhattan has the highest actual fees for most procedures, Montana the lowest.)

The CRVS lists a partial mastectomy as worth 15 points, a simple (or total) at 30 points, and the Halsted radical at 70 points' worth of dollars. Interestingly, it does not even include the modified radical, but presumably this would fit somewhere between the simple (or total) and the Halsted—at about 50 points.

A look at the CRVS point system and a random sampling of medical insurance companies' fee schedules does make it look as if surgeons here might be deliberately doing the Halsted to earn a few extra dollars. Could Dr. Crile have been right? After interviewing many general surgeons, however, I have decided that the "economic incentive" is not as much of a factor in their choice of the Halsted as are habit and training. The big profits come from those little twenty-minute operating-room biopsies, not from the lengthy mastectomy surgery.

A medical education has always been very expensive, and the tuition fees are still rising. Becoming a surgeon takes three or four years of undergraduate work, four years of medical school, a year of internship, and another one or two years of residency. Although interns and residents are paid, it is barely enough to make ends meet, as a rule. The result is that a surgeon has invested some ten years and thousands of dollars in learning his trade, and must do a lot of cutting just to recover his investment. So the "economic incentive" is very powerful in the United States.

My brief twenty-minute biopsy earned the local surgeon who did it $200, not counting another $30 he got for my office visit and his attempt to aspirate the tumor. (The same fee is charged regardless of whether the tumor is malignant or benign.) Although only two lumps of every ten turn out to be malignant and require a mastectomy, ten biopsies are performed to find those two. Based on my surgeon's fees, that adds up to $2,000 for about 200 minutes of work—or $10 per minute. No surgeon in his right mind will give up that kind of easy money without a fight—especially if he has the myth of "implantation by scalpel" or "seeding by knife" to use as his excuse.

While he may make an extra $100 or so by performing a Halsted instead of a modified, either kind is difficult and time-consuming surgery. The average mastectomy takes over three hours—a minimum of 180 minutes in which the surgeon could be earning far more doing quick and easy biopsies. No, Dr. Crile, it is not the Halsted mastectomy that is the basis for the "economic incentive" in breast-cancer surgery; it is the surgical biopsy.

Changes are on the horizon, however. In the torrent of publicity that followed Betty Ford's and Happy Rockefeller's operations, people who had never questioned physicians' procedures
began to do so—and to demand some answers. One question was
why always such a rush to mastectomy? Condemnation of the
one-stage procedure by *some surgeons themselves* has been the
most important outcome.

In the February 15, 1975, issue of *Modern Medicine,* Drs.
Edward C. Saltzenstein, Robert W. Mann, Thomas Y. Chua, and
Jerome J. De Cosse, all affiliated with the Mt. Sinai Medical
Center and Medical College of Wisconsin, in Milwaukee, suggested the time had come to end the old tradition. In addition
to citing all the psychological and physiological reasons for doing
the diagnostic biopsy on an outpatient basis, these surgeons gave
another one: that many women refuse to be examined at all
because of their intense fear of being hospitalized for the
biopsy and then perhaps "mastectomized" while still unconscious.

In the March 1975 issue of *Medical Opinion,* another surgeon,
Dr. Gordon F. Schwartz, of the Jefferson Medical College, in
Philadelphia, addressed to his colleagues "A Plea for Sensible
Breast Biopsy." Dr. Schwartz's plea was for surgeons to abandon
the anachronistic diagnostic methods used in this country today.
Even before that furor, Dr. George Rosemond, also of Philadelphia, a former president of the American Cancer Society, had
urged an end to routine surgical biopsies in all cases. This was in
a 1973 issue of *Cancer,* a journal for oncologists.

Maybe, with some surgeons now on our side, we women will
be able to put an end to the barbaric biopsy business.

9

Surgery: Toward Freedom of Choice

"A whole book about breast cancer? I don't believe it." I had just turned down her third party invitation. "What's there to say you haven't already said? You've written articles about the different operations. What in the world will you fill a book with?"

"The mastectomy is just the beginning." I tried to break into her flood of questions. "It's nowhere near as important as—"

"Losing a breast isn't important?" she cried. "You must have forgotten what *you* went through or you couldn't say that."

She was right. I had forgotten. In less than a year, I had forgotten my horror at being suddenly confronted by the prospect of losing a breast. The awesome, awful ordeal—the mammograms, the thermograms, the research into choices of surgery, the rush to Sloan-Kettering, and finally the flight to Buffalo, to Roswell Park. The pain of the surgery, the agony of that first moment naked and unbandaged before a mirror, stuffing cotton balls into bras, the first time Harvey saw the incision—how could I have forgotten so much so quickly?

But, as I wondered, my belly tightened and I felt the fingers of dread creep along my skin. No, I had not forgotten. Those clammy conditioned reflexes will probably be with me forever. But the mastectomy itself had become less important. In learning so much about breast cancer, I had put the surgery itself in its proper perspective, as only the beginning of treatment.

The blazing "breast-cancer controversy"—lumpectomy versus mastectomy, modified radical versus Halsted radical—is not the real burning issue of breast-cancer treatment in the United States today. As Ann Scott had said so poignantly in her televised interview, most women believe that choosing the kind of mastectomy is the end of their problems. Afterward, they think, as soon as they have bought the "stupid prosthesis" and learned some cosmetic tricks, life goes back to normal. Few women realize that mastectomy simply marks the beginning of at least five years of intensive care and examination, five more years of close medical supervision, and a lifetime—a long and healthy one, it is hoped—of constant vigilance for signs of recurrence or metastasis.

I called my friend back to explain. "There are so many other things wrong about the way women with breast cancer are treated," I told her, "that the kind of mastectomy just doesn't seem as earth-shaking as it did."

"Like what?" She needed convincing.

Ann Scott was uppermost in my mind. "There's not enough good follow-up," I told her, giving details.

She remained quiet for such a long time that I thought we had been disconnected. Then she spoke. "It does make 'What kind of mastectomy?' sound like a huge tempest in a small teapot, doesn't it?" She forgave me for again missing her party.

Burning issue or not, some kind of surgery must be the first step. Here is a brief description of the possible alternatives, from the least extensive to the most.

1. *Lumpectomy, tylectomy, and local excision.* The entire lump is removed, along a little surrounding tissue. Unless the tumor is very large, the breast involved should look the same as the other one afterward.

2. *Partial mastectomy, segmental resection, and wedge resection.* The tumor and a considerable portion of the surrounding breast tissue are excised, along with overlying skin and underlying fascia. The axillary lymph nodes may also be removed, making this a "partial radical" mastectomy. The breast will be somewhat smaller, but still there.

Important note: Neither the lumpectomy nor the partial mastectomy can be done in every case.

3. *Simple (or total) mastectomy.* Both terms describe the same surgery; many doctors nowadays prefer "total." The breast is removed, but the axillary nodes and pectoral muscles are not. Some surgeons also routinely biopsy the last lymph node in the "tail of the breast," the one closest to the axilla, to see if it has been invaded; others do not. If the node is found to be malignant, either the axilla is irradiated or a radical mastectomy is done.

4. *Modified radical mastectomy.* All tissues of the breast and the axillary lymph nodes are removed. The pectoral muscles are kept intact.

5. *Halsted radical mastectomy.* All tissues of the breast, the axillary lymph nodes, and the pectoral muscles are removed.

6. *Supraradical mastectomy or extended radical mastectomy.* The breast, axillary lymph nodes, pectoral muscles, and the internal mammary chain of nodes are removed. To get at the internal nodes, some sections of rib must be taken out as well. A few surgeons even remove the supraclavicular nodes, which are in the angle where the neck joins the shoulder. This operation is rarely done today.

7. *Subcutaneous mastectomy.* All the internal breast tissue is scooped out, with or without the axillary nodes. The nipple is preserved, if possible, by grafting it temporarily elsewhere, and enough skin is left to accommodate a silicone implant (*not* an injection), which is inserted several months later. If the nipple must be removed, a new one can be created, from the labia or from the second nipple. This kind of reconstructive surgery is "custom-tailored" for each case.

Except for the first and third options, all these procedures permit the surgeon to excise and examine at least some of the axillary lymph nodes—even if not all of them are removed. There is no way to know a breast-cancer patient's real physical condition without the "radical" part of a mastectomy, but oncologists have

been battling for decades over whether or not removal of the
nodes is always the best operating procedure. Many distinguished
scientists insist that survival rates are just as good if only the
breast is removed. Curiously, patients themselves give little
thought to their nodal watchdogs. To them, it is the visible
breast that counts.

"My lump was only about a centimeter long on the mammogram," a woman cried over the telephone. "But my doctor insists
that I must have the whole breast taken off if it's cancer. And he
said something about needing a radical. What do you think?"

What do I think?

My opinion should be obvious. In my own case, I decided to
go ahead and have a modified radical mastectomy, having a
tumor only slightly larger than hers. For her? I think it should
be her decision, not mine or the doctor's. But first she must
know why a radical mastectomy is usually the recommended
surgery, even when the suspected cancer is tiny.

Earlier, in describing Dr. Dao's laboratory, I compared his
sophisticated gadgetry with what we see in the Mission Control
Center in Houston during moon shots. But the similarity ends
there. Space scientists, with their electronic equipment, can
eavesdrop on astronauts in the lunar module hundreds of thousands of miles away. We have no such miraculous machines
that can peer a few centimeters into a woman's axilla to "eavesdrop" on her nodes. The only way to know whether they have
become cancerous is to cut them out and put them under a
microscope.

I explained that possible lifesaving treatment for her would
depend on the diagnosis of her nodes. Painfully, my caller accepted the hard facts and went to surgery not knowing if she
would awaken with one or two breasts. It was cancer; she was
mastectomized while still unconscious. Luckily, all her nodes
were free of disease. But when she went to sleep she didn't even
know she had cancer.

"If that happened here, I should think we would all be sued,"
Dr. Trevor Powles, of London's Royal Marsden Cancer Hospital,
responded when I described this routine. "It may even be against
the National Health Service laws, for what I know."

The only patient he could recall who had had a mastectomy

without being informed of it in advance was a twenty-nine-year-old African woman who had no clinical symptoms of cancer. He explained that patients at Royal Marsden are examined by a team, composed of a medical oncologist, a surgeon, and a radiologist, not just by a single physician. "We were all agreed her tumor could not possibly be malignant," Dr. Powles insisted. "The odds were a thousand to one against, and we assured her that it was certainly benign. To make the situation even worse," he continued, "it was a carcinoma that required immediate mastectomy. Otherwise, I would have closed the incision, let her awaken, and then told her about the absolute need for further surgery later. In this case, it was not possible."

After I returned home, I realized I had neglected to ask Dr. Powles what kind of cancer it was that had made immediate mastectomy necessary. Dr. Dao also was curious about it and asked me why "this case was so special." Unfortunately, I did not have the answer. The explanation may be that the cancer was so widespread in the breast or so intertwined with other tissues that it could not be removed intact. I know from my reading and personal interviews that many surgeons insist on removing the entire breast immediately when they discover a tumor that cannot be isolated and excised.

Dr. Powles seemed to shudder at the memory. "You can imagine how upset she was when she awoke!" Again he stopped. "I don't mind telling you, we shan't forget that young woman for a very long time. It was awfully, awfully bad for all concerned."

He said that he does prefer to do the surgical biopsy, if this is necessary, and the mastectomy in one procedure when it is certain beforehand that the breast will have to be removed, and when the patient knows and is expecting it.

"No woman who has been told she will lose a breast is ever disappointed and grieved to awaken and discover our preoperative diagnosis was wrong." He grinned. "But if the patient is not psychologically prepared for mastectomy, I certainly think the two procedures can and should safely be separated."

Dr. Powles also thinks the patient has the right to decide what kind of surgery she will have, although he uses all his wiles and charm to persuade her to change her mind if she refuses to give up her breast. "I do believe some kind of radical mastectomy is the best we have at this time, and I do everything I can to be positive that patients know all the risks of doing less."

It was encouraging to discover that Dr. Powles did not consider it outrageous of me to have insisted on the two-stage procedure. As a matter of fact, at Guy's Hospital, also in London, the practice is actively encouraged. Most biopsies at Guy's, in the heart of the city (Royal Marsden is in Sutton, a London suburb), are done on an outpatient basis, in the clinic, and do not require a hospital stay at all.

One of my reasons for visiting European cancer centers was that I suspected breast-cancer surgery would not be as extensive in countries where there are more women practicing medicine than in the United States. Also, I wanted to see if care was better under socialized medicine than under our fee-for-service system. Both hunches were right, but in reverse order of the importance I had given them. The "economic motive" has *much* more to do with the amount of surgery performed than does the number of women on the medical staff.

But having more women on hospital staffs does have an effect on the women patients and on male doctors. It cannot be a coincidence, for example, that Moscow's oncology institute—where an all-female medical staff directs breast-cancer research and treatment—is now in its fourth year of clinical trials of partial mastectomies. Although Professor Sviatukhina thinks radical mastectomy offers the best chance for a cure, she is nonetheless willing to do lesser surgeries on women who want them and whose tumors meet certain criteria. Her male boss, academician Professor Nikolai N. Blokhin, the director of the institute, has apparently given Professor Sviatukhina carte blanche to do as she sees fit.

At the Royal Infirmary in Edinburgh, the chief of the breast service is Professor A. P. M. Forrest, whose concern for his patients is as sensitive and sympathetic as any woman's could be. (In staff conferences, he invariably asks about patients' husbands, children, and family problems, as well as about their medical status.) Under his direction, the breast-service staff, three-fourths female, does no radical mastectomies at all. The practice here is to do simple (or total) mastectomies, with ir-

radiation of the nodes postoperatively if there is reason to think
the cancer has spread beyond the breast. The results are, I was
told, as good as those from radical mastectomies, where the axillary nodes are removed surgically. Professor Forrest had tested
the treatment for seven years in Cardiff, Wales, before moving
to Edinburgh, and those patients are still being followed.

At Stockholm's Karolinska Institute, Dr. Westerberg, of the
Breast Section (a two-thirds female staff), told me the custom
there is to try to persuade reluctant women that radical mastectomy is best in terms of a possible cure. She smiled. "However,
it is, after all, their bodies to do with as they see fit. If we do
not succeed—and often we do not—we do as the patient wishes.
Over the years, there have been quite a few young women who
have had only the tumors removed, and most are doing well.
While we do not advise it, we most certainly do permit it."

The attitude at Royal Marsden and Guy's hospitals, in London,
is the same.

On the other hand, in Leningrad's oncology institute, the chief
of surgery, Professor Riurik Melnikov, is a staunch defender of
the Halsted radical, and so are all the other men on his surgical
staff. Their salaries are paid by the government, and they earn
nothing extra for doing more extensive surgery. Professor Melnikov told me he had used the modified radical several years
ago, but had poor results and returned to the Halsted. Naturally,
his younger surgeons followed their chief's preference.

So, even where women predominate on the breast staff, some
kind of mastectomy is the preferred operation everywhere. The
feminine influence is seen mainly in increased interest in experi-
menting with lesser operations and in more awareness of the emotional problems the patient faces. Now that I have made my
peace with my silicone-gel falsie and am more concerned with
other problems related to breast cancer, I no longer have the
same fears as I endured during that horrible month in June 1974.
But it is not difficult to revive them. Whether it makes sense or
not, knowing a breast must be amputated is terrifying. Having
physicians who can empathize and sympathize because they, too,
have breasts must be very supportive. There are many decisions
to be made, many benefit-risk ratios to be weighed, and having
a knowledgeable, understanding woman to explain and answer

questions helps many patients with cancer face the loss of a breast more calmly.

Why, for example, must the axillary nodes be cut out if none can be palpated—do not appear to be "clinically involved"?

"Clinical axillary node involvement" means that the nodes can be felt manually in a physical examination, and, unfortunately, many errors occur in such checks. Dr. Robert Shirley, assistant clinical professor of obstetrics and gynecology at the Harvard Medical School and director of the Breast Clinic at the Boston Hospital for Women, says that manual examination of the nodes is "like flipping a coin." Enlarged nodes may just be bigger or inflamed, not cancerous; nodes that feel normal can be malignant.

Is it safer to remove the pectoral muscles, too, just in case some malignant nodes may be hidden by or even attached to them?

Although the National Cancer Institute has been comparing radical mastectomies with simple (or total) mastectomies followed by postoperative irradiation of the axillary nodes, no controlled study had ever been done comparing the Halsted radical to the modified radical. Finally, Dr. Dao and an associate at Roswell Park, Dr. Takuma Nemoto, published the results on 109 women whose pectoral muscles had ben left intact and 121 women who had had Halsted radical mastectomies. They had been followed more than five years, and at the time the report was written (March 1975) there was no difference between the recurrence and survival rates of the two groups.

What are the survival statistics if the nodes are negative? Suppose some are positive?

Statistics from the National Cancer Institute's 1974 "End Results" data (based on figures from Connecticut's tumor registry) show that a woman whose nodes were negative has about an 85-per-cent chance of living as long as a woman who has never had breast cancer. (The difference is due to the possibility of a metastasis via the lymphatic vessels or blood stream.) However, national statistics indicate that a success rate of three out of four —75 per cent—is a more accurate ratio throughout the country.

What does the American Cancer Society say about the different surgeries available?

The ACS, our volunteer watchdog over all phases of all

cancers, issued a policy statement at the end of 1974 clarifying
its stand on the question of breast-cancer surgery. "Pending clear
proof," the statement said, "that equally good results can be
achieved by limited procedures less than mastectomy, the American Cancer Society believes the public should not be misled into
accepting less proven methods." These "proven methods," according to the pronouncement, are the Halsted radical and the extended radical, or supraradical, mastectomies. Almost grudgingly,
the society admits that the modified radical might be all right,
too.

What is the difference between the Halsted and the modified
as far as the patient is concerned?

On paper, the Halsted radical does not seem to be much
different from the modified radical. In the body, there is an
enormous difference. The Halsted operation "seems to have
been designed to inflict the maximal possible deformity, disfigur-
ation, and disability," according to Dr. Crile. "The incision," he
wrote, "extends nearly vertically up over the shoulder so that the
scar is impossible to hide. The removal of the muscles of the
chest wall causes a depression below the collarbone that cannot
be concealed unless a high-necked dress is worn." Dr. Crile continues, in this gruesome vein, about "skin paper-thin," "sloughing
of the skin," ad infinitum.

For all the unnecessary ugliness and discomfort of the Halsted,
the results of these two radicals—in terms of years—are about the
same. I must mention that many of the women I interviewed
said their Halsteds were not as horrible as Dr. Crile paints them.
A great deal of the cosmetics, apparently, depends on the surgeon.

Mammoplastic reconstructive surgery, by the way, is not even
mentioned in the American Cancer Society statement, which goes
on to declare that "recommendations for treatment of a breast
cancer should be made by the physician" and that "the patient
and selected members of the family should be thoroughly advised
by the physician about the proposed surgery and its rationale;
this being the essence of informed consent."

Nowhere does the policy statement hint that the patient might
have opinions or desires different from those in the satement or
from those "advised by the physician," and that she has the

absolute right to decide for herself. While I chose to give up my breast and nodes, to have a better chance of surviving longer, every woman—once told of the differences in risk—should be allowed to have a lumpectomy or anything else she wants, even if her surgeon or her husband or family disapproves.

If the axillary nodes are invisible and removing them doesn't show, why do specialists feel that leaving them in the body is so important?

This puzzled me for a long time. The major question among oncologists for decades has been whether the radical part of the mastectomy is necessary. Do the axillary lymph nodes have to be removed, or is the simple (or total) mastectomy, which leaves them intact, just as effective? This behind-the-scenes struggle got some public airing immediately after Mrs. Ford's operation, but it disappeared as quickly as it had come. In the medical literature, however, it is very much alive.

About thirty years ago, Professor Sakari Mustakallio, a Finnish radiologist, began removing the breast but leaving the lymph nodes, using irradiation to destroy any suspicious ones. Occasionally, if the tumor was very small, he removed only the growth. After twenty-five years of these conservative procedures, Professor Mustakallio analyzed his results and found no difference between them and those of the various radical surgeries.

In 1948, Dr. Robert McWhirter had begun doing the same kind of nonradical mastectomy with irradiation at Edinburgh's Royal Infirmary, and with the same results: no significant difference in either the five-year or the ten-year survival rates. Then, in Wales, Professor Forrest began his clinical trials with simple (or total) mastectomy plus irradiation, the treatment he is continuing at the Royal Infirmary in Edinburgh.

Dr. Roberts explained the Royal Infirmary practice. "When the breast is removed, one node—the one that is in the tail of the breast, closest to the axilla—is removed and examined by serial dissection." This, she said, means that the entire node is sliced and examined, instead of only a sliver or two. "If that node is negative," she continued, "the patient is discharged and nothing more is done. However, if the node has a carcinoma, she is given X-ray therapy. Our results have been equal to or perhaps a bit better than at hospitals where radical surgery is the rule."

I asked if the irradiation caused any harmful aftereffects, and Dr. Roberts insisted that a temporary reddening and peeling of the skin were the only problems. She emphasized, however, that the Edinburgh "four-field" X-ray technique is special and cannot be compared with ordinary irradiation treatments.

"If I were to develop a breast tumor," she told me earnestly, "I would never submit to a radical mastectomy. To me, it would be unthinkable. There's no justification for it whatsoever."

Across the North Sea in Stockholm, Dr. Westerberg felt just as earnestly that the lymph nodes must be removed. "It's absolutely necessary," she insisted. "The reason is really quite simple. The nodes must be examined to know if the disease has spread and, if so, how far. Future treatment depends on having this knowledge, and there is no way to be certain unless at least twenty or twenty-five are removed and studied."

Nodes are not invaded by cancer in any particular sequence, she explained. There are "skipped nodes" and "transverse nodes" and other ways for cancer to by-pass the one in the tail of the breast. "It's quite possible that the node removed and studied would be free of disease, while others were malignant," she said. "One node is not enough."

The controversy about the nodes is still far from resolved. Data pro and con keep pouring out of cancer hospitals all over the world. When I first learned about this medical argument, the conflict made no sense. "Who cares about them?" I asked Dr. Bernard Fisher, one of the National Cancer Institute's consultants, at a press conference. "The nodes are invisible. The important parts are the breast itself, first of all, and then the pectoral muscles, second."

Since then, I have learned one good medical reason for the concern about nodes. I met a woman with "milk arm"—lymphedema.

This serious complication of any kind of radical mastectomy is due to two factors. When removing the axillary nodes en bloc—in a continuous section—the surgeon must also cut out the lymphatic vessels connecting them. This is unavoidable if the axilla is to be thoroughly cleared. In addition, other, uninvolved lymph vessels in the region must be severed. The degree of circulatory damage resulting from this part of the operation can be limited if the surgeon is especially skilled and well trained in doing axillary dissections. The vessels, if not realigned properly, will not be connected well afterward, and the lymphatic fluid that should be pumped from the hand up through the arm and to the heart is blocked. With nowhere to go, it simply fills the vessels of the arm.

The woman I met was so grotesquely misshapen she did not want to show me her arm. Confined to long sleeves forever, she also suffers from a twisting, grinding pain that has persisted long after her mastectomy.

Unfortunately, the lymphatics must be cut in any radical operation, and some blockage is inevitable. No surgeon can align every tubule with its severed mate so that the joining is as it was before the operation. But some surgeons are better at it than others. As far as I am concerned, avoiding milk arm is only one more reason to find a surgeon who specializes in breast diseases, rather than one who may do only two or three mastectomies a year. But, since most mastectomies *are* done by surgeons who do not specialize in breasts, the danger of milk arm is one reason operations that salvage the nodes are being studied so intently.

There is another important reason for wanting to leave the nodes intact, if this can be done safely. They are the first line of defense, the "local militia," for fighting disease in that part of the body. They protect us against many other invaders besides cancer cells. Bacteria shooting up the arm from an infected hangnail or a cut finger, for example, would have to tangle with the nodes before they could infect the rest of the body. As far as the cancer is concerned, Dr. Crile, in defending lumpectomies and partial mastectomies, feels that once the primary tumor has been removed, the nodes are freed to attack stray neoplastic cells that may be left wandering in the lymphatic system or blood stream.

Opponents of this theory argue that thousands of lymph nodes are scattered throughout the body and that—like our other duplicate mechanisms—they take over the work of the excised ones. But this is still an unknown of immunology.

The morbidity of radical mastectomies—complications and side effects such as those just described—is why oncologists are so vitally interested in avoiding as much surgery as possible.

In Finland, there are now thirty years of follow-up results on the operations that left the nodes in place; in the United Kingdom, twenty years, including Professor Forrest's work in both Cardiff and Edinburgh. In Denmark, in Canada, and even at some medical centers in this country, it has been shown that simple (or total) mastectomy plus irradiation brings the same results as radical mastectomy. Finally, in 1971, controlled clinical trials were begun in thirty-four hospitals around the United States to compare the two procedures.

On September 30, 1974, Dr. Bernard Fisher, professor of surgery at the University of Pittsburgh Medical School and chief of the National Cancer Institute's National Surgical Adjuvant Breast Project (NSABP), sponsor of the study, reported the preliminary findings to an international conference.

After three years of follow-up, Dr. Fisher said, there were no significant differences in the survival rates of the two kinds of mastectomy.

I wrote Dr. Fisher to ask why experts here were redoing trials that have been done in Europe for years. His answer came in an inch-thick pile of articles reporting on work that has been done around the world in breast-cancer treatment. Apparently, none of the foreign studies were controlled trials. In other words, the women compared often were suffering from different stages of disease; some of the hospitals were more selective than others in choosing eligible patients; X-ray equipment and irradiation methods differed widely from hospital to hospital. Some surgeons thought that the removal of fewer nodes—eight or ten, rather than the twenty to thirty usually found in the axilla—made the surgery a "simple" mastectomy.

"As a result of these divergent responses," Dr. Fisher wrote, "there arises a pertinent question, 'What does one do with data?'"

In the United States, scientists had decided to use the data accumulated abroad to construct a rigidly controlled series of clinical trials in which patients and procedures were matched as closely as possible. After three years, Dr. Fisher's data showed no significant difference between the results of simple (or total) and radical mastectomy in "patients *without* clinical axillary node involvement" (the emphasis is Dr. Fisher's). The study is continuing.

What about having only the cancer removed, or a partial mastectomy? Are these procedures really much riskier than other mastectomies?

When I called Dr. Jerzy Einhorn, the director of the Karolinska Institute's Breast Section, his secretary told me immediately that the policy there is to remove the whole breast, not merely the tumor. "Perhaps this is not the place you want," she said. "We do not advocate simple removal of the tumor here."

I asked Dr. Westerberg, the following week, if many women came to Stockholm thinking that liberal Swedish doctors specialized in this operation. She laughed. "Why, no, I don't think we have been inundated with requests for lumpectomies," she told me. "We do them only if patients insist. The multicentricity of breast cancer makes it far too dangerous." To be honest, I had assumed that Sweden would be far ahead in doing all the lesser surgeries. I was wrong. Moscow is doing more than Stockholm.

As I mentioned earlier, Professor Sviatukhina is in her fourth year of clinical trials of partial mastectomy. Although she gave me no preliminary results, I assume that continuation of the trials is itself an indication of at least some success.

Partial mastectomy in selected cases is being done in many hospitals and clinics in the United States. But the data available from such small samples of highly selective cases are not too meaningful as guides to all women. I knew, from the book written by Dr. Crile, Jr., that the location of my cancer on the edge of the nipple meant I could not be a candidate for this surgery. Several women I interviewed had been examined by Dr. Crile or by other surgeons experienced in partial mastectomies, and were also told the procedure was not for them, for other reasons. Because of this selection process, women interested in the lesser surgeries must get individualized, personal advice.

Although there have been no controlled studies comparing the success of radical mastectomy with that of lumpectomy or partial mastectomy, statisticians estimate that the survival rates of the lesser surgeries are probably, over all, about 15 per cent lower than those of radical mastectomy, except for the special cases. Converted to flesh and blood, that equals about 1,200 additional deaths every year.

When considering a lumpectomy or a partial mastectomy, the multicentricity of breast cancer cannot be forgotten. On the other hand, multicentric tumors are not invariably present. If a woman is so anxious to keep her breast that she is willing to risk a multicentric growth, she can still have a mastectomy later, if a microscopic spot does grow into a full-sized cancer. Especially for a young woman, buying a few years in this way might be enough to prepare her for the loss of a breast. The same is true if one or more of the axillary nodes subsequently become malignant. They, too, can be cut out later.

However, women must also be warned that they are taking a chance on having a cancer cell float off in the blood stream or lymphatic channels to start a new colony. It is benefit versus risk from beginning to end in dealing with all cancers.

I have a friend, now in her mid-fifties, who took the risk and absolutely refused to have a mastectomy fifteen or so years ago. She had only the tumor removed, and was given X-ray treatments afterward. She is fine. Obviously, every woman must compute her own benefit-risk ratio. For those to whom two breasts are the prime factor, partial mastectomy or lumpectomy may be the answer.

But why do women have to calculate the benefit-risk of the lesser surgeries by and for themselves? Why have we not had controlled trials here comparing lumpectomies and partial mastectomies with the routine extensive surgical procedures?

In these United States, where almost everything is studied by one independent testing laboratory or another, it seemed strange to me that lumpectomies or partial mastectomies had not been evaluated scientifically. I was so puzzled by this enigma that asking about it became a standard question in all my interviews with surgeons. Such trials must certainly be held sometime soon, they all agreed. But who would do them? And how many women, apprised of the relative risks of radical mastectomy, which are known, and of partial mastectomy or lumpectomy, whose risks are a total blank, would give their informed consent for the so-called lesser surgery?

"I would certainly never do a lumpectomy," Dr. Dao declared

flatly. "I do not think it is the best thing for a patient, and I would not participate in any trial that required me to do this kind of operation." That was one answer, and a frequent one. Usually, it was followed by a question. "How, in good conscience as a physician, can I randomly assign a woman to be treated by a technique that is unproven and could be very dangerous? There is, after all, a time-tested alternative—radical mastectomy."

The dilemma is quite different from the ethical questions involved in testing new anticancer drugs on humans. "We know all tumorcidal agents, or drugs, are potentially lethal," I was told. "In some cases, we may be able to find one that does not have the side effects of another, but, basically, little is known about any of these substances. The situation is very different with surgery. Radical mastectomy has been around a long time, and we know its results. So, even if partial mastectomy or lumpectomy is just as effective as a radical, there's no way to know from the scattered samples available now."

It is a vicious circle. How can women be thrown involuntarily into random slots labeled "partial" or "lumpectomy," which may be very dangerous, when a known safer alternative is available? It reminds me of the euthanasia controversy. I have known many physicians who believe, in principle, that severely ill patients reach a point where the kindest thing the doctor can do is to give them overdoses of painless lethal drugs. But I have met no one who is willing to push the plunger of the hypodermic syringe.

Many surgeons I talked to feel that reconstructive plastic surgeries, like the subcutaneous mastectomy, are also risky. "We have to preserve the skin and other tissues of the breast, as well as the nipple," I was told. "Suppose there are cancerous centricles hiding in them?"

Of course, this is an added risk. But reconstructive plastic surgeries should not be banned by the surgeon. They should be explained—and their risks carefully outlined—to women who want to keep both their breasts. Reconstructive surgery is new and constantly changing. Specialists in mammoplasty who keep up with these advances can be found in most large cities. In considering any plastic-surgery procedure, however, a woman must remember that the silicone insert could make a recurrence or metastasis difficult to detect.

Earlier, when I described the various kinds of breast cancer, I mentioned the rare inflammatory carcinoma, a disease whose symptoms are swelling, intense pain, and redness. Many doctors consider this to be inoperable because it is so widespread throughout the lymphatic system. However, I have found references to several cases of inflammatory carcinoma in which the breast was treated with irradiation or drugs, which alleviated the symptoms enough to make mastectomy possible. None of the women had very long lives after the surgery, but they did gain a few comfortable years. Any woman with any kind of "inoperable" breast cancer—any person with cancer—ought to be given the chance to opt for some extra time on earth. Freedom of choice does not apply only to the *kind* of surgery, but to the right to have surgery at all. When doctors automatically pronounce someone "inoperable," they are playing God. And they do play God too often.

Not long ago, many surgeons would not perform a mastectomy on a woman under thirty. According to statistics going back to 1851, young women had shorter survival rates after mastectomy than older ones, so why operate? This do-nothing attitude persisted for decades. In 1958, a controlled study was finally done of 550 women under thirty on whom mastectomies had been performed. Some differences were found that made their cancers more lethal, but many of them did live a long time after surgery. Happily, since then surgeons have been giving young women their fair chance at life.

For decades, surgeons refused to operate on women during pregnancy or while they were nursing. Breast cancers are so well fed by hormones at those times, the argument ran, that the pregnant woman would probably die before her baby was born. Another reason for declaring these women "inoperable," Dr. Dao told me, was that the extended radical, or supraradical, mastectomies done routinely in the past were so "formidable" as to make the surgery itself too dangerous to consider. Sometimes, with an early pregnancy, abortion was recommended instead, in the hope that a sudden reduction in the hormone level would stop the cancer's fast growth. It was found, however, that an abortion, without mastectomy, made no difference.

The problem had never been studied experimentally. Then mammary carcinomas were induced in mice, half of which were impregnated, half not, and mastectomies were performed on all of them. While the over-all survival rates of the pregnant mice were lower, some of them lived long enough after surgery to show that mastectomies are worth doing during pregnancy. As a matter of fact, some of the experimental animals lived to a ripe old mouse age. Most breast-cancer specialists now treat pregnant and lactating women exactly as they treat all their patients.

Many surgeons also feel that an elderly woman should not undergo a mastectomy, especially a radical. Some only irradiate the tumor and axilla; others remove just the breast and irradiate the nodes. Here again, I think the woman should make the decision herself.

Curiously, while surgeons in the United States seem to have no qualms about declaring certain patients "inoperable," in other cases they do mastectomies when the surgery is clearly useless—when the cancers have already metastasized to other organs. As Dr. Roberts, in Edinburgh, stated so emphatically, "If a cancer is found to be metastasized during the preoperative staging examinations, the woman should be put on chemotherapy immediately and no mastectomy should be permitted at all. There is *absolutely* no medical justification for these procedures." Those were the only unnecessary mastectomies I found in my months of research.

People who are furious over automatic resort to the Halsted radical get absolutely apoplectic about the extended radical, or supraradical, mastectomy, which cuts out everything Dr. Halsted did plus the internal mammary chain of lymph nodes, under the ribs. To do the operation a "window" must be sawed in the rib cage, and afterward the "defect of the chest wall" is patched with a graft from somewhere else in the body. Just reading about this procedure is enough to make the skin crawl. According to doctors I interviewed, such surgery might be justified when the tumor is right over the breastbone and seems to be firmly attached to the muscle and bone underneath, but not otherwise. Luckily, most cancers appear first in the outer quarters of the breast and travel by way of the axillary nodes, not the internal ones. And, according to the "end results"—survival rates—women so extensively cut fare no better than those of us who are relatively intact.

Believe it or not, it was once common surgical practice (and not so long ago, either) to remove the second breast "prophylactically" along with the cancerous one. To a surgeon, I suppose the reason makes sense, of a sort. About 1 per cent of patients with a breast cancer also have an undetected one in the other breast. Sometimes these are even "mirror-image" tumors, found in exactly the same place in both breasts. In addition, 10 per cent of the women who have had a cancer in one breast subsequently develop a second in the other. But a cancer cannot occur where there is no breast, and so some surgeons used to advocate routine removal of the second organ by simple mastectomy at the same time as they were amputating the malignant one radically.

This barbaric practice has become unfashionable in surgical circles in recent years—albeit for scientific reasons, not humanitarian ones. Many of the women died of metastases from their first cancers long before a new cancer would have had time to develop in the second breast. Moreover, these women lived no longer than those who did not have the unnecessary second mastectomy. There are still a few die-hards today who advocate the prophylactic second mastectomy, but they are disappearing.

Many surgeons routinely perform an ovariectomy on premenopausal women immediately after mastectomy if the pathological examination of their axillary nodes shows that more than three were malignant. However, top breast-cancer specialists no longer do so unless they are certain that the cancer is hormone-dependent. Dr. Edward Lewison, at Johns Hopkins, for example, prefers to "reserve this procedure for the treatment of recurrent or metastatic disease when and if it should occur."

The rationale is that removing the ovaries immediately takes away a valuable clue to the hormone dependency of the cancer. If the ovaries have been left in and a new tumor develops, removing the ovaries at this stage can tell a lot about the tumor. When the loss of the ovaries has *no effect* on the size of the tumor, the doctor knows that it is hormone-independent and tailors his therapy accordingly. Improvement in the patient's condition after removal of the ovaries means that the tumor is hormone-depen-

dent, and future treatment would most likely involve some kind
of hormonal manipulation.

Not everyone agrees that removing the ovaries should be postponed. I learned that this is another controversial gray area. Dr.
Dao, for example, said it was an "old approach and is rather
dubious and inaccurate." However, he must keep in mind that
Roswell Park has the equipment, and he has the expertise, to test
for hormone dependency at the time of mastectomy. Therefore,
he has no need to wait for clues. Most surgeons and their patients
in the United States are not so fortunate.

This hormone assay (also known as an estrogen-fixation assay)
is available in only a few hospitals in this country as yet. Since
the test must be done immediately after excision, the tumor
cannot be bottled and sent elsewhere for analysis. To my regret,
my tumor was not assayed. My biopsy, remember, was performed near my home, because the mammogram had said the
tumor was benign. Although the lump, preserved in a jar of
formaldehyde, was clutched in my hand all the way to Buffalo,
it was too late to do the test. Dr. Dao is sorry he did not do
my biopsy, so that he would know about the hormone dependency. If I should have a recurrence or metastasis, he would have
no alternative but to take out my ovaries, unless the second neoplasm could be removed surgically. If this should be the case,
an assay might again be possible.

He explained the test's importance to me. "Only about one-
third of all breast cancers are strongly hormone-dependent," he
said, "even though there is evidence that there are some hormone
receptors in all the other tumors, as well. But that one-third has
so many hormone receptors, we know positively that these women
will be vastly improved by oophorectomy."

In a recent interview in a medical journal, Dr. Robert L. Shirley,
the Boston breast-cancer specialist, recommended that a hormone
assay "become an essential method for studying breast-therapy
options," because the test can predict if removing the ovaries will
help or not. It is regrettable that so few hospitals have the necessary equipment or personnel. I hope the test does become "essential," as Dr. Shirley feels it should.

At the end of all my research and interviews, I was suddenly hit with a devastating thought. All surgical innovations in the treatment of breast cancer—including Dr. Crile's—use radical mastectomy as the yardstick for measuring "success." To be as good as, or even better than, the radical is the goal—from Professor Mustakallio in Finland in the 1940s right down to the experts at the National Cancer Institute in September 1974. It would seem as if the results of radical mastectomy were truly spectacular, to make it the criterion all other procedures are measured against. Unfortunately, the over-all survival rates of radical mastectomy are far from spectacular: a fifty-fifty chance of living longer than ten years after surgery.

I remember the precise moment the idea chilled me. I was in the Edinburgh air terminal, with Professor Thomas Symington, of the Chester Beatty Research Institute, waiting for the shuttle flight to London in early December 1974. I turned to him, shaken. "Isn't anyone looking for something with *better* results than radical mastectomies?"

He seemed stunned by my question. He pondered it for a few minutes before answering.

"It's probably that surgery has gone as far as it can, my dear," he said softly. "The place to look for an end to breast-cancer death is not to the scalpel."

It was a sobering thought, which put all the controversies about "What kind of surgery?" into proper perspective.

The treatment of breast cancer with the knife has gone as far as it can go.

10

After Surgery: Physical

"I didn't have five minutes' worth of pain. My years of periodontia hurt me a helluva lot more than the mastectomy did, that's for sure."

The booming, hearty voice coming over the telephone sounded as if it were coming from a large, athletic woman. I guessed right on the sports.

"Three weeks after the stitches were out, I was knocking buckets of golf balls all over the driving range. Nobody could believe it." She laughed, a deep, jolly belly laugh. "And, believe me, everybody was looking at me, too. I think they were all trying to decide which one had been cut off, but I fooled 'em. Nobody could tell a thing, even with that skimpy golf shirt on."

"How long ago did you have your mastectomy?" I asked. Quickly I grabbed the notebook I kept ready on the corner of my desk to record the answers to a questionnaire I was circulating to women who had had mastectomies.

"Seventeen years ago next July," she told me happily. "That pretty much puts me in the clear. I hope the same for you."

Seventeen years. No wonder she could not remember the post-mastectomy "discomfort" as accurately as I could, after less than a year.

I had been warned about this so-called telescoping phenomenon. "The longer after the mastectomy," several surgeons told me, "the less traumatic it was. The first couple of years, the operation is remembered as excruciating. Then it diminishes to very painful. Then, somewhere along the line, the 'very' disappears, and ultimately a mastectomy is remembered only as uncomfortable or even altogether pain-free."

The surgeons were using the telescoping phenomenon as a defense against the traumatic psychological shock women experience when they do not know in advance that a breast will be amputated. "The same kind of defensive memory mechanism," I was told, "protects women from suffering too long from the shock of losing the breast without advance warning."

I decided to see if telescoping worked in this ebullient former patient. "Did you know ahead of time that you would lose your breast?"

"Hell, no!" she yelled. "Knocked the Captain for a loop, too. It was done in a navy hospital," she explained. "My husband was in the service then, stationed out in California. The Captain told me afterward he could have sworn he'd be done and finished in half an hour." She laughed at the memory. "He was madder than a hornet, he was. He was a tennis nut and had a big match scheduled that morning. Had to miss it on account of me."

"How did you feel when you woke up and discovered one of your breasts was missing?"

"Well, being in the service, and being a navy brat to begin with," she told me, "you sort of get used to being knocked around. When my husband came in to see me, he grinned and said something about getting brassieres at a discount from then on, because I wouldn't be needing half. I guess that pretty well sums up what both our attitudes toward the operation were—a bad break. The main thing was to be finished with the cancer, and that took a long time to know."

After seventeen years, telescoping had worked with this woman. I had not yet passed seventeen months, and the memory was still very clearly in focus.

On awakening in the hospital recovery room, the first thing I remember feeling was an intense burning in my throat and in the area of the incision. The throat problem did not last long; it was a local irritation from a tube inserted in my windpipe. I had been warned that I might have a lot of mucus and that a bubble-blowing machine would be used to clear my pipes. As it turned out, it was not necessary. However, it is common to need to blow some bubbles after such anesthesia.

The burning in the incision was caused by two vacuum drains that had been left there to draw out serous fluid, which would otherwise accumulate and cause pain and swelling. The drains were attached to a pouch called a Hemo-Vac, an ingenious gadget that exerted just enough reverse pressure to prevent the unwanted build-up of fluid—important in preventing postoperative swelling and pain.

Except for my throat and the spots where the drains were, I was totally numb in the left side of my chest and in most of the upper left arm. My first thought was that I was paralyzed. Then I realized that most of the nerves had been cut during the surgery and would need time to reknit. Naturally, I would be numb in the meantime.

"Your sensation will gradually return. Don't worry," Dr. Dao assured me. What he did not explain was that when the sensation came back, it would come as pain. But that was several months later for me, and I have learned that the time varies from woman to woman.

For the moment, the drains were my only problem, and they were removed on the third or fourth day. My chest did not hurt, but I felt as if a huge, tight rubber band were squeezing me from the armpit to below the rib cage. There were slight pins and needles, tingles, and occasionally a short, sharp, darting sensation, which came unexpectedly and disappeared just as quickly. The area involved was not only that part of me around the incision and the armpit, but also the shoulder, the adjacent part of the back, and the inside of the arm. These are not painful now—less than a year after mastectomy—but all women are different in their responses. Sometimes a sudden, intermittent, mild electric shock strikes me unexpectedly, but that is all.

The weirdest sensation—or, rather, lack of sensation—was trying to shave under my left arm. Normally, this cosmetic job can be done without even looking; the nerve endings guide the razor to the proper spot. After a mastectomy, these nerves are temporarily deadened, and for a while I had to look to be sure I got all the stubbly patches.

These sensations, I later discovered, are perfectly normal in all postmastectomy patients. The length of time for the nerves to be restored varies with the kind of surgery, the surgeon's skill, and the woman's speed of healing.

A mastectomy is major surgery, and it involves a good bit of cutting, regardless of what kind it is. The breast is exceedingly vascular—chock-full of blood vessels—so there is considerable loss of blood. Some surgeons give routine transfusions afterward; others, like Dr. Dao, do not if these can be avoided. Also, every surgeon has his preferred anesthetic.

Depending on the speed of his scalpel, the operation can take from three to as long as seven hours. Probably the less time the patient is unconscious, the better for her. However, I found no mention of duration of surgery as a factor in success or failure.

Most surgeons make a horizontal incision, with the idea that it is more easily hidden by a conventional bra. Some make diagonal incisions. Mine is vertical, beginning about five inches below the shoulder and ending just where the bottom edge of my bra can hide it.

"I like a vertical incision," Dr. Dao told me, "because I like to think of a woman being able to wear a plunging neckline. But it is purely a matter of personal preference with the modified radical. It makes no difference medically."

I had not given a moment's thought to any kind of incision. Who had ever thought of mastectomy at all, much less how the breast would be cut off? Most women still know little, unless they are personally affected.

What they might have learned recently has come from the numerous magazine and newspaper articles that appeared after Betty Ford's and Happy Rockefeller's operations. And whenever these famous patients were asked how they felt, they were always "just fine." Once the spate of publicity about their surgeries was over, they were banished from the front pages and exiled again to the women's sections. There, both were back in the social swim of official Washington—giving out Halloween candy, appearing at luncheons, parties, confirmation hearings, and congressional sessions. All there was to it, one society columnist wrote, was "a little foam rubber."

In an article that appeared in February 1975, Mrs. Ford did confess she tired more easily and that she rested her arm on pillows whenever possible. But pain? Swelling? Not a word. The only problems either woman would admit to were some fatigue and discomfort.

I knew it could not be true. On the other hand, my own experiences were probably not typical, either. To get a broad picture—physical and psychological—I somehow had to find a way to reach many women of different ages, marital status, and socioeconomic situation. I called a friend at the National Cancer Institute's breast clinic for advice and, I hoped, help.

"You know," she said, "no matter what you do, you're going to get a very biased sample."

"I don't want to know their names or anything."

"That doesn't make any difference," she said. "Women who are having troubles, either physically or psychologically, will not have anything to do with you, your book, or anything else. They want to block out the whole business and forget it."

I thought for a moment. Of course she was right. A woman would have to be well adjusted to her mastectomy to be willing to talk about it to a total stranger, anonymously or not. Maladjusted women, naturally, would refuse.

"How about talking to psychiatrists?" I asked.

"They would give you an opposite bias," she countered. "You'd be hearing about women so badly adjusted they needed psychiatric help. You would get the two extremes. There's no way I can imagine to get at the women who can't accept the loss of a breast but aren't in bad enough shape—or good enough financial condition—to get help from a shrink. There's no way I can think of to get around this."

I thanked her and put down the receiver. The problem was unexpected, but, after thinking it over, I realized I should have anticipated it. Certainly, women who had never been able to accept the loss of a breast would be unwilling to talk to me or to answer a written questionnaire.

Reach to Recovery! That was the natural organization to help me. An important branch of the American Cancer Society, the program enlists volunteers who try to visit every mastectomy patient in the country, right after her surgery, to give advice, answer questions, and lift her morale. Once again I was disappointed.

"We didn't want Reach to Recovery to become a crutch," a representative of the program told me, when I called the office of the Washington ACS chapter. "After all, the whole point of Reach to Recovery is to convince women they do not have a disabling handicap. We talked about having a mastectomy club, like the various ostomy clubs and laryngectomy clubs. But that would have defeated our whole purpose. Having a mastectomy is *not* a permanent handicap, and even the worst of scars can be hidden by a well-fitting prosthesis and the right clothing. So we decided we would help the patient for just a few weeks, and then leave her to her own psychological recovery."

It made good sense from her point of view, but for my purposes I wanted to talk to women who were not immediately "postop." I needed women who were far enough beyond the surgery itself to have some perspective on what they had gone through.

The logical people to help—surgeons—were not likely to be too co-operative. In the widely syndicated article I had written for the *Washington Post,* I had made it crystal clear I did not think general surgeons should be doing mastectomies, and that had not endeared me to members of the American College of Surgeons.

I was still in a deep quandary when a department-store ad appeared in the newspaper announcing a week-long visit by the representative of a prosthesis manufacturer, the Airway Surgical Company. That might be the answer, I told myself. Immediately I called the representative, explained my problem, and asked if she would mind giving my name and telephone number to the women who came to her to be fitted that week. The representative, Mrs. Loretta Marsh Crowell, agreed without hesitation. On the first day one woman called; the second day, none; the third day, none. The fourth day I went to the store myself, to be sure she hadn't forgotten me.

"No, I haven't," she said. "I'm really surprised that only one woman called you, because there were about fourteen who wrote your name down and said they would."

As long as I was in the store, I asked if I might park in one of the fitting rooms for the afternoon, so that her customers could come in to talk if they wanted to. Of the number who were fitted during those few hours—I do not know how many it was—only three came in to be interviewed. As I had expected, all three had made good adjustments, were open, requested no anonymity, and were positive in their attitudes about the surgery. Two of them were grandmothers and had been postmenopausal when their tumors were discovered. The third was younger, but very down-to-earth and sensible.

After they left, I talked with Mrs. Crowell. She agreed that I would get a distorted picture going this route. "For one thing," she said, "a lot of women don't ever get adjusted enough to buy a prosthesis in the first place. The little bit of confidence or whatever it takes to face me or any other fitter just isn't there. Even to come to this department, she first has to admit she needs an artificial breast, and that is more than some women can do. There are women, I am sure, who live all the rest of their lives with cotton batting or even Kleenex stuffed into the cups of their bras." (And, judging by the response, of those who did make it to the fitting room that week, only a few were willing to be interviewed.)

Before Mrs. Crowell left the Washington area, she said that she and her firm would do anything they could to help me reach mastectomees in other cities. Thanks to their help, the questionnaire I had devised was circulated via the lingerie departments of stores around the country.

CONFIDENTIAL

1. Age when mastectomy was performed?
2. How long since the surgery occurred?
3. What kind of mastectomy, e.g., Halsted, modified radical, simple, etc., if information is known?
4. What was foremost in your mind when the suggestion of cancer was told to you?
5. Were you aware before the actual mastectomy that your breast would be removed?

6. If the diagnosis was made in a separate procedure, what was this technique?

7. Was the physician a male or a female?

8. Were you visited by Reach to Recovery volunteers of the American Cancer Society? Did these women help?

9. What were the attitudes toward you by other patients?

10. What were the attitudes toward you by hospital personnel?

11. What were the attitudes toward you by relatives and friends?

12. How did you deal with your immediate family? Children, if any?

13. What was husband's attitude or boyfriend's response? This is a critical question, of course, and I would like as much information as possible, especially anecdotes, if any. Unfortunately, I must also pry into the bedroom and ask if there were any differences after your mastectomy. Forgive me!

14. Did you consider having a so-called lumpectomy or other lesser operations in order to save your breast?

15. Did you require postoperative irradiation, chemotherapy, or other treatment?

16. What kind of follow-up care are you being given?

17. Has your physician warned you not to take oral contraceptives?

18. Has the mastectomy made any difference in your life? If so, kindly detail. I am especially interested in your own feelings of womanliness and femininity, male attitudes toward you, and any economic problems you might have encountered. An important aspect is also whether you feel it is a matter you keep privately to yourself or whether you have no qualms about having others know about the surgery.

Any additions that you may think pertinent, based on your own experiences and not covered in this questionnaire, will be appreciated.

At the other end of the spectrum, I asked several psychiatrists with postmastectomy patients if they would have these women call me, and all said they would recommend it. One cautioned that such a sample would represent patients who had serious problems and might slant the results.

"That's what I expect," I replied. "I can't seem to strike a happy medium, so I'm using psychiatric patients to illustrate poor adjustment—if that's the way it is—and, at the other end, women who voluntarily answer questions and seem to have no problem." I described my questionnaire and told him how well adjusted all my respondents had been so far. "These women are slanted in the opposite direction," I said. "I don't know how to get to the ones in the middle—women too adjusted or too poor to see psychiatrists, but not adjusted enough to go to a store to buy an artificial breast."

I never did find a way to reach this group. But I know they exist.

One other group got into my survey—about thirty-five women, some of whom I had known for years, who phoned after my article appeared to ask questions or simply to welcome me into "the club." And, of course, I received dozens of calls and letters from women who had read my article and wanted more information.

Altogether, I spoke with or received responses from about 130 women as of the time this book was completed, but the questionnaires are still coming in. The respondents were young, middle-aged, and older. Most were married, but some were divorced, some widowed, and some had never been married. As I expected, most of those who telephoned were very well adjusted, at least according to what they said. None of the telephone interviewees asked for anonymity. Several of the women I knew asked me not to tell anyone else, just as they had never told me anything before the story about my own mastectomy was published. Of the mailed questionnaires, less than half had no name or address; the rest of the women were candid and said I could communicate with them if I needed more information.

Of the women who were referred by the psychiatrists, most said their problems had nothing to do with the mastectomy but had simply been aggravated by it. Several said they had been in treatment when the cancer was discovered, and I verified this with the psychiatrists. Incidentally, I discovered that they had asked more women to call than actually did.

In keeping with surgical practice in the United States, most of the women had had Halsted radicals, and most had not known in advance they would have a mastectomy, although many said the possibility had been mentioned "in passing."

The questionnaire did not ask about education or the kind of work a woman did, and I was sorry later it did not. In the conversations, both subjects came up, and most of these women, I found out, had gone to college for a year or two. While I do not think education or a job has anything to do with making the kind of adjustment I was interested in, I do think it indicates (1) the kind of woman who reads the editorial section of the *Washington Post*'s Sunday edition; (2) the kind of woman who seeks psychiatric counseling; (3) the women who are financially able to afford an expensive, lifelike prosthesis and special brassiere, if needed. Therefore, my random and unscientific poll was less random and more unscientific than I thought. I do believe, though, that it gave me a fairly good idea of the physical and psychological problems encountered after mastectomy. I also learned how the women had accepted the knowledge of having a potentially fatal disease.

In all the flurry of articles that followed the first and second ladies' mastectomies, this grim side of the breast-cancer story was somehow understated. The media seemed to concentrate only on the cosmetics of breast cancer. Jacqueline Susann's death after a secret and silent fourteen-year battle, coming as it did during that period, did not dispel the aura of sexuality and fetishism surrounding the mammary glands.

The surgery that can stop the disease *is* disfiguring, but breast cancer kills. Except in selective Stage I cases, mastectomy of some kind is the only treatment now known that gives a woman a good chance to live in spite of it. If I were to compose the questionnaire today, I would include a question about how it feels to be alive, putting much less emphasis on what doctors call "cosmesis." At the time, however, I myself knew so little about the seriousness of the disease that, once I accepted amputation, I was most concerned with questions of discomfort and disability —not of death.

The amount and intensity of pain immediately after the operation and during the months that follow vary considerably. Some women whose surgeries were fairly recent told me they still felt nothing at all except numbness in most of the affected area. One young mother of two girls, who was only thirty-four years old, was hitting tennis balls at a public court less than six weeks after her stitches were removed—and introduced me to friends who had witnessed the feat! I could never have done that. When I interviewed her (about a year after the mastectomy), she still had no pain. All she felt was tightness across her chest.

I was then just a few months postop and still tender in most places; other places really hurt. However, apparently my nerves had healed quickly. Otherwise I, too, would not have felt anything as early as I did. But tennis? I doubt it.

Much depends on the kind of surgery done. Most of my respondents, who had had the Halsted radical, said it was difficult for them to re-educate auxiliary muscles to take over for the pectorals, which had been removed. For them, regaining the full use of the arm had top priority; pain and cosmetics were secondary.

Also, quite a few post-Halsted women required skin grafts (which are usually taken from the thigh) to patch up the breast area. The grafts caused complications of infection, sloughing—the word used to describe grafted skin that refuses to stay put—and itching. But the last is a problem after any surgery. The nerves in the top layer of skin are not functioning and cannot transmit a helpful scratch to the miserable itch.

Marvella Bayh, the wife of Indiana's Senator Birch Bayh, had had a modified radical, and had no trouble with grafts or with her arm muscles. "But that postoperative X-ray therapy made me so sick," she told me. "I remember that as being worse than anything about the surgery." Mrs. Bayh's recollection was typical of women who had had diffuse "prophylactic" irradiation as soon as their incisions were healed enough for them to undergo it. Invariably, the weakness, fever, retching, and nausea—as well as the burned skin—that usually accompany high-dosage radiotherapy are remembered more clearly than the mastectomy itself. X-ray treatments can also cause additional swelling and pain by damaging the lymphatics even more than the radical mastectomy did.

Many women complained that their treatments caused their hair to fall out, often to the point of real baldness. In checking with experts, I was told that, properly done, X-ray therapy for spots of metastasis after radical mastectomy should not require doses large enough to cause hair loss. "Or possibly their entire bodies—including their heads—were irradiated," one therapist explained. "But I don't know why anyone would do that after radical mastectomy."

I found other differences in physical condition during the first months and years, all seeming to depend largely on age, number of small children, and economic status. For example, all the women who were over sixty at the time of mastectomy complained that they had a hard time bouncing back to their preoperative physical condition and energy level. "If I go to the grocery store or to the library," one of them told me, "I am finished for the day." At the time she was eight months postop; I was four. I attribute the difference between us simply to the fact that older women in general do not bounce back as easily as younger ones do.

Having young children still in diapers, who must be carried or who crawl all over their mothers, is also something I did not have to cope with. I learned from younger patients that, as happy as they were to be able to look after their babies or toddlers, they had serious physical problems if they had to care for the children by themselves. That is where economic status came into the picture. Those with higher incomes could hire help, and the convalescent mother had a more comfortable recovery.

Another postoperative problem, which in some women is temporary and in others permanent, is milk arm, or lymphedema. As I have said, the surgeon's skill in dissecting the axilla is probably the most important factor in the seriousness of this complication. Three of my respondents had had simple (or total) mastectomies. Since their nodes and lymphatic vessels were not removed or cut, they, of course, had no swelling at all. Some women have such mild lymphedema that it cannot even be seen; they feel only a tightness in the upper arm. Others must wear elastic bandages occasionally; some are sentenced to a lifetime of wearing a postmastectomy sleeve.

This helpful medical accessory is a long elasticized glove minus the fingers, which comes in different sizes. It extends from the upper part of the hand to the shoulder and resembles the long opera gloves that were fashionable for prom wear when I was a teen-ager—gloves with fingered mitts that could be removed without taking the whole glove off. The sleeves are made of the same flesh-colored material as support stockings for varicose veins and act the same way the hosiery does—they squeeze the arm to stimulate circulation.

Many women had some limitation of shoulder motion. However, because of variations in surgery, postoperative treatment, age, and probably the stage of the disease (only about half a dozen had had enough time between biopsy and mastectomy to have been staged, however), the women I interviewed had only three common physical problems: (1) the very tight, binding feeling across the chest, a constriction that lasted for months for almost everyone, but with different degrees of discomfort; (2) the strange, eerie business of having to crane the neck to shave under the arm; (3) the refusal of an itch to go away after being scratched.

Everything else I personally experienced seemed to differ considerably from one patient to another. So I will just describe my own postoperative physical sensations, which may or may not be typical of women my age (forty-five) after a modified radical mastectomy.

The site immediately around the incision was numb for about five months. Once, I developed a small infection in the incision, and Dr. Dao told me, via long-distance telephone, to use hot compresses. The temperature that was comfortable to my fingers was hot enough to print a neat red square on the skin of my chest, although I could not feel anything there. I remember staring in horror as the color appeared—I had not realized that the water was too hot for new skin. My shoulder and arm, however, were exquisitely sensitive if touched. It was not a constantly present pain, but even a light brush with a feather felt like a lighted match. To bump the shoulder or put any pressure on the upper arm was agony.

To anyone interested in my sex life, I must point out that fondling from the waist up was out of the question. I was not one to whip off my bra as soon as I got my husband into the bedroom alone, but even if I had been, it would have been strictly no touch anywhere near the left arm.

As for swelling, I still have occasional tightness, but nothing that can be seen or measured. I discovered that anything that had made me puffy before the mastectomy still did. For example, I habitually retained fluid before and during the first few days of my menstrual period, and this pattern is persisting. If I eat too many salty or highly seasoned foods, I feel the salt in my upper arm the next morning. Maryland's hot humidity has always made me swell and continues to do so now. (The humidity is one of the reasons a Washington-area job is considered a "hardship post.") I found the effect of the weather on my new incision to be the same as it had been after my appendix was removed. For me, pulling or twisting in the incisional site is a better barometer than the weather bureau's.

Because I had my operation away from home, I was hospitalized for more than two weeks, so that Dr. Dao could be certain the incision was healing well and there were no complications before I left Buffalo. For this reason, all my stitches had been removed by the time I was discharged. The normal practice, however, is to stay in the hospital about a week. The stitches (sutures) in the parts of the chest subject to the least stress are removed first, usually in the hospital. Then, a few days or a week later, the rest are taken out in the doctor's office.

Exercises are begun as soon as the recovery from anesthesia and the patient's general condition permit. Roswell Park has a physical therapy department, and I was taken there the morning after my surgery. It is vital, after a Halsted radical mastectomy, to begin exercising immediately, to strengthen the auxiliary muscles of the arm that take over for the removed pectorals. It is also important after a modified radical, even though the chest muscles are intact. As I have said, the "radical" part of a mastectomy is the removal of the nodes and some lymphatic vessels and the cutting of other vessels. Exercises help get the blood and lymph circulating through the damaged area. If the arm is pampered, the temporary blockage could become permanent, resulting in ugly and painful milk arm. In addition, in the modified radical the pectoral muscles must sometimes be pulled aside (retracted), or even cut, to enable the surgeon to see and remove all the nodes. Getting the pectorals quickly back into shape prevents later stiffness and soreness.

The most useful and universal exercise is the spider walk. The healthy arm is stretched as high up a wall as it will go and a spot is marked at the tip of the longest finger. The trick is to walk the index and middle fingers of the affected arm up the wall, a little farther each time, until they can touch the same spot. Spider walking is done in two positions: facing the wall and at a right angle to it.

Another helpful exercise is to pull a rope about four feet long back and forth across a high horizontal bar. The shower rod is high enough for a short woman, but a tall one might have to install something different. Women who have had Halsteds also find that squeezing a rubber ball in the palm of the hand strengths the auxiliary muscles.

A rope, a ball, and a "lounger"—a temporary prosthesis—are given to mastectomy patients shortly after their surgery by Reach to Recovery. At the surgeon's request, and with the patient's approval, a volunteer comes to the hospital the second or third day after the operation to present the kit, a manual of exercises, and a list of dos and don'ts, and to give general moral and psychological support. Naturally, Reach to Recovery volunteers must themselves have made a good adjustment in order to qualify. I did not have the visit, but those patients I interviewed who did were full of praise for the help they got from these volunteers.

Besides squeezing the ball while reading or watching TV, another exercise that can easily be done at such times is hairbrushing. It is not only good for the hair, but good for the shoulder and arm as well. At the beginning, a mirror is essential, because the arm is sore and the reflex is to bring the head down to the brush, instead of vice versa. However, a few sessions before the mirror quickly train the head to stay erect.

Swimming is excellent exercise after a mastectomy, especially the backstroke.

After any radical mastectomy, women are warned—or should be warned—that *never again* must the affected arm be used for taking blood-pressure readings or for inoculations, vaccinations, or injections of any kind. Some surgeons even ban manicures and underarm shaving on that side.

It is also a good idea to avoid exposing the arm to too much sun, although this problem probably varies greatly from one person to another. In my own case, I found out the hard way. Dr. Dao had told me, when I got my final instructions, to be careful of sunburn, but the warning somehow did not sink in adequately. After I spent a day basking on a Caribbean beach, his words emerged from my subconscious as my left arm began to develop strange swollen curves and to twist and grind.

"I didn't remember," I wailed to Harvey, my arm propped up on three pillows. "I remembered no blood pressure, vaccinations, shots, or inoculations, but I forgot all about the sunburn warning."

"So now you've had a good lesson," he comforted. "You won't do it any more."

When the arm is injured, by either infection, trauma, or sunburn, the underlying tissue generally fills with lymphatic fluid, as protection against further damage. If the lymphatic vessels have been cut, the fluid cannot circulate normally and sometimes backs up in the arm. The result is lymphedema and pain. Of course, the fluid did filter back into my system, and my arm was fine after a day on the pillows, far from the beach. But the rest of my sunbathing was done wearing long sleeves. The problem may not bother some women at all; it is also possible that the blockage would not have happened to me if my tanning had been gradual, in small doses, rather than in a full day under the blazing Caribbean sun.

Another curious physical aftereffect of that trip was a reaction to altitude. The cabin of the airplane we flew down in was pressurized to about 6,000 feet at a cruising altitude of 32,000 feet. As we ascended, I noted a gradual tightening in my chest and arm, a sensation that disappeared within an hour or so after we landed. The same thing happened on the way home.

An airline pilot I questioned said he could not understand why a higher altitude should have an effect on only one part of the body, regardless of its condition. But a physicist thought this was possible. "It's like having some leaking tin cans of water," he explained. "You change the air pressure on the outside, reduce it the way you do up at 6,000 feet, and you'll have more force pushing from the inside outward than you would at sea level." According to him, even a minor blockage of a few lymph channels would be enough to turn them into "leaking tin cans," which would be more sensitive to changes of external pressure than normal vessels would be.

But that was months after the mastectomy. Immediately afterward, when I first returned home, my main physical reaction was exhaustion. In the hospital, I had been in great condition in comparison with most of the other patients, and of course I had had nothing much to do but brush my hair. My meals were served to me, I enjoyed daily naps, and physical therapy was the only activity that called for any energy. Back home, it was different. Just clearing the breakfast dishes was fatiguing. What had happened to all the vim and vigor I had had in Buffalo?

The vim and vigor were the same. It was only that my home life was taking more of them than my life in the hospital. This is perfectly normal after a mastectomy, especially if no blood transfusions have been given. The operation costs a lot of blood, and that leaves the patient weak, though not necessarily anemic. The important thing to know is that it takes time to get back to a normal energy level, and she must be careful not to overdo at the beginning. This does not mean she has to be pampered, though. Mastectomy is not a disabling operation. A woman should get back into her old routine as soon as possible, judging how soon by how she feels.

In addition to the hairbrushing, the spider walk, swimming, and pulling a rope, certain household jobs are excellent therapy. For example, the movements of washing windows and walls are very helpful—and leave the house shining in the bargain. Anything that requires reaching or stretching is good. There really are no household chores that have to be avoided altogether. During the first month, the one important rule is moderation. While all women have different problems and all surgeons give different instructions, in my case the only restriction was not to lift anything heavy and not to pull or push anything with a lot of weight attached—like an upright vacuum cleaner through a thick shag rug. Other than this, I was encouraged to do anything I wanted to, as long as it did not overtire me.

I have already said that as soon as the bandages were removed I put on a loose-fitting bra and stuffed the empty cup with absorbent cotton. Later, I called my local Reach to Recovery office and was given one of their loungers to wear temporarily.

A surgeon usually does not want his patient to have a permanent prosthesis until her incision is well healed and beyond any possibility of complications. For this reason, most reputable firms require a prescription for the permanent form. That is one case, by the way, where needing a doctor's prescription can help the purse. Medical insurance usually pays for prescribed surgical appliances.

There are many permanent prostheses on the market, ranging from inexpensive Dacron-filled ones to specially weighted, latex-covered, silicone-gel shapes that feel as natural to the touch as a real breast. My strong opinion is that economy should be thrown out the window at this time (especially if the insurance will pay most of the bill). From my interviews as well as my own experience, I can say without hesitation that nothing is as important as knowing both breasts look alike, are symmetrical, and "only her corsetière knows for sure."

The silicone-gel prosthesis costs almost a hundred dollars, but mine has been worth every penny the insurance company paid. The latex cover makes it adhere to the skin, so that it does not shift out of position but stays where it belongs. The slick, silky coverings of other prostheses I tried often moved when I moved; occasionally I would discover the "breast" up near my shoulder or somewhere under my arm, instead of on the left side of my chest.

The reason for the weighting is simple physics. The smallest breast—even my A cup—does weigh something, and when the weight is removed that shoulder will ride high. A bra stuffed with cotton is not heavy enough to pull the shoulder back to its normal position. Until I got my permanent form, I had sudden and strange neckaches, backaches, and headaches. All disappeared as soon as I was fitted with the weighted prosthesis. I had been walking around for more than a month with my shoulders askew, and the resulting stress had brought on the nagging pains. So a weighted form is a medical necessity for me.

Women with large breasts may have to have special brassieres as well. There are also different shapes to accommodate different kinds of surgery. Women who have had the modified radical or simple (total) mastectomy will be uncomfortable wearing the shape designed for the Halsted. It has a short "tail" intended to fill any cleft left in the axilla. If the surgery has been less extensive and there is no such cleft, the tail feels lumpy.

Because the Halsted is by far the most common mastectomy, my biggest problem was to find the shape manufactured for the modified radical in my size. Most surgeons in the United States do not get involved in advising patients about prostheses. Once they write a prescription, they count on Reach to Recovery volunteers or on the expert fitters found in the lingerie departments of most good stores to take care of it. Surgical-supply houses in larger cities also have well-trained personnel.

Other countries I visited, by the way, have no Reach to Recovery, and American women should consider themselves lucky in this respect. Mrs. Betty Westgate is attempting to get a similar program started in England and has already begun a Mastectomy Association. In Scotland, Sweden, Finland, and the Soviet Union, doctors or nurses give advice about prostheses, and all stress the importance of having a good postmastectomy form.

The silicone-gel forms are not new; they have been available for nine years. At first, I thought I was fortunate to have had my mastectomy after their invention. In interviewing several women who had had their operations years ago, I was told again and again what a blessing they are. "I fought many a battle with a bulge," one fourteen-year veteran said, laughing. "These new jobs are marvelous! You don't know what you missed." One woman, who was only thirty-two (and four feet, ten inches tall) when she lost her breast eleven years ago, complained bitterly about the ugly surgical-support brassiere she had worn for years. Even the golfing navy wife, who was neither young nor tiny—she weighed in at 176 at the time we talked—waxed eloquent over not needing a "garment" any more. "It has made all the difference in the world to me," she boomed. "Now I can wear see-through blouses without worrying that that hideous old thing with five hooks and two-inch straps will look like hell underneath."

The reason all these women thought silicone-gel forms were "new" is simply that they were never promoted by the manufacturer, Mrs. Crowell told me. Like breast cancer itself, the prosthesis was unmentionable.

With bathing suits, or with dresses that cannot be worn with a bra, I have found an easy way to hide the absence of a breast. I bought some inexpensive Dacron fiber fill in an upholstery store and made several forms by packing this fluff into the feet of old nylons. The shaping is not important here, because the form will take on the contour of the garment. (At least, my garments are contoured, because I have never had enough natural shape to fill them.) Then I stitched the nylon covering of the form about a quarter of an inch from the edge of the built-in bra cup, so that to notice it someone would literally have to lean over and peek inside my cleavage. When the tan of the stocking might show, I simply covered the "prosthesis" with a patch of fabric the same color as the dress. Using such devious disguises, I have been able to wear my premastectomy bikini and a dramatic dress with one bare (naturally, the left!) shoulder, which I had bought a week before I found the lump. I can also wear plunging necklines.

Unfortunately, all this may not be helpful to those who have had a Halsted radical mastectomy. I know of no clever, ingenious ways to camouflage the scars left by that operation except sleeves and high necklines.

Aside from the cosmetic aspects, the physical problems of a mastectomy are very like those following any kind of major surgery. Everyone heals and recovers at a different speed and experiences different reactions. Because the woman around the corner was playing tennis six weeks after her surgery does not mean that anything is wrong with a woman who, like me, could not. As long as her doctor is satisfied, there is no cause for worry. The aftereffects of the surgery will not last forever, and inevitably the mastectomy will stop being a good excuse for getting out of club or committee work. Enjoy it while it lasts.

One very unfortunate aftereffect of mastectomy does not go away for a long time, however. That is job discrimination. Since I had worked on my own for years as a free-lance writer, it had never occurred to me that having had a mastectomy could hurt a woman's ability to get a job. Then, in the *New York Times,* on November 28, 1974, it was reported that Mrs. Joyce Arkhurst, a New Yorker, had been denied a job at the United Nations because she had had a mastectomy in April 1973.

Her cancer was cured, according to her doctor, but the personnel office at the UN, where she had applied for a job supposed to last two years, would not hire her. Although everyone who had interviewed Mrs. Arkhurst thought she was qualified, she could not get the necessary medical clearance. The United Nations, she was told, does not hire cancer patients until five years have passed since their last treatment.

Mrs. Arkhurst came to the National Conference on Cancer

Management, held in New York, to demonstrate to the physicians attending that the problems of a cancer patient are not only medical. Dr. Robert McKenna, a cancer surgeon, who was also at the meeting, reported on fifty other cases of employment discrimination against cancer patients he knew of in California alone, and said that most government agencies and many private companies have employment practices identical to the United Nations'.

Certainly it is hard to think of any major surgery less handicapping than a mastectomy. Except for a job as a go-go girl, a strip-tease dancer, or possibly a lingerie model, I cannot imagine why any employer would argue against hiring a mastectomy patient. I called the personnel offices of several firms in my area, as well as the United States Civil Service Commission, to ask about it.

"There's no way to know if a cancer patient is cured for five years," I was told. "Suppose we invest a lot of time and money in training the person, and they get sick with cancer again. All that goes down the drain."

"Suppose you invest all that time and money in training someone, and the person walks into the street and is hit by a car!" I responded in disbelief. "Anything can happen. If you hire a young secretary, how do you know she won't get married and leave because her husband is transferred? What about getting pregnant?"

This practice does not make any sense at all. But it is a fact of life. Hiring someone who has had cancer apparently presents problems. First of all, a large number of firms have insurance and pension plans that will not cover such employees. The union—if there is one—requires that all employees be covered by whatever plans are in force, and the result is that firms simply ban the hiring of former cancer patients. Second, there is that ridiculous but nonetheless persistent superstition about cancer's being contagious, and many firms are afraid of losing employees who have this unspoken, subtle fear of cancer. Another reason is the worry over absenteeism if the disease recurs. Finally, there is in this country an over-all, general, grossly unfair discrimination against hiring handicapped people of any kind in most of government and industry.

Dr. McKenna made the point that cancer of the breast is considered very curable today and that, whether the personnel director knows it or not, one of every thousand job applicants is a "closet" cancer patient. He also calculated that such discrimination against cancer victims means about a $500 million annual cost to the United States economy in taxes, welfare, and other financial assistance. In October 1974, the American Cancer Society had formed a study group on the problem of job discrimination, with Dr. McKenna as its chairman.

One way to get around the persecution, of course, is for the former patients not to tell their employers. However, they would then have to pay their own medical bills, in most cases, since they could not collect anything under a firm's group plan. This would be an enormous—and obviously unfair—hardship. Another suggestion is to initiate a mass-education program aimed at personnel officials in industry and government, with the goal of convincing them that a former cancer patient is no higher risk than any other employee. Still another approach being considered is to give special tax benefits to employers who hire the handicapped —cancer patients and all others. So far, it is mostly talk.

Coincidentally, shortly after I learned of Mrs. Arkhurst's problem with the United Nations, I was invited to a party given by someone in my husband's company. One of the other guests, a senior employee—a very sharp, highly trained, competent woman of perhaps fifty—took me aside and told me she envied my being free to talk about my cancer openly without fear of a penalty.

"What do you mean?" I asked.

"Exactly what I said," she whispered. "I had a mastectomy last April and went back to work half days after only two weeks, just to be sure my supervisor didn't suspect I had anything serious."

I stared at her in disbelief. This was, after all, the same place where Harvey worked—presumably a sophisticated, enlightened, well-educated bunch of people. "They couldn't possibly have refused to give you back your job, you know," I told her. "There are laws now—"

"I wasn't worried so much about this job," she told me quietly. "I do know my rights, and if I had been fired I would have gone to the EEOC [Equal Employment Opportunity office] before they could have blinked. No, I was worried about my prospects for getting another job. Who knows? Something might happen here, and I'd be out of work. Where would I get a new job with a fresh mastectomy printed on my personnel record? That's the big problem I face—getting a new job. We don't have to worry about hanging on to the old ones. We're protected there. But getting a new one is different."

"But don't you think you could accomplish more by going public and fighting?" I asked.

She shook her head sadly. "I've got three kids in college, and a lot of expenses. I'm afraid I'm just not in a financial position to do any fighting for this cause." She smiled and patted me on the shoulder. "But right on to you, for anything you can do."

She got up and looked around to see if anyone had overheard us. "Please keep my secret. I really have to go on working."

Since then, I have read and heard more such stories. Dr. McKenna's committee is trying to get employment policies changed for former cancer patients. Other organizations are working hard to change them for all handicapped people. Undoubtedly, there are many jobs that victims of certain handicaps cannot manage. But having one breast instead of two? I doubt it would handicap even a prostitute.

Everything I have said so far about postmastectomy care is important, but the most imperative information concerns early detection of a recurrence (the appearance of a second cancer in the general area of the first) or a metastasis (the malignant spread of the cancer to another organ).

There is not much we can do for ourselves here, but those few things must be done religiously. The monthly BSE should include a careful palpation of the area around the incision. Frequently, a recurrence appears in the incisional site itself. Menstrual irregularities or changes should be reported, and so should lingering coughs or hoarseness and signs of possible liver problems.

To review what was said in the section on proper follow-up care, quarterly examinations are needed during the first two years and semiannual examinations for the next three, along with the X-rays and blood studies mentioned, and the mammograms twice a year if over forty. (As I have said, there is controversy about semiannual X-rays under this age, but one each year is imperative.) A patient who moves to another city during the five years must not neglect to check in with a new doctor right away, and to have all her records forwarded, so that earlier X-rays, blood studies, electrocardiograms, and so on will be available as a base line for measuring any changes.

Breast cancer is a chronic disease, just as diabetes is a chronic disease. Like diabetics, women with breast cancer must always be on guard for symptoms. That may be a cruel and heartless thing to say to a woman who has gone five years or even more without trouble and thinks she can stop worrying forever. But to lie would be more cruel and heartless, because it could result in unnecessary deaths. The years without recurrence or metastasis are called disease-free years; cancer specialists do not speak of cure rates but of survival rates. Women who have had breast cancer must face the facts.

We can relax and breathe easier after two years—the period when more than half of the recurrences and metastases first show up. And we can breathe even more deeply after five years. But the definitive time for measuring breast-cancer survival is now ten years. The five-year period formerly applied to all cancers is under no circumstances valid for mammary carcinoma. We must be on guard, although not as intensively, for ten years.

I hope that by the time I am ten years postop, "mastectomy" will come right after "leeches" in the medical-encyclopedia listings of quaint old surgical practices that have been abandoned.

11

After Surgery: Psychological

"Do you still feel attractive and appealing?" the young host of the TV talk show asked.

I squinted at him angrily. The subject of sex, I thought, had been laid to rest during an earlier off-camera break for a commercial.

"I don't feel any different from the way I did before," my fellow guest began to explain. "I've always thought too much of myself to think that everything I am, my personality, my intelligence, had anything to do with whether I had one breast or two." A sensible explanation, but a totally unnecessary one.

We had been invited to appear on the local daytime show to talk about the problems of mastectomy after both of the top Washington ladies—Betty Ford and Happy Rockefeller—had their operations. My partner was attractive, in her late forties, fourteen years postop, and she seemed to have been subjected to that kind of question before. She also had had enough mutilation from her surgery that I could see a dip in her upper chest, even though she was wearing a high neckline.

Our host was a young blade-about-town with a reputation for smart-alecky wit and an ability to get to the heart of a panel's subject quickly. To him, the heart of breast-cancer problems is sex.

"Now, I'd like you to talk about the differences in your relationships with your husbands after the operation," he had instructed us during the commercial. "This is what our viewers are interested in, you know—the changes it has made in your marital situation."

"That's ridiculous!" I had snapped. "Women watching this show have more sense than to be curious about our sex lives when we've had operations for cancer."

Then the light flashed, signaling we were about to return to the air. From his first question, it was obvious that he either had not heard or had not paid any attention to my comment. Even after my partner did her best to close the subject politely, he could not let it pass.

"If you've seen Coke ads since the age of eight," he continued, "you obviously have to dwell on the fact that having breasts is part of our culture."

I stared at him, through what I hoped were narrowed, angry slits, and did not answer. My partner, however, continued womanfully to try to mollify him without prostituting the principle that sex has no place in any intelligent discussion of breast cancer.

"It really has nothing to do with—" she began.

I thought he was about to break in with a more pointed question, and, television or no, I could not hold back any longer. I remember leaning so far toward him that the microphone hanging from the cord around my neck jerked to one side. "Just a minute!" I interrupted. "The thing you're forgetting is that we're discussing a fatal disease, and the important thing is that the doctor get rid of the cancer, and are you going to live? Unless a woman is unbalanced, the first thing she worries about is her life."

He didn't seem to understand. "But once she wakes up, and she doesn't have her breast, but she has her life—" he broke in.

"The first thing she says is 'Did you get it all out?' " I completed his sentence.

It must have seemed incredible to him. "It is?" he asked softly.

"You better believe it," I snapped.

I don't think he believed me.

In my questionnaire I had reluctantly asked a question about sex, because people do want to know. I did not like it, however;

it seemed wrong. Evaluating the replies made me realize how very wrong. To almost all the women who wrote or telephoned, sexiness and being appealing and attractive to men *were* unimportant. They had more significant things to worry about.

Evaluating postmastectomy psychological attitudes was complicated. The psychiatrists I queried pointed out that there is no single psychological problem, but, instead, separate stages of anxiety and fear, which begin the instant a lump is found. These are: (1) the interval between discovery and going to the doctor; (2) the interval between the doctor's physical examination and confirmation of the diagnosis by mammogram and biopsy; (3) the interval that should exist between biopsy and mastectomy (unfortunately, for most women in the United States this interval is actually between mammogram and mastectomy); (4) the interval immediately after surgery—especially traumatic to women who have had no warning or definite advance knowledge; (5) the interval after discharge from the hospital and the resumption of a normal life.

In addition to the five stages of psychic trauma, I discovered—from my biased sample—several variables that affect women differently: extent of the disease; the woman's age; her marital and family status; the condition of the marriage; whether she has young children, or older ones still living at home; and unrelated premastectomy psychological problems.

Please bear in mind that my poll was based on replies only from women well enough adjusted to talk or write to me about their mastectomies and was not a scientific study, by any means. For example, unmarried women under forty-five seemed to be in better psychological health than the postmenopausal unmarrieds. But only eight women in the younger group responded (as of April 1975), and only three of these were under thirty-five—a sample that is out of proportion with the over-all incidence statistics. Many such young women, I suspect, just could not call or return their questionnaires. After all, most of the current clamor here for lumpectomies and reconstructive mammoplasties seems to be coming from women in this category. In both Stockholm and Moscow, I was told that young women were involved in the trials of lesser surgeries; in those countries, too, the young unmarrieds apparently think two breasts are essential for finding husbands.

I immediately discovered a dramatic dichotomy between the attitudes of women who had already gone five or ten years with no recurrence or mestastasis and those who knew their cancers had not been stopped by mastectomy. The difference was so stunning that the two groups seemed almost to represent completely separate diseases.

Women whose doctors "did not get it all out" or who were too advanced for mastectomy to help had little interest in discussing the kind of surgery they had had. They usually couldn't even recall the details. Their worry about the spreading cancer overshadowed such relatively minor woes as ugly scars, lymphedema, disability, and all the other things we have been led to believe are the major problems after mastectomy. This applied to all ages. The youngest woman in this group had her surgery when she was thirty-three, only six months after her youngest child was born. The oldest, sixty-seven when I interviewed her, has since died. None of these patients cared much about skin grafts or Halsted versus modified versus lumpectomy. They had left these concerns behind them long ago.

"What I couldn't understand," the youngest of them told me, "is why everyone in the media—including you—thought it was so important that Betty Ford had a Halsted instead of something else. What the hell's the difference, if the surgery cures her?" Now forty-two and a practicing architect, this woman has survived nine years of flare-ups and hospitalizations. Today she is adjusted to living with recurrences and metastases and to the knowledge that she will always have cancer. "But nobody even hinted at the time of my surgery that it was going to be a chronic disease," she said. "All my lymph nodes were fine. I was cured, they told me."

Her first metastasis, to the lung, was not discovered until her chest was X-rayed for pneumonia almost three years after the mastectomy. "I *have* gotten better examinations since I had that first metastasis," she said ruefully. "Before that, it was just a quick examination of my other breast. I'm getting much more attention now." She paused. "But not as much as I think I should have. Sometimes I have to insist that I *know* something is wrong before anything is done."

Nine years after surgery, her mastectomy itself is as buried in her memory as her own birth. This attitude is typical of women not cured by mastectomy. Again and again, over and over, I heard the same lament from them. Doctors did not examine carefully or often enough to find the recurrence or metastasis early, when they might have been able to stop the cancer from spreading farther.

When I pointed out that many treatments being used so effectively today—especially new drugs—were not available even five years ago, most long-term survivors seemed to feel better. But nothing assuaged the bitter, sometimes violent, rage of an Ann Scott, whose metastases, if found early, could have been helped by drugs already on the shelves of cancer-hospital pharmacies.

"What kind of checkup do you get at Roswell Park?" I was asked repeatedly. As I described the procedures there, I could often hear a pencil or pen taking quick notes. Several women even asked me to slow down a bit. Only one of those I talked with had been scanned before the metastasis was found. None were having semiannual mammograms; some had not had any postoperative mammograms. Most had had chest X-rays, but as part of a routine physical by the family doctor, and several had had occasional X-rays of the spine, ribs, and skull. As with the architect, most of the doctors did become more careful after the metastasis appeared.

Without question, women who know their breast cancers have not been stopped by their mastectomies have totally different emotional problems from those who either are "waiting" or are breathing more freely after ten years.

"I wish all I had to worry about was whether my scar shows in a bathing suit or if I can pick up a ten-pound bag of sugar," one woman told me. "It depends where you sit how you stand, I guess." She roared with laughter when I told her about the questions I had been asked on the television program. "Now, that has got to be the epitome of insanity," she finally spluttered. "Who in her right mind would be worried about being appealing when she finds out she's got cancer?"

Unless a woman is so insecure or neurotic that having two real breasts means more to her than staying alive, her main concern after a mastectomy should be "Does the surgeon think it was caught in time?" and not "What will my husband think when he sees me naked?" Who cares what he thinks? If he loves her, his first concern also will be for the cancer, not for the imbalance in that part of her under the shoulders. A man who throws over a woman because of a mastectomy, or even two, is not worth having.

Television talk shows and the worry about being appealing notwithstanding, the single biggest psychological adjustment a woman must make is to the sudden knowledge that she has a chronic, potentially fatal disease and that removing the breast is only the first step in trying to stop the malignant spread.

Her family and friends know it, too, but are helpless to do much about it. In order to keep them from falling apart, the woman tries to keep her chin up and a smile plastered on her face—at a time when she herself is most defenseless and in need of support.

Being in another city, I had no friends visiting me at all, but it was supportive for me to be in a hospital devoted exclusively to the treatment of cancer, as Roswell Park is. My first room-mate was a retired librarian who had had miscellaneous skin cancers for thirty years. When I arrived, shaken and trembling, almost a week before the mastectomy, she was just waking up from her latest bout of skin grafts. Her grogginess lasted only a short time, and then she was bouncing around cheerfully, bandages swathing her face.

"You're in the best place there is in the world," she assured me. "I found my first cancer thirty years ago, and now I'm seventy-four and still going strong. It's because I have Roswell Park to come to. If anybody can keep us going, they'll do it here." With that kind of person as an introduction, I could not fret and cry. It was impossible.

"If you've got to have cancer"—she grinned weirdly through her bandages—"the best kind to have is what I've had all these years. Skin. But the second best is your kind, the breast. If it's caught in time, it's the easiest to cure. So what if you lose a breast? There are a lot of patients in this hospital that would change places with you in a second." She looked at her watch. "It's almost time for dinner. I'll introduce you to some of them afterward."

Next to Betty Butterfield, Larry Bohne, who died early in December 1974, did more to adjust me to living with cancer than anyone else. When I met Larry, he had already been declared terminal three times, and many of the drugs that had pulled him through had had their first human trials on him.

"I guess I'm the first person after the gorillas," he quipped. "It's been fifteen months now since I should have gone, and I'm still here. Every day is worth while. It's not the quantity of life that counts, it's the quality. Remember that."

With so much courage from a thirty-year-old man whose first child was born just before he became ill, how could I weep and wail about my small breast tumor? And there were others, whose first cancers had been discovered years before and who came regularly to Roswell Park for checkups or treatment.

True, it was difficult at times. I had to tread delicately with patients who were seriously ill, and not rub salt in their considerable wounds by appearing to be so hearty and healthy. The first few hours were hard, too. It was painful to look around at people with amputated organs, skin grafts, missing hair, and miscellaneous pipes and drains, and to accept the knowledge that I belonged here, that it was not just a ghastly mistake. On the other hand, it was enormously helpful, in more important ways.

Cancer had always been a scare word to me, an automatic signal to order a cemetery plot and a tombstone. Meeting people who had lived for years with as many as fourteen tumors made it much easier for me to hear that I now had a chronic disease to take care of for the rest of my life. The only long-term survivor of breast cancer I had ever heard of was Theodore Roosevelt's daughter, Alice Longworth, Washington's *grande dame*. While there was no breast cancer in my own family, as far as I knew, I kept remembering the close relatives on Harvey's side of the family who had had breast cancer, none of whom had survived.

These first days at Roswell Park made me realize that the

kind of surgery performed, how ugly the scar would be, whether I could wear low necklines and bikinis—everything that had concerned me earlier—were frivolous worries. After talking to Betty, Larry, and others on my floor, I was glad I would be cared for by a breast-cancer specialist in a cancer hospital. But for a far more significant reason than the one that took me to Buffalo in the first place. Never mind the beauty of a modified radical mastectomy. Suddenly, quite suddenly, I was surrounded with proof that having an oncologist could save my life.

On her morning television show, *Not for Women Only*, Barbara Walters asked Marvella Bayh why she had been so public about having a mastectomy, and not secretive, as Jacqueline Susann had been.

"I really had no choice in the matter," Mrs. Bayh replied. "Birch had already declared himself to be a candidate for the presidency in 1972, people had already begun working on his behalf, and money had been collected. He could not have dropped his plans without explaining the urgent reason for withdrawing." She said that afterward she had been happy there was no choice. She had discovered how much good she could do by telling about it and letting people see that she was well enough to lead the busy, active—often frantic—life of a senator's wife. Mrs. Bayh, who looked radiant, said she hoped her example, like Shirley Temple Black's, Betty Ford's, and Happy Rockefeller's, would help get rid of some of the fears that keep women away from early-detection clinics and doctors' offices.

In my case, there was no urgent reason to tell the world. I simply discovered that I, like most writers—especially those of us in and around Washington—abhor secrets. To us, a secret is something to dig out and tell to the public. It never occurred to me to keep my mastectomy quiet. In fact, I began keeping notes the night I found the lump. It may seem macabre, but that's the way it is with people whose job is communicating—we have to communicate. With these notes, jotted down as I went along, I have been able to reconstruct very accurately the changes in my attitudes throughout the whole dreadful business. Without them, I am certain I would have suppressed a great deal.

Everything—the first panicky terror at finding the lump, the confusion and conflicting points of view about what to do, the inaccuracy of the diagnostic techniques available, the ignorance of the average doctor, who nevertheless is sure he knows everything, and, finally, the subtle but sudden switch in my thinking during that first bull session in my room at Roswell Park—all is inscribed not only in my memory but also on paper.

The two days after my admission were busy with preoperative tests and X-rays, to let Dr. Dao know if I was an eligible candidate for mastectomy. Everyone was rooting for me, and when the good word finally came, Betty, Larry, some of the other patients, and I had a wild evening over a pint of Scotch (permission requested and granted). Who would have thought, just a few days earlier, that I would be celebrating the prospect of losing my breast?

There were other moments, not of jolly celebration. Frequently I would realize I was cuddling my left breast as if to say a last good-bye. On the weekend prior to the surgery, I was given permission to leave the hospital, and Harvey and I drove to Niagara Falls, which neither of us had ever seen. The gaudy, honky-tonk Wonder of the World was filled with people old and young who had come to see the spectacle, and often I found myself looking at some particularly ugly, grotesque, or obnoxious woman and thinking bitterly, enviously, "Why me and not her?" It was not a nice thought to have.

I was so ashamed of myself for having it that I am sure my mind would have blanked it out if it had not been written down at least a dozen times, in different notes. Later, when I began interviewing postmastectomy patients, I found this jealousy was not unique to me; everyone had felt it at one time or another. And everyone had been ashamed, too, and had never mentioned it, even to husbands, friends, or close relatives.

The questionnaires and telephone conversations taught me how wrong my ideas had been about other aspects of breast cancer. For example, I had automatically assumed that younger women—especially unmarried ones—would be hardest hit psychologically by the loss of a breast. My poll said this was a false assumption, but, on the other hand, only eight younger women responded, while about thirty older ones did. According to the responses I got, older women who are widowed or divorced suffer far more, and even the older married ones have greater problems adjusting—particularly those whose husbands are going elsewhere for sexual solace.

Of the eight premenopausal unmarried women I interviewed (please remember, a biased sample of well-adjusted women), *none* spoke of any problems with sex after mastectomy. One wrote that—while she was already engaged before the surgery, and her fiancé had not been disturbed by it—she had been unsure she would be attractive to a new man. To test her appeal, she invited an "admirer" to her apartment. Apparently, he was not at all fazed by her single-breastedness, for, she wrote, her self-confidence was completely restored.

My first encounter with the special difficulties of a postmeno-pausal widowed or divorced woman came the night of that tele-vision program. "It's easy for you to sit up there in front of a television camera and tell everybody the important thing is that cancer is fatal, and that losing a breast and sex come second," an anonymous caller reprimanded me over the telephone. "You're married, you said the 'baby' of your family was almost sixteen, and you had more than a week between the biopsy and the operation to get adjusted to the idea. You're really nobody to talk."

My caller was very angry and, of course, rightly so. It was easy for me to say what I said five months after the shock of the mastectomy was behind me. But she had more on her mind than the television program.

"I'm sorry if it got you upset—" I tried to apologize.

"I'm not upset. I'm just mad. Are you old enough to remember the movie *King's Row?*"

"I even read the book."

"Do you remember that scene when Ronald Reagan woke up and began screaming to Ann Sheridan, 'Where's the rest of me?' "

"Yes," I replied. "I even remember that Claude Rains was the doctor."

"Well, that's exactly how I felt and exactly what I yelled when I woke up in the recovery room and found myself wrapped tight

in bandages," she said. "The doctor had told me all I would have
was a Band-Aid and that I didn't even have to cancel a dinner
party I had planned for that night."

"He never told you he might have to do a mastectomy?"

"No, absolutely not. Never! The word cancer was never mentioned. He said it was a cyst and that it ought to come out—
that's all."

Poor woman. "What kind of surgery did you have?" I asked her.

"What else? The bad one—the kind that cut all the way into
my armpit and left my rib bones sticking through the skin like
spikes. That didn't happen to you."

"Are you having trouble with your husband because of it?"
I asked gently.

"That bastard!" she spat. "We were separated almost a year
before the operation. I called him afterward and asked if he would
mail some checks for me and go up to Bowdoin to tell our boy,
so he wouldn't have to hear about it first over the telephone. He
told me that when the judge gave me custody, he gave me custody, and I'd have to take care of everything myself. He's re-
married now, and his new wife is pregnant. Imagine!" She almost
moaned with pain. "A fifty-eight-year-old man able to get a
twenty-six-year-old wife and starting a whole new family. If the
situation was reversed . . . but it wouldn't ever happen."

"I'm sure you'll be able to find somebody—"

"Oh, sure, I'll be able to get somebody else, with a chest like
this," she cried. "Who would want to look at me now? If I had it
to do over again, I would do what you did—sign the paper only
for the biopsy. But if the verdict came back that it was cancer,"
she said angrily, "I would take my chances."

What could I say? I had had so many advantages. I could not
imagine going through the long ordeal without a loving, reassur-
ing husband to hang on to, to have at my side all the time, and,
in addition to his emotional support, to do chores like filling out
hospital admission forms, getting airplane tickets, and managing
general logistics. How had she managed? Now, apparently, she
felt alienated from everyone because of the mastectomy. "It really
isn't that important how you look if someone loves you, is it?"
I said.

Her voice became harder. "Sweetheart," she said evenly, "it's different if you already have someone who loves you. Then it probably doesn't matter. But I'm fifty-five years old and have no one in sight. Getting someone new to love me at my age would have been hard enough." She laughed, almost a cackle. "Look at my ex-husband, getting a woman less than half his age. Have you ever heard of that happening with a woman, unless she's rich or something? I've never been a beauty. Now I'm completely shot." She began to sob and could not finish the conversation. I heard the receiver quietly put back into its cradle.

I cannot adequately convey the psychological trauma mastectomy must be to these women. I could think of little to say to those I spoke with, except that men need a lot of educating about the unimportance of a missing breast. I can only record the problems of these women, so that they will know they are not alone. For—extrapolating from my unscientific sample of the luckier, well-adjusted women—there must be thousands in this cruel situation.

Young unmarried women were also upset and shaken, but, according to my poll, were third from the top in the degree of severity. However, I did receive only eight responses; such a small number can hardly be typical. There is more trouble smoldering quietly than these examples indicate. With the eight I interviewed, the major complaint was the extent of the surgery and the fact that they were not offered any choice. (All were free of disease, as far as they knew.)

"I probably would not have taken any chances with my life," one twenty-nine-year-old secretary told me. "I'm positive I would have agreed to the mastectomy. I'm not so uptight about having two breasts that I would have risked dying of cancer." A sharp edge came into her voice. "But I feel I was duped. The surgeon didn't mention even the remote possibility of needing a mastectomy before the biopsy. He told me later that the odds were so much against it, because I was under thirty, he was surprised at the diagnosis himself. But he did a Halsted," she continued, "and never mentioned any other operation. I didn't know there was another kind until the publicity in the newspapers after Betty Ford's mastectomy. The s.o.b. never said he could have saved my muscles." Now she sounded very angry. "Athletics have always been the big thing in my life, ever since I was a little kid," she explained. "And tennis has been sport number one for me. It took me months to get that arm back, and it still isn't as good as it was."

She paused. "After I read about the modified radical Happy Rockefeller had, I called the surgeon and gave him hell. He tricked me, pure and simple. There are no two ways about it."

As I have said, I was surprised to discover that young married women were not as horrified by the loss of a breast as postmenopausal married women, whose youth and sexual attractiveness have begun to fade (or so they think). These women are far more vulnerable to psychological problems, because they tend to have emotional troubles at this time of life even without the loss of a breast. Their children may no longer be living at home; husbands may show little concern for their wives. Then the pain and strain of breast cancer and mastectomy are added.

The emotional condition of the older married women seemed to depend on the status of their marriages. If their relationships with their husbands had been rocky—if he had been adventuring around, or was a "workaholic" who was never at home—losing a breast was a more severe psychological jolt than for women who had good marriages.

"It's just one more thing to keep him away from me," a very wealthy fifty-eight-year-old woman told me. While she had no financial worries and was still covered by the security blanket of her husband's name, social status, and reputation, she did not have him. "He's alway traveling or working overtime," she complained. "And when he is home, he's upstairs in his office with that briefcase. This awful scar is just another reason for him to want his own bedroom."

Psychiatrists assure me that the mastectomy is not the problem here, and seldom is when divorce follows soon after the surgery. "Those marriages were on the skids long before," they agree. "The mastectomy was only an excuse to get out of a situation that was already bad." Without exception, none of the psychiatrists or other physicians I talked to knows of a sound marriage that has been destroyed because the wife had a mastectomy. Other problems, especially work and other women, have probably already shaken the marriage. To these older wives, losing the breast meant losing any chance they might otherwise have had to reattract their errant husbands.

An interesting sidelight is that none of the young married women I heard from had any worries about other women. "They're secure in the inherent sexuality of youth itself," a psychiatrist explained. "They have enough sexuality not to fear their men will go away because a piece of themselves had to be removed."

Young women with good marriages seemed to have few problems adapting to the silicone gel in their future. They were primarily worried about having cancer and being incapacitated. "Who would take care of the kids if I had to go in and out of the hospital for treatments?" one thirty-four-year-old mother of seven asked. "My mother is dead, and my husband's mother can't manage even two of 'em, much less the whole brood. That's my main worry, the kids and dying, not losing a breast." None of the young married women I interviewed had considered removing only the lump, even for a moment. "I've got four kids to worry about," one explained realistically. "They need a mother, not a second breast."

One young married woman had to have a second mastectomy the year after her first. She told me—though I did not believe her until she explained—that she had been delighted! "My real ones were so enormous." She laughed. "Before my first mastectomy, I could never wear a store-bought dress from the racks. The top of me was size 44, and the bottom a size 10. I spent my whole adult life in skirts and blouses, except for a couple of things I had custom-tailored." She grimaced. "I even had to have the blouses altered, because the shoulders of the size 44 reached my elbows. My own sewing ability stops at buttons, and I had to pay a dressmaker to take darts in the shoulders of everything I owned. When I had to buy my first prosthesis, I had trouble finding one big enough to match my right breast. And I had to wear a horrible surgical brassiere, with thick straps that dug into my shoulders. Now," she continued, "I'm a perfect 34B—just what I've always wanted to be."

Older women who had never been married seemed to have the least emotional trouble getting used to having only one breast. Their major concern, like that of the young married women, was over having a possibly fatal disease. They usually had a large circle of friends, who rallied around to give aid and comfort, and also had maintained close ties with relatives. But all the responses I had, written or telephoned, showed they were terrified that the cancer might not have been stopped.

"Taking the breast off didn't bother me at all," a retired school-teacher told me. "But I'm sixty-seven, and I've had so many friends, now, go through with the mastectomy and die anyhow. So many of my friends over the years. That's what I am really most frightened of." Such women have long ago made their adjustments to living alone, and the mastectomy seems to have little effect on their attitudes, except for the fear of cancer itself. The schoolteacher explained her feelings. "Maybe I'd think differently if I were thirty, or even forty, but at my age the fuss they're calling the breast-cancer controversy makes no sense at all."

Wise woman.

It was very different with the women who were still hoping to find someone to occupy the empty side of their double beds. Suddenly, with the sharp precision of a surgeon's scalpel, they saw their hopes for catching another man slashed away.

All the women who had not known they would have mastectomies complained about the absence of information before they were wheeled into the operating room, although most seemed to have rationalized it by the time I talked to them. "I was furious with the doctor then and there," one woman told me. "But it would have had to happen anyhow. This way, I got it over with in one operation instead of going through it twice. Now I'm glad I didn't have all that worry and aggravation in advance."

Everyone who had had the Halsted radical mastectomy said she would have chosen the modified radical had she been asked. "I'm just sorry it wasn't invented fourteen years ago," one woman said, smiling. "But I guess that's true with everything in medicine, isn't it?"

Actually, the modified radical mastectomy was "invented" as long ago as 1900, when Cleveland's Dr. George Crile, Sr., and some courageous colleagues challenged Halsted's routine removal of the pectoral muscles. Thirty years later, in England, Mr. David Patey introduced a similar operation. In most countries, the

Halsted has virtually been abolished in favor of some kind of modified radical mastectomy.

As I said earlier, all the women who complained about disfigurement or the loss of a breast were among those who had not suffered recurrences or metastases. Such women made up about three-fourths of my poll, and the biopsy, mastectomy, and associated psychological shocks were the main themes of their conversations. The one-fourth who had developed new cancers did not mention the original surgery at all unless I brought it up, and then they were usually vague about the details.

So, in terms of age and marital status, the women who took the mastectomy hardest were, according to my poll, in their fifties or older and were either widowed or divorced. Their desire to ignore the tumor completely, to have only the tumor removed, to have a lumpectomy or partial mastectomy, or to investigate plastic-surgery procedures was greater than I found in any other group I interviewed—although I must repeat that I think this is a reflection of the bias of my responses.

Second on the list of badly adjusted postmastectomy respondents were the older women whose husbands paid little attention to them, for various reasons (usually the suspected reason was another woman). All but one of these had passed the menopause or were going through it, and all had grown children who no longer needed a mother's care and attention. Most of the children were gone from home entirely; five women still had children living at home, commuting to college or working. For this group, finding a cancer in the breast had been an additional emotional shock at a time when their womanliness and motherliness were at an end.

The third most affected group, my sample indicated, were premenopausal unmarried women. None of the eight responses I received reported any differences in "self-esteem," "self-worth," or "inherent sexuality"—to use the psychiatric jargon. While I would like to believe this is universal, I'm afraid the statistical odds are against it.

Premenopausal married women (most in my poll had young children) were most concerned over dying and leaving their children motherless. As far as their marriages and their husbands' attitudes toward the mastectomy, all replied that the experience had brought them closer than before. Older women who had never been married were similarly most affected by their fears of the cancer itself, the pain, and possible imminent death.

Returning to the five separate stages of emotional trauma that accompany mastectomy, as I said earlier, the first phase begins the moment a lump is found. The woman will behave in one of four ways. She might make an appointment immediately with her doctor; unfortunately (at least, until the fall of 1974), this has not been common. She might watch the lump and hope it goes away; many of these women finally do go to a doctor, but often a cancer has been spreading during the "watching" interval. A third group acknowledges the presence of the lump, but, instead of going to a doctor, resorts to prayer, faith healers, or a variety of superstitious, nonsensical cures like rubbing it with a raw potato or parsnip which is then buried. The fourth group simply suppresses all thought of the lump. Somehow or other, this mental trick can be so successful that a woman may actually be incapable of feeling the tumor!

Doctors hope the examples set by Betty Ford and Happy Rockefeller will change these delaying actions. It is too soon to know, yet, if the rush to early-detection centers will be permanent or only temporary—no more than a statistical hook in the breast-cancer incidence curve.

The second phase of psychological anxiety begins when the doctor confirms that something may be wrong and orders further tests. Dr. Edward Lewison, of the Johns Hopkins breast-cancer clinic, deals with this psychological anxiety in a sensitively written textbook for doctors. Aware that two of every ten women wheeled into an operating room for a simple twenty-minute operation will awake some hours later to find themselves plugged with drains, he insists that surgeons must take the time to warn every woman, in advance, of the possibility of mastectomy and prepare her to face it.

While Dr. Lewison prefers to combine the surgical biopsy with the mastectomy in a single procedure, he admits that the prospect of breast loss may be one of the reasons women procrastinate before submitting to the diagnostic procedure. Therefore, he would agree to separate the two for a patient psychologically unable to agree to a biopsy because of the possibility of waking up an amputee.

Most surgeons in the United States follow neither of Dr. Lewison's suggestions.

Of course, the one-stage procedure does have the virtue of eliminating the third phase of psychological trauma—the time between a definitive diagnosis of carcinoma via a separate biopsy and the mastectomy itself. By combining them, surgeons spare their patients these few additional days of anxiety. But how many women avoid the earlier anxiety by never going to the doctor at all, because biopsy is virtually synonymous with mastectomy in their minds?

The fourth traumatic phase comes immediately upon awakening from the anesthesia and finding the breast gone. While I knew in advance this was going to happen, the utter and absolute totality of the amputation was still a chilling shock. It is impossible for me even to try to imagine what it must be like for women with no advance knowledge.

All the problems discussed earlier in this chapter constitute the fifth phase of postmastectomy psychoemotional problems. My poll, however, cannot and must not be taken as an accurate summary of the psychological troubles that follow a mastectomy. Few of the poorly adjusted women responded, but I did receive some replies. One, for example, admitted changing her life style drastically because of the mastectomy. "If this may be my last five years," she wisecracked, "I'm entitled to live it up." She had gone on a wild shopping spree and, along with an expensive wardrobe, had bought a fur coat—none of which her family could afford. She had also gone alone on a Caribbean cruise. "I don't care if I do leave debts behind me," she insisted. "He'll be alive, after I'm in the ground, to work and pay them off. I don't want another woman spending my money later when I'm doing without now."

But she was an exception in her bitterness about her husband and her worries about a possible successor. She was, by the way, one of the women referred to me by a psychiatrist, one who had already been in treatment when the cancer was discovered.

The major symptoms of disturbance I found in my poll were

relatively minor from a psychiatric point of view. Primarily, these were intense bitterness that it had happened at all ("Why me?"), a deep jealousy of women with two healthy breasts, rage at the surgeon for mutilation later found to be unnecessary, and fury about poor follow-up care that resulted in not finding recurrences and metastases until these were far advanced. If these can legitimately be called "disturbances."

By and large, even these were muted, however. Except, of course, for the women with metastatic disease, almost all my respondents had accepted their mastectomies—mutilating or not—and had found that the surgery made little difference in their lives. Their main problem was worry about the future. But even here there were rationalization, resignation, and reconciliation. The general philosophy (my own, too, I should add) seemed to be: "You never know when your number's up. I could walk out and get hit by a car in front of my house."

Because I am an insider and know very well that I have changed many of my ways, I knew the right questions to ask about what changes others had made. (These, by the way, were not on the written questionnaire. I was afraid that too many answers to write might mean no response at all from many women.)

"Haven't you found that you have reordered your priorities?" I began. "Isn't it less important now whether the beds are made every day than it was before?"

"Well, when you put it that way, I guess I have changed," one mother of five told me. "I was always after the kids to do this and that, or not do this and that, and now I sort of let it all pass me by. In the end, what difference does it make if they spill juice on the floor or get fingerprints on the wall? The house will be here long after I'm gone."

"Do you feel as if you want to go places and see things now that you might have postponed, even if it means borrowing money?" The answers to this question seemed to be related to the family's standard of living.

"Well, my husband and I did talk about going to Scandinavia someday," one thirty-two-year-old told me. "But we were going to wait till the kids were old enough to really appreciate traveling. Then, after the mastectomy, we decided what the hell. So

we packed them up and went last summer. The doctor told me I
had six positive nodes, and there is a very good chance I might
develop another cancer within the next few years." She laughed.
"But we didn't really borrow. We did the whole trip with credit
cards."

Women who had no yearning to travel to other countries did
admit they were visiting relatives or taking holidays and vacations more frequently.

To my surprise, I discovered that the United States is not the
only breast-conscious country in the world. On the basis of my
tour abroad, I think Sweden outranks us, and even in the Soviet
Union women are very reluctant to lose their breasts, although
perhaps for a different reason. The Intourist guides for my group,
for example, were young women, and I asked them how they
would feel about having a mastectomy. They said their reactions
would be not so much sexual as maternal.

"When I was growing up," one told me, "a woman's breasts
were a symbol of fertility and motherliness. This is not important
in big cities like Moscow and Leningrad, but if I return to my
home town, it would be a real reason for hiding such an operation." She explained that centuries of superstition, folklore, and
mythology might tag single-breasted women as freaks in rural
areas. Also, she added, cancer itself is highly feared in the
countryside as something unnatural, as a disease that might be
"catching."

In the oncology institutes of Moscow and Leningrad, I learned
that *no* cancer patients are ever told the disease for which they
are being treated. The oncologists deleted the word cancer even
in our discussions; it was always mammary carcinoma.

"But what do you tell a woman when she has her breast removed nowadays?" I asked. "Even in the country, women must
know that breasts are removed only for cancer."

"I do not know what they think," Professor Melnikov, in Leningrad, said. "I know only that in the Soviet Union the word cancer
is never mentioned, by doctor, patient, or family. If a woman
suspects it is a mammary carcinoma, she will not speak of it."

Since the plaque on the wall of the hospital clearly said INSTI-
TUTE OF ONCOLOGY, I wondered what the patients thought they

were there for. On the other hand, I also know how people can block, suppress, repress, and lie to themselves. At Roswell Park, I spoke with several patients who hastened to tell me they were not being treated for cancer, that their presence in the hospital was a dreadful mistake. This trick of the human mind may well be the reason the word cancer can so easily be avoided in the Soviet Union.

In Sweden's Karolinska Institute, Dr. Westerberg told me that the Breast Clinic had once conducted a psychological experiment to ascertain how Swedish women felt about mastectomy. Dr. Jerzy Einhorn, the chief of the Breast Section, had agreed to the survey, although confident it would show sensible Swedish women to be more concerned about the disease than about preserving the organ intact.

"Dr. Einhorn was shocked," Dr. Westerberg said, "and he said so repeatedly. He was shocked to discover that almost all the women were very much afraid of losing the breast and wished to do whatever possible to preserve it." She laughed. "He was indeed very, very surprised."

Dr. Westerberg explained the procedure. As women came into the clinic, they were asked if they could spare the time to meet with a psychologist and several other women for about an hour a week to discuss their attitudes about the loss of a breast. But the sample, planned to be random and consecutive (the first hundred women who came into the clinic, regardless of age, marital status, and other factors), could not be done as planned. Many worked, had large families, or for other reasons could not participate. So all the women involved in the survey were those who were relatively free of other cares. Nonetheless, Dr. Westerberg feels it was a good enough sampling to give the psychologist an idea of how Swedish women felt about mastectomy.

"As I said, Dr. Einhorn was shocked to learn that almost all the women would do anything to avoid it." A lovely example of Swedish womanhood herself, Dr. Westerberg chuckled again at Dr. Einhorn's astonishment. "As a matter of fact, one of the most difficult cases I can recall was persuading a very attractive woman of about fifty-five or sixty that she should not risk a simple removal of the lump. She was divorced and had a fiancé who would, she was quite certain, leave her if she underwent a mastectomy. Ultimately, I was able to persuade her that life was more important than her breast or the man, but it was very, very difficult to do so." Again, as in my sample, an older unmarried woman was most resistant.

At the Royal Marsden Cancer Hospital, in London, and the Royal Infirmary in Edinburgh, there was no language barrier, and I was able to talk directly to patients. Four women I interviewed were still bandaged, carrying their drains in little knitting bags. All had known in advance they had cancer, and all were primarily worried about whether the disease had been stopped by the surgery. None was concerned about the lost breast, and all said their husbands had been more tender and attentive since they became ill than they had ever been before in their years of married life.

And that brings us to sex. Apologetically on the written questionnaire, and even more apologetically over the telephone, I asked if there were any before-and-after differences. Women who had good marriages said the surgery had brought them and their husbands even closer. "It's a subtle change that I can't put into words," one woman explained. "But the difference is for the better. We have never enjoyed each other so much."

One caller confided over the telephone that she was a member of the rare breed whose nipples are so generously endowed with erotic nerve endings that kissing and caressing them can produce an orgasm. "I've gotten so used to that," she laughed, "I'm not sure I'd be able to enjoy sex without it."

"Well, you still have one," I reminded her.

"I know, and as long as I've got it, I'm okay," she said. "But what in the world will I do if I have to have another mastectomy? I think I'd lose my mind."

As for my own psychological feelings after the mastectomy, I seem to be typical of the premenopausal married women with older children. While the idea of leaving them motherless is not as poignant in our case as it is where young children are involved, none of us want to die without seeing our children into full adulthood, married, and happy in their work. Many women, including me, would like to be around to baby-sit with their grandchildren.

I confess that I did not let Harvey see the incision immediately.

Because I'm a small person and do not have much skin to spare, Dr. Dao had pulled the edges of the cut area very tightly together so that I would not need a skin graft. The immediate postoperative appearance of the incision was a puckered, ugly slit—like a fiery red shirred seam, not a pretty sight. Even I had trouble looking at it without flinching. In a few months, though, new skin grew, and the repelling wrinkles disappeared. I stopped being shy. But there was no blare of trumpets, like Salome shedding her seventh wisp of cloth. I was in the tub, and Harvey came in to get something from the medicine cabinet. That was that.

He probably misses my left breast just as I sometimes miss his once thick head of curly hair. When we were first married, I wore a 36D bra, and he broke a comb in his thatch every week. Neither of us is the same as we were twenty-four years ago.

One woman described her husband's attitude beautifully and eloquently on the questionnaire. "My husband is now, if possible, more tender and loving than he ever was before," she wrote. "Our love life has a brand-new dimension that wasn't there until I had the mastectomy. It's as if he suddenly realized that I was something very precious that he almost—and could still—lose. This feeling of being 'cherished' like something very valuable, a treasure, is what has been added to our love." If I were asked properly about my love life, that would be my answer as well.

Immediately after surgery, I had other problems, although these pale to insignificance in comparison with some I have been told about. Nonetheless, they were (some still are) serious to me. The first one I encountered, after coming home, was living with—enduring—the doom and gloom of friends and relatives. Many came through the door and immediately burst into tears. Men treated me as if I were a fragile, very delicate piece of rare Meissen porcelain, or a vase from the Ming dynasty, to be handled with great care. I could not reach for a Kleenex without having six people jump to get it for me. At first it was funny, then tedious, and finally oppressive.

During the spring, my daughter, Lesley (who planned to work every summer after that one), had persuaded me to rent a beach apartment for her, one of her friends, and me for this last free vacation. When I became ill, I called the landlord and explained my predicament. "If you can rent it at this late date, I'd appreciate it," I said. "If you can't, I'll honor the contract." Luckily, it had not been rented. The week after returning from Buffalo, I was finished with all the tea and sympathy. I called my daughter's friend's mother, extended the invitation to include her, and we packed off for two weeks on an ocean beach. Between sessions of the House Judiciary Committee's impeachment hearings, I began to assemble my notes.

The surgery had had an immediate impact, by the way, on Lesley. A few days after the operation, the same friend's mother had called me in Buffalo. "Lesley doesn't think you're telling her the truth," she said. "She's scared about your having cancer and is sure the reason Harvey hasn't brought her to Buffalo to see you is that things are worse than you and he are saying."

The reason no one except Harvey had come to Buffalo was pure practicality. But as soon as I put down the telephone we decided Lesley had to fly up. We also brought Todd from Cambridge (where he had a summer job in a chemistry lab). I had called our older son, Gantt, a rock-and-roll musician then playing in a Denver club, to assure him that the only difference was a little more flat-chestedness, which he would probably not even notice. He was twenty-two then and did not frighten easily. He seemed to take it well. Once Lesley and Todd came to Buffalo, went with us to Niagara Falls, and we had a little time together, both were confident nothing was being withheld from them. They were also reassured by Dr. Dao's explanation of what had been done to their mother and why.

Remembering to include older children in their parents' problems at such a time, I found, is important for *their* psychological well-being. Having lost both my parents when I was young, I had sometimes worried that my children would have secret fears of my dying early, too. What could I do to reassure them? The only route I could see was to be open and candid, and answer every question.

After a week or so at the beach, Lesley got so used to protecting my left arm from bumps and flying Frisbees that it became an automatic reflex. Later, after I had begun the research for this book, I heard her tell Harvey that she was "sick and tired of hearing about breast cancer night and day. I wish she'd finish and get on another subject." What had been a horror word just a few months before had become a subject, like manic-depression, Tay-Sachs disease, and some of my other total-immersion projects.

Both boys were and are, at least outwardly, adjusted to having a mother with breast cancer. Todd calls or comes home with the latest immunological data on the disease from MIT labs. Gantt, back from Denver now, is very matter-of-fact about it. As he put it once, "So when did I ever have a well-balanced mother?"

As for my feelings about still being attractive to other men, it has never occurred to me to wonder about my appeal to anyone other than Harvey. I am not sure if this is because I am sedately married and older, or because I have been too busy since my surgery to think about other men. To find out, I would have to experiment with an admirer, as my respondent did, and the idea does not appeal to me or to Harvey—even for the sake of science. But I have had a couple of experiences since my mastectomy that have shaken me into thinking that my attitude about my desirability may have changed. Someday I will have to analyze these episodes.

When I was in Moscow, in December 1974, an American businessman, quite attractive and much younger than I, invited me to dinner. I had already eaten, with the group I was traveling with, and so I told him no. He tried to change my mind, arguing that our dinner had been meager (it was not) and that I would be hungry again in a few hours. But it had been a long day, and I still had work to do before I could crawl into my fluffy featherbed and go to sleep. "No, thanks." I smiled gratefully. "I've got too much to do."

Then we met again in the elevator and discovered we were both on the seventeenth floor, only two rooms apart. He had told me he had been away from his wife almost two months, and now he made a remark about the convenience of our locations, but I pretended not to hear. Suddenly, fleetingly, a picture flashed into my mind. What would his reaction be, I giggled inwardly, if I invited him in, whipped off my bra, and confronted him with the still blazing scar where he expected a breast? It was only a momentary thought, leaving as quickly as it came. But it may be significant to a psychiatrist.

One change that I know would be tagged as significant is a strange feeling of being "protected" by the mastectomy.

In Stockholm, I was fast asleep one night when there was a knock at my door. "Who is it?" I asked, completely unafraid.

"Jeemee." I could hear him trying to jiggle the lock to open the door.

"Jimmy who?" I called, still totally unpanicked.

"Italian Jeemee," he said, in heavily accented English.

"I don't know any Italian Jimmy," I answered.

He went away.

In my travels as a free-lance writer I have had a number of similar nocturnal visitors. Apparently it is customary for Jimmys to watch hotel lobbies for single women and call on them later in the night. Always before I had been petrified, but not this time! Again, the same thought had flown across my mind. Suppose I had opened the door and pulled off my long, baggy thermal nightgown? What would his reaction have been? Would he have fainted? Would he have screamed with shock and run away?

I hope all this does not mean I no longer consider myself worthy of seduction. Quite honestly, I don't know. I only know there *is* some difference in the way I now react. None of the women I interviewed mentioned similar feelings of being "protected" from unsolicited ardor, by the way. On the other hand, I didn't ask.

From my 130 interviews, I discovered that my experience was not a typical one, from the very beginning. For example, because I have been a medical writer for a long time, I can understand doctors' jargon and can read "the literature" without its being simplified in the popular press. Also, I had the advantage of being ten minutes away from two of the finest medical libraries in the country—the National Library of Medicine and the library of the National Institutes of Health. Most women do not have either piece of good luck. They must rely on their doctors to explain. The word most of my respondents used to describe their feelings was "helpless." One said she "suddenly became a shivering bit of jello who followed my surgeon like a toddler following mommy on the first day of nursery school." And, of course, I knew in advance that I would have a mastectomy. Only one of the women in my poll was so well prepared for the shock.

As I have stressed, I knew of no way to contact women who refused to have a mastectomy at all and chose to risk death instead. Nor did I find a way to reach those who will not bare their bosoms to a prosthesis fitter. And, of course, many women did not call or return their questionnaires. Psychiatric patients referred to me had problems totally unrelated to the mastectomy, although the surgery had made these troubles more difficult for them to manage. All I know about the thousands of unreachable women is that they *are* there, suffering secretly, only occasionally becoming ill enough to need serious psychiatric help.

A report published in April 1975 by the National Cancer Institute says there are about 677,000 women living in the United States with a known history of breast cancer. Yet the number I found accounted for by either Reach to Recovery, psychiatrists' records, or news articles cited 300,000 to 350,000 at most. What has happened to the rest of the 677,000 women? Are they suffering—secretly and silently?

Yes. And their suffering is known. A January 1975 report in the *American Journal of Psychiatry*, "Psychoemotional Aspects of Mastectomy," lists twenty-two different studies in its bibliography—not enough really to examine the psychological troubles, but certainly enough to signal their widespread presence.

The *American Journal of Psychiatry* article gives a faint glimmer of what is going on in the minds of unreachable women. According to the author, Michael J. Asken, only a few think in terms of having a potentially fatal disease (remember, these are women who are written about in psychiatric journals). "While mastectomy performs a gratifying service by saving a woman's life," he says, "her appreciation is muted by the price she must pay for that service—the loss of a breast and permanent disfigurement. Within the value system of American society, that price is a considerable one."

Asken refers to "mastectomized women" and calls their anxiety and depression "psychological morbidity." On his anxiety scale, their fear of death ranks below "concern over sexual desirability, interpersonal and sexual relations, and, if the woman is married, dangers to her marriage." She feels herself to be "untouchable,"

Asken says, and fears that she did something at some time to cause the cancer.

Looking for someone or something to blame is not confined to women in psychiatric journals, however. I have spent many hours wondering what I have done or taken or been exposed to that might have caused the cancer. My suspects have ranged from estrogens to our microwave oven and the color TV. One of the psychiatrists who was helping me said his patients usually blamed people, not things. They often blamed themselves and felt the cancer was a retribution for past sins. Other disturbed patients blamed husbands, children, or others. In holding things responsible, I assume I am in comparatively good mental health.

Another point Asken makes in his article is the effect of the woman's personal psychiatric problems on the rest of her family. She is apt to feel less feminine, less sexy, ugly, and so on, and to pass this drop in self-esteem along to her husband and children. Asken calls it a "distorted self view as a person unworthy and unable to re-adapt to her normal role." Her husband, of course, cannot help her, and he begins to feel guilty because of this failure. The same pattern occurs with the children, possibly showing up in their schoolwork. Life at home is hell, husband and children walking on eggs whenever the mother is nearby. She, in turn, considers their behavior to be rejection, and the circle goes around again, aggravated.

Much effort is being expended on ways to reconstruct the breasts by plastic surgery as one way of preventing the more severe postmastectomy psychological states. When this is not feasible, for either financial or medical reasons, many psychiatrists are urging that postoperative counseling be done routinely, on an individual basis or in group therapy. Psychiatrists would like more co-operation from surgeons, Asken writes, but "the surgical role presents practical problems that inhibit the surgeon's ability to respond as a palliative psychological agent. Heavy caseloads and demands of surgery preclude the establishment of more than a fleeting relationship." It is kind of Asken to forgive surgeons on our behalf. I am afraid I cannot share his sympathetic viewpoint.

The article in the *Journal* ends with words that are a fitting end for this chapter as well: "To save a woman by surgical intervention and then deny her emotional support necessary to form a different life style and accept an altered body image is a contradiction in terms."

Those words should be engraved in every surgeon's office, in a spot where he can never miss seeing them.

12

When Mastectomy Is Not Enough: Chemotherapy

About six years ago, a friend of mine was diagnosed as having cancer of the breast. She went through the usual general-hospital routine of mastectomy, ovariectomy, and weeks of intensive X-ray treatment. For almost three years, she managed to hang on to life, although she had to go through periodic, increasingly frequent stays in the hospital for "shots of cobalt."

One night Harvey and I met a mutual friend at a business party. "How's Lil?" I asked. "She sounded so bad the last time I talked to her that I've been afraid to call again."

He shook his head sadly. "She's back in the hospital. They've put her on chemotherapy. That's the last resort."

We shook our heads in agreement. "When they start using drugs," Harvey said, "I guess that's the end of the line."

Less than a decade ago, chemotherapy was the end of the line for breast-cancer patients, the last resort, in general hospitals in the United States—although the treatment was being successfully used in specialized cancer clinics and hospitals. But we have come a long way in a few years. Now, when a radical mastectomy has not stopped the disease or if many positive nodes are present in the axilla, chemotherapy has become the first resort—even in general hospitals, by general practitioners. But it took a long time for the word to filter down.

Dr. Paul Ehrlich, inventor of the "magic bullet" against syph-

ilis, was the scientist who opened the first door to cancer chemotherapy. In 1910, he proved that alkylating agents—substances
that affect DNA duplication—could destroy cancer cells. But he
thought carcinoma was caused by invaders like the infectious
organisms that run rampant in the blood stream, and he tried
to kill them in the same way—as if they were microbes that
lived separately outside healthy cells. Without the technical
know-how provided by the electron microscope, it was impossible for him to know that this theory was wrong, that malignant
diseases are not caused by the same kind of foreign invader as
syphilis and smallpox are.

The first "drugs" used to fight breast cancer were estrogens.
But it was a negative use of the female hormones. Women's
estrogen factories, their ovaries, were removed surgically. Ovariectomy, or oophorectomy, was not considered chemotherapy (and
it still is not, by most doctors and patients). But decreasing
the level of estrogens by removing their producers is as much
chemo- a therapy as giving a drug like androgen—the male hormone—to neutralize the female hormones in the blood stream.
Accurately, therefore, the age of chemotherapy for breast cancer
began in 1896, when Sir George Beatson discovered that removing the ovaries sometimes retarded or even regressed the
progress of the malignant disease. This operation became a
routine postmastectomy procedure, but it was done empirically—
no one knew why it worked. The results were unpredictable.
Some women improved; some did not.

The work done by the University of Chicago's Dr. Charles
Huggins, a 1966 Nobel laureate in medicine, provided a clue
regarding the unpredictability. He wondered why some young
women whose ovaries had been surgically removed still had
enough estrogens in their bodies that they continued to have
menstrual periods. His research showed that the adrenal glands
also produced female hormones, and he suggested these, too, be
removed, by adrenalectomy, in breast-cancer patients who developed recurrences or metastases after mastectomy.

As the years passed, it was found that many women did not
respond at all to the surgical estrogen manipulation. The theory
—now a known fact—evolved that not all breast cancers are
stimulated by estrogens, that is, not all are hormone-dependent,

and only the definitely hormone-dependent tumors are affected by surgical removal of the ovaries.

But surgeons had no way to know in advance what kind of tumor it was, and therefore most of them, immediately after radical mastectomy, routinely performed ovariectomies on all premenopausal women with three or more positive nodes, in hopes of preventing recurrences or metastases. However, many breast-cancer specialists began to feel the procedure should be held in reserve until a metastasis or recurrence actually appeared. Their reasoning was that if the ovaries were removed then and the second tumor's growth was retarded by the operation, this would be an indicator that the cancer was hormone-dependent and that the patient would probably benefit from adrenalectomy, too. On the other hand, if the tumor showed no signs of being affected by ovariectomy, there was no point in removing the adrenal glands.

Today, in those specialized cancer hospitals and clinics that can do hormone assays of a tumor as soon as it is removed, surgeons know its nature within a few days of the mastectomy. Where this is not possible, they must still make decisions about whether and when to perform ovariectomies according to guess-work.

Often, however, even ovariectomy plus adrenalectomy did not reduce the estrogen in the blood stream to zero. The pituitary gland, deep inside the brain, still continued to release another hormone, prolactin, which scientists knew was important in the growth and nourishment of a breast cancer in the presence of estrogens. But, at that time, they did not understand how or why, since this hormone is always present in a woman's body and is secreted in very large quantities after childbirth to trigger milk production. Yet lactating women, even with their elevated pro-lactin levels, rarely develop breast cancer. Because of this contradiction, scientists theorized that there must be some kind of blocking factor in a woman's system during breast feeding, an inhibitor that prevents prolactin from causing neoplasms to occur.

In addition, scientists think there is an extraglandular mechanism in many cells of a woman's body that produces estrogens. This means that such cells are themselves minuscule hormone factories, manufacturing and releasing estrogens into the system independent of the pituitary gland. Going one step further, some investigators, notably Dr. deWaard, in the Netherlands, think that all cells have the same capability to manufacture estrogens. This is the foundation of his theory that tall as well as obese women, because they have so many more cells in their bodies, have a much higher risk of developing breast cancer.

Until the extraglandular concept was theorized, many experts felt that a breast-cancer victim's pituitary gland should be removed, by an operation called a hypophysectomy. However, this requires major cranial surgery—a very considerable risk. And, anyhow, an extraglandular system would not be affected by removal of the pituitary. There had to be another way. The most obvious alternative was to prescribe androgens—male hormones—in the hope that they would counteract the effects of the estrogens. These helped in only about 20 per cent of breast-cancer patients, not enough to make the treatment routine.

Meanwhile, however, scientists discovered that, while hormonal manipulation improved about one-third of all breast-cancer patients, it was totally useless in another one-third, and the remaining third responded unpredictably. Only recently have researchers developed the technical know-how to find out why. All breast cells (and those of the other female organs) contain bits of protein called estrogen, or hormone, receptors. As blood circulates within the breast, estrogens from it filter through the membranes of the cells and attach, or bind, to the receptors. Naturally, the more receptors a cell has, the more estrogens will remain locked tightly to the receptor molecules. This explains why some tumors are more hormone-dependent than others; their cells have more receptors and therefore get and retain more estrogens from the blood. (The binding mechanism, and its variability from woman to woman, also explains why the monthly cyclical changes of estrogen secretion affect women differently.)

Within the last few years, the technical know-how has developed to analyze newly excised tumors for their hormone dependency—the hormone assay. This examination, when it has been done, has prevented many unnecessary ovariectomies, since there is no reason to send a young woman into a sudden, precipitous artificial menopause if her tumor is hormone-independent. Unfortunately, the technical expertise required to evaluate hormone dependency is available in only a few specialized cancer hospitals and clinics in the United States. When the assay cannot be done, urinalyses, vaginal smears, and certain blood tests can give estimates of estrogen levels. Unless they know how badly a cancer needs estrogens for its nourishment, surgeons still have no alternative but to cut out the ovaries of premenopausal women when second cancers develop.

At the Royal Infirmary in Edinburgh, I spoke with biochemists who—using complex equipment and techniques—have developed a sugary concoction to trap estrogen receptors. On the basis of their experiments, they have concluded that *all* breast cancers are hormone-dependent to a greater or lesser degree when the tumors are young. Thus, in their opinion, ovariectomy would help every woman with early breast cancer. These results are not definitive or widely accepted, but they are apparently solid enough to have convinced the biochemists of the Royal Infirmary. "If my wife developed a breast cancer," one of them told me, "I would not hesitate for a second before asking that her ovaries be excised."

Some women with breast cancer improve when they are given additional estrogens. Others respond to hormones like cortisone and prednisone, a type of cortisone. Some specialists say these steroid hormones help improve breast cancer because they suppress the production of estrogen by the adrenal glands, a theory that would be true for premenopausal women. Others think that postmenopausal patients are helped because the steroids are somehow converted into estrogens by the body.

The contradictory actions of steroids on breast cancer in the two age groups are added support for the view that there are two different kinds of the disease, depending on age.

It must be remembered that hormone therapy—like any therapy —must be tailored to the specific situation. Because one woman did well on androgens, estrogens, or prednisone does not mean someone else will benefit, too. But women who regularly add large quantities of estrogens to their systems should think about their hormone receptors. To me, these are red, flashing stoplights.

Learning about the role of hormones and estrogen receptors in the breast was not to be the end of the hormone story, just

another clue. Even women who improved after ovariectomy ultimately reached a point at which their cancers grew at about the
same rate as those in women who did not have the operation.
Such clinical evidence, plus laboratory data from animal experiments, showed that all breast cancers eventually become auton-
omous—hormone-independent. This would account for the many
cases in which breast cancers regress after the ovaries and
adrenal glands are removed, only to begin thriving again later.
Thus, even with strongly hormone-dependent tumors, estrogen
manipulation was not enough, and the search for "something
else" continued.

Basing their experiments on Dr. Ehrlich's original ideas about
alkylating agents, pharmacologists began to test drug after drug,
hoping to find one that would destroy malignant cells with minimal side effects. The major discovery grew, as I have said, out
of war, and the development of nitrogen mustard as a biological-
warfare weapon. In 1946, scientists discovered that mustards
shrank cancerous tumors in mice. Then, in 1948, it was found that
leukemia victims were helped by the first of the antimetabolites
—aminopterine.

Everything on earth has probably been tested at one time or
another for its effect on cancer. Certainly, few substances have
not been used on animals, to see if they can destroy the cancer
without also killing the host. Unfortunately, most that are effective are so lethal they fail this critical test. Going back to the
analogy of cancer and the war in Vietnam, the "medicine" we
gave that country to fight off its malignant insurgency was too
strong to attack only the invaders. B-52 bombers, massive artil-
lery, napalm, and defoliants were too random and indiscriminate
to hit just the "enemy"; hundreds of thousands of helpless, in-
nocent Vietnamese were killed or wounded as well. In the end,
the body was destroyed by the medicine.

There are, however, about thirty deadly drugs that have been
found safe to use in small doses in cancer treatment. Of these, a
dozen or so are effective against different breast cancers. So, in
addition to hormones of one kind or another, our pharmacopoeia
now includes alkylating agents, antimetabolites, mitotic inhibitors,
antibiotics, enzymes, and miscellaneous "random synthetics."

Most of the drugs that affect cancer cells either stop cell reproduction altogether or kill the malignant cells during that one vulnerable time, the period when the DNA molecules are twinning—the only time most scientists believe healthy cells can become malignant. I stress that to show the vital importance of timing in the use of any anticancer weapon.

The alkylating drugs widely used now on breast cancer include phenylalanine mustard (L-PAM, Alkeran) and cyclophosphamide (cytoxan). Thio TEPA, once a popular alkylating agent, is no longer used much in the United States, although I found it was still prescribed in some of the European countries I visited. All are cell poisons, whose molecules have many electrons that attach themselves easily and quickly to various substances inside the cancer cell. Alkylating agents act so much like radiation that they are often called radiomimetic agents—radiation imitators. Their effectiveness stems from the fact that malignant cells twin so much more frequently than the normal cells around the tumor that they can be killed more rapidly. Drugs can get to the tumor without affecting as much healthy tissue as X-rays do, and therefore quite potent drugs can be used to treat breast cancer without *as much danger* of causing other cancers elsewhere. There *is* danger, however; no anticancer agent is safe.

In a telephone conversation with Dr. Bernard Fisher regarding the National Cancer Institute's trials of L-PAM, he told me of having received calls and letters from doctors all over the country who "wanted to know where they could get the drug." He sounded annoyed, as if it were the exaggerated media coverage of his announcement that had caused all the trouble. Then he remarked that it was nothing for pharmacies to dispense as they do aspirin, since the compound was still under clinical trial. This made me curious to see what potent anticancer alkylating drugs are available on drugstore shelves. While no pharmacist I called stocked L-PAM, other mustards are generally available, by prescription, to be taken orally or in solutions to be injected by any physician.

The second most popular group of drugs used for breast cancer is the antimetabolites. Methotrexate and 5-fluorouracil (5-FU) are the most common. These are "Trojan horses"—counterfeiters that sneak inside a cell's membrane disguised as nutrients and "fool" the cell into using them. Since they are fake foods, they cause a massive indigestion that interferes with DNA duplication and either kills or sterilizes the cell. These drugs destroy healthy cells as well, if they are in the process of division. Thus the anti-metabolites are also potentially lethal and should be given only by cancer experts. The physicians' label (patients do not see it) says of 5-FU, for example: "It is recommended that FLUOROURACIL be given only by or under the supervision of a qualified physician who is experienced in cancer chemotherapy and who is well versed in the use of potent antimetabolites." This paragraph is set off from the rest of the material on the instruction sheets by a box and is labeled "Warning," in boldface type.

Random calls to several local pharmacies told me the warning is being ignored. "Most of our 5-FU supplies go to general practitioners and some internists," one pharmacist told me. "As far as I know, the specialized chemotherapists work out of hospitals, and we wouldn't be filling their orders in drugstores." A second pharmacist told me cytoxan (an alkylating agent) and metho-trexate (another antimetabolite) were also popular items with general practitioners. "They want to take care of the patients as long as they can, I guess," a third explained. "Then they send them to specialists." Sales of all such anticancer drugs, I was told, were "very good." Yet both alkylating agents and anti-metabolites are so potentially dangerous that expert chemothera-pists often interrupt their administration with an antidote drug to halt cellular destruction after a certain interval.

Another way to attack a cancer cell is simply to prevent it from beginning to split. The substances that do this are the mitotic inhibitors (from mitosis, or cell division). Two descendents of the common periwinkle plant, vinblastina sulfate (Velban) and vincristine sulfate (Oncovin), are such drugs. By preventing mitosis, these substances sterilize the cancer cell, but they do not necessarily kill it. Therefore, the tumor may not grow much more, but neither will it shrink, as cancers do when their cells are destroyed. For this reason, and because many women cannot tolerate their toxic side effects, the mitotic inhibitors are not used for breast cancer as frequently as the other drugs.

A fairly new and very potent tumorcidal antibiotic—adriamycin

—was approved for general use about five years ago. Since then, it has been shown to be remarkably effective against a large number of tumors that were among the most stubbornly resistant to chemotherapy, and these include advanced breast cancers. "Until the advent of adriamycin," said Dr. Stephen Carter, acting deputy director of the Division of Cancer Treatment at the National Cancer Institute, "these malignancies had been considered almost totally unresponsive to chemotherapy."

NCI experts recommend that adriamycin be given in a "chicken soup" formula (explained later). But, unlike most of the other drugs, it can also be given as a single course of treatment for breast cancer if radical mastectomy shows that more than three axillary nodes were invaded. One advantage in this is that a single injection can be given every three weeks on an outpatient basis, instead of the multiple injections requiring several days of hospitalization every month or six weeks, as is the case with other drug therapy, properly administered.

But there is nothing good in cancer therapy that is without some bad side effects. Adriamycin can cause cardiovascular problems, and a weekly blood test and monthly electrocardiogram must accompany treatment. Moreover, chemotherapists recommend that the drug not be given more than nine times, at three-week intervals—a period of just over six months. The only patient I interviewed who had been given adriamycin verified its "spectacular effect" on her disease. However, she told me sadly, as soon as the six months were up—she had no cardiac complications and completed the course of treatment—she relapsed and was soon back where she had been before taking the new drug, then experimental. (I reminded her she did get six pain-free months from adriamycin—no small benefit.)

She had also told me the adriamycin was given to her as a single agent. According to Dr. Carter and Dr. Paul Carbone, also of NCI, as well as other experts in cancer chemotherapy, adriamycin is far more effective when combined with cyclophosphamide and 5-FU. The dosages have not yet been worked out with precision, but Dr. Carbone said the drug has "given higher rates of partial and complete responses and improved survival times" when combined with other anticancer agents.

The toxicity—harmful or uncomfortable side effects—of all

known anticancer weapons is a major medical problem. It obviously does no good to stop a tumor from spreading if the patient must spend most of her time plugged into intravenous contraptions in a hospital or bald, vomiting, and feverish at home. But toxicity is only one of the problems encountered in chemotherapy. For reasons that are not really understood, most patients become less and less sensitive to a particular drug as time goes on, and eventually a point is reached at which a formerly effective drug does no good.

How do doctors know when this happens? One of the best ways is to ask the patient how she feels. When a drug is working, the patient can usually tell the difference before any test results do. In addition, scans, blood tests, urinalyses, and even manual examinations, in the case of certain tumors, can indicate progress or lack of it. These objective tests are also needed when a drug's side effects are so severe that the patient feels worse even though there has been improvement in her cancer. The usual procedure, when there is no improvement as measured by the tests, is to switch to another drug.

Because of the severe toxicity of large doses of anticancer drugs, as well as the temporary nature of their effectiveness, specialists not long ago were facing an impenetrable stone wall. One part of this wall is the problem of timing. To do its lethal work, a tumorcidal drug must attack a malignant cell while its DNA molecule is twinning. But single doses of single drugs can injure only a relatively few malignant cells at a time. Simple arithmetic indicated that a broader spectrum of drugs, each having a different toxicity and *modus operandi,* would have a greater impact than single drugs used one at a time, and another approach in breast-cancer chemotherapy was developed.

The answer turned out to be the "chicken soup" recipe: a combination of drugs that would work either simultaneously or sequentially, drugs with different side effects, different lengths of effective time, and different routes of attack.

The idea evolved from a study of chemotherapies used on children with leukemia. At the National Cancer Institute, in the 1950s, clinical trials had shown that smaller doses of several drugs used together or in sequence were better than a single drug in a larger dose given alone. New data regarding the importance of hitting the cancer cell precisely when its chromosomes are twinning added to the arguments in support of this multimodal approach.

In the clinical trials with the young leukemia victims, the chicken-soup attack worked. Several drugs were given in smaller doses—some together, some in sequence—and an unexpected number of the children improved. If the technique was successful with leukemia, why not with breast cancer? Dr. Carbone, a top chemotherapist at NCI, set three criteria a drug must meet to be considered as an ingredient in a breast-cancer chicken soup.

1. It must be an effective anticancer agent by itself. In larger doses, each drug in the "soup" must be able to kill cancer without help from any other agent.

2. There must be no overlapping toxicities; that is, no two drugs whose major side effects—liver damage, for example—are the same can be included. This is essential to prevent the possibility of one drug's compounding the toxicity of another.

3. All drugs must be able to do their killing job on an intermittent or interrupted basis, so that continuous administration will not be required. The patient must have time between doses to permit her body to recoup and regain strength.

Several chicken-soup recipes are currently going through clinical trials in cancer centers around the country. The preliminary—*preliminary!*—results are encouraging. Fewer and more easily tolerated side effects are being reported, and patients are living more comfortable lives—not always the case when a single drug is given in large doses. (Adriamycin taken alone is apparently an exception. The cardiovascular side effects of large doses of this drug, when they occur, seem to show up in tests but not in the way the woman feels.)

The drugs most frequently used in the chicken-soup trials are simultaneous or sequential combinations of methotrexate, 5-FU, and cytoxan. Combinations of other drugs are being evaluated, as well. Recipes will undoubtedly be changed as new substances are developed and proven effective. Adriamycin, for example, is now being added in many cancer clinics and hospitals.

Women who suffer from metastatic disease of breast cancer can be treated by ordinary intravenous injections. But usually chemotherapy is given by infusion. The drugs are slowly dripped into a vein and travel through the system for several hours or even days, depending on the extent of disease. Certain modifications can supply more of the drug to a particular area, if necessary, by means of a pump that pushes a continuous, uniform flow to the tumor. As I said earlier, when large doses are used, it is often necessary to minimize toxicity by giving an antagonist, or antidote, to counter the side effects. This is most often done with antimetabolites like methotrexate or 5-FU.

The drug L-PAM requires no injection at all. It is a tablet, taken by mouth, once a day for five days every six weeks. Phenylalanine mustard, L-PAM's real name, is currently undergoing controlled clinical trials in thirty-seven institutions around the country. A relative of nitrogen mustard, it would be a boon to breast-cancer patients if the good results (dramatic in premenopausal women) of the first two years of trial stand the test of time. In addition to the advantage of oral administration, L-PAM seems to have fewer side effects than other anticancer agents. According to the first reports, L-PAM does not cause the baldness or severe gastrointestinal upsets associated with other drugs.

The development of this anticancer drug is an excellent illustration of a very touchy and difficult medical problem. How are new chemotherapeutic agents to be tested in humans? On September 30, 1974, Dr. Bernard Fisher, at an international conference at the National Cancer Institute, gave a preliminary report on L-PAM's effectiveness after two years of trial. The study involved 250 women, all having positive axillary nodes. They were divided into premenopausal and postmenopausal groups, and half in each group were given the drug, the other half a placebo. It was a double-blind study—neither the women nor their doctors knew who was getting what. When the "code" was broken, a difference was seen in the recurrence rates of the women who had received L-PAM and those given the placebo. The impact was greatest in the premenopausal group, although older women also had fewer recurrences.

Immediately a great hue and cry was raised in the press, a storm of criticism about the medical ethics of such a study. Those poor, persecuted women who were given the placebo had recurrences because they fell into certain slots in random studies, the critics charged, while the lucky women who accidentally fell into the L-PAM slots benefited at the expense of their less lucky trial mates. I have been told (but have not been able to verify) that several of the women in the placebo slots have threatened lawsuits against NCI, despite having given their informed consent and having been told all the details of the clinical trial before it began.

Of course, no one knew for two long years that L-PAM would have such successful results. The outcome could just as easily have been the opposite: the persecuted victims could have been those who got the drug, not the placebo. For that matter, the real results are still not known, and will not be for years. It is possible that the women receiving L-PAM will have harmful long-term effects the others will escape.

No one who has read this far can believe I am an apologist for the medical profession. Nor am I unaware of the fraudulent ways by which informed consent often is and has been obtained in medical trials in various institutions in the United States. However, three women who had been involved in various breast-cancer clinical trials were among the respondents to my questionnaire, and all of them spoke of the great pains taken and the time consumed to explain every facet of the study they were participating in. (I must add that all were at NCI and were describing what was done in only this institution.)

Still, there are limits to how informed any woman's consent may really be, no matter how clearly the details are told.

"What are they giving you?" I asked one patient, five months after her mastectomy.

"I don't know," she said. "All I know is that I'm B."

A double-blind study, I thought. Naturally, she would not know what she was getting. "Are you getting pills or shots?"

"Pills. I take them a couple days every six weeks."

"How many nodes did you have?"

"What are nodes?"

"Didn't they tell you what nodes are?" I asked.

There was a momentary silence. "Now that you mention it, the word sounds familiar. I guess they told me all about that the day I signed the papers."

"What was in the papers?"

"Oh, I really didn't read it all," she said. "The social worker, or whoever she is, told me what was in it."

"What did she say?"

"She told me they don't think they got all my cancer out. That's where I guess that word you said—what is it, now?—came into the talking. And she said if I wanted I could be taken care of at the Cancer Institute for nothing."

"Is that all she said?"

"No." The patient continued. "She told me that I would be taking a brand-new medicine—I didn't know then I'd be B—and there'd be three other kinds of medicines compared with what I was getting. I guess they're A, C, and D."

"Did she explain anything else?"

"She said I didn't have to do it if I didn't want to, if that's what you're driving at. But I talked it over with my husband and daughter, and we decided that as long as it wasn't going to cost me anything, and I had cancer anyhow, I might as well do whatever I could to help somebody else."

She paused. "The social worker did tell me that nobody knows anything much right now, so the medicine they're giving me is as good, or could even be better than the stuff they're giving the other three women." Again she paused. "She said it could get worse, too. It's a chance I'm taking, and I know it. All I can do is hope that the B pill is the best pill."

This is probably typical of the attitude of women involved in clinical trials. I know I would feel the same way. So much is unknown about the treatment of breast cancer that it is almost like flipping a coin. Unfortunately, to be a guinea pig, in the hope that whatever is being used in a specific medication will be the best the "state of the art" has to offer, is sometimes the only choice a woman can make.

Certainly clinical trials are the only way specialists will learn which are the most effective drugs against breast cancer. The point comes when animals can no longer be used for testing, and the first trials must begin on humans. If this is not done, no drug will ever be found.

Reporters' outraged outbursts and letters to the editor that I have read protesting the "ethics" of clinical trials leave me cold.

These people are complaining in the abstract. They themselves are not faced with the helpless horror of a disease that is destroying their bodies while doctors know of nothing that will stop it. It is easy to complain about ethics in the abstract; I have done it myself often enough. But abstract is abstract. When a patient with cancer is faced with inevitable death unless something is done, and doctors want to use an untried and unproven drug, in the hope it will help, the situation becomes very concrete.

I can say this because I would do it myself, and at this stage my consent is very informed. If there had not been other L-PAMs in the past thirty years, chemotherapy would still be languishing back in the ranks of last resorts, instead of being up front where it is and should be—the most promising hope for curing breast cancer on the horizon today.

All the chemotherapeutic agents and techniques I have described are used on women who have recurrences or metastatic disease, or who had three or more positive axillary nodes and therefore have a high risk of developing another cancer. But what about those who, like me, were staged at $T_1N_0M_0$? No nodal involvement was seen during my surgery, and Dr. Dao and the pathologist feel the cancer was confined only to my breast, yet the dreadful "end results" show that women like me are not at all immune to developing new cancers. During my interviews with mastectomy patients, I learned that many who later developed recurrences or metastases also had had only negative nodes at the time of their surgeries. Is there no safe drug for us?

Unfortunately, no. Every drug now known to be effective against cancer, including L-PAM, has some possibly serious side effects. L-PAM, for example, has caused certain blood disorders in mice that did not show up until a long time (in a mouse's life) after the drug was discontinued. If it is certain, or very likely, that a woman will develop an early recurrence of cancer, then the benefits of taking a drug having possible long-term harmful effects must be weighed against the high short-term risk of a new cancer. In a benefit-risk situation like this, it might make sense to risk perhaps developing leukemia in fifteen or twenty years, instead of facing almost certain death from breast cancer in five or ten.

But no responsible doctor will prescribe such a drug for a

patient who shows no sign of being so high a risk. The best
sign doctors now have is the number of positive axillary lymph
nodes found during a radical mastectomy. If three or more nodes
were malignant, the woman is known to be a high-risk candidate
for another cancer. Having fewer than three positive nodes re-
duces the risk considerably. But even when all the nodes are
negative, the risk does not drop to zero.

It is a difficult doctor's dilemma, according to Dr. Dao. He
feels—and I assume his views represent those of his colleagues
—that he cannot give a potentially harmful drug unless he has
good reason to think the cancer will spread. "In your case, for
example," he told me, "you have almost a 90-per-cent chance of
being cured. How can I give you something that might cause
trouble? And besides, if you did not get a recurrence, I would
still not know if it was the drug that had prevented it, or if you
would not have gotten one anyhow. Giving you any kind of a
preventative agent at this point would not prove anything at all,
and might be harmful to you."

He said that most breast-cancer specialists do feel women
with negative nodes might benefit from something given immediately after surgery to prevent a recurrence. But how could
such a drug be tested? As Dr. Dao pointed out, negative-nodes
patients have relatively few recurrences or metastases anyhow,
and it would be impossible to know with scientific certainty
whether it was the drug that had prevented them. And, of
course, there is the worry about unknown, possibly serious
long-term aftereffects. So, while almost all the experts I talked
to thought it would be a good idea to give a woman with negative
nodes a prophylactic drug of some kind, they had too many
good reasons for not doing so.

In the European cancer centers I visited, by the way, the
same drugs as are used here are known and in use. To my surprise, in Leningrad I learned that Professor V. M. Dilman, an
endocrinologist, has been testing certain neurological drugs as
breast-cancer treatments. One is L-Dopa (L-3,4 dihydroxyphenyl-
alanine), a medication used to control Parkinson's disease, and
another is dilantin, an antiepileptic medication. Neither has
effected a cure, but Professor Dilman told me he had had some

success in relieving pain and reducing the size of breast tumors. The professor said he thought the reason these drugs have such effects is that both inhibit the secretion of prolactin, the female hormone that is to a cancer cell what gasoline is to a fire. If these drugs and others like them help breast-cancer patients, while other mind-bending drugs, like reserpine (a tranquilizer before it became a reducer of high blood pressure) and chlorpromazine, prove harmful, a whole new Pandora's box in breast-cancer drug treatment would open up.

The reason is that L-Dopa and dilantin work through the hypothalamus, the part of the brain that governs emotions, such as anger, fear, sexual drive, and who knows what else? If the hypothalamus should be an important factor in the development of breast cancer, that might well mean psychological factors are involved in the cause of the disease.

Often, in my research, I had stumbled across references to the role of stress and the influence of many of the same adrenal hormones that are known to be involved in certain psychiatric disorders. Dr. Lawrence Le Shan and Dr. Richard Worthington, two California psychotherapists associated with UCLA, began to study the personality patterns and life histories of cancer patients as long ago as the early 1950s. During the first five years, about 450 patients were tested and interviewed. Dr. Le Shan found that 72 per cent of his subjects had personality problems and life-history patterns that were apparent in only 10 per cent of a control group without cancer. The cancer patients had a great deal of "psychic pain"—repressed anger, loneliness, hopelessness, self-hatred, rejection.

It is known that the hypothalamus controls a woman's hormonal secretions and therefore has an effect on her breast tissue. Since the emotions are also hypothalamically controlled, a possible interplay of the hormones—or antagonisms between them—resulting from emotional upsets and stress may be involved in the development of breast cancer.

Some doctors I have discussed this with feel that Dr. Le Shan's research harks back to the medieval "black bile" theory of cancer—that there is an association between neurotically depressed women and breast cancer (melancholia equals an excess of black bile). Psychiatrists I spoke with invariably thought the idea made sense, but physiologically oriented doctors scoffed at Dr. Le Shan's conclusions.

Nonetheless, the theory could be true. It is well established that many hormones in the body influence the emotions and that these same hypothalamically controlled substances—the adrenal gland's steroids, for instance—interact with other hormones to cause physical changes and disease. Not enough is yet known about the roles hormones play to be able to say that they have nothing to do with cancer—especially breast cancer.

In the past, no matter how Freudian they were, psychoanalysts usually were cautious about suggesting that cancer could be a psychosomatic ailment. The evidence incriminating the hypothalamus may make this attitude ancient history.

What a field day psychoanalysts will have if a definite link is ever forged between the emotions and breast cancer!

13

When Mastectomy Is Not Enough: Radiotherapy and Immunotherapy

RADIOTHERAPY

"Would it be accurate to say that X-ray treatment has absolutely no place in managing breast cancer after a radical mastectomy?" Again I was calling Dr. Gerald Johnston, the chief of Nuclear Medicine of the Clinical Center of the National Institutes of Health.

"Let's have that again?"

I repeated the question.

He pondered it for a moment or two. "This is for the record, isn't it?"

"Yes," I told him. "You're a top authority in the best United States research center. What you say would be a definitive quote to end all quotes."

"Hmm. That means I have to be very, very careful." He laughed. "You did say treatment, not diagnosis, didn't you?"

"Treatment," I repeated. "I know mammograms are X-rays, and I know they have to be done for diagnosis."

"And you're only referring to a primary breast cancer after a radical mastectomy? I do think X-ray therapy has a place as a palliative in metastatic disease."

"No, I don't mean X-rays to kill pain," I explained. "I'm asking about the prophylactic drying-up X-ray treatments women are given even after they've had all their axillary nodes cut out."

Another short silence. "I think, then, it is an accurate statement to make. No radiation treatments for primary localized breast cancer are justified after radical mastectomy, under any circumstances."

"Suppose there is a sign that the cancer has spread to a couple of spots in the bones?" I pressed. "Would you recommend X-ray treatments for those places?"

"If there is any sign of bone metastasis, the patient should be put on drug therapy immediately—not X-ray, except to alleviate pain," he answered quickly. There was no pondering silence about this answer.

"So you would not advocate post-radical-mastectomy X-ray therapy at any time for any reason except to relieve pain?" I repeated the question, to be positive I had not misunderstood his reply.

"You can quote me as saying I think all radiotherapy in the postoperative treatment of all cancer will be as obsolete as the buggy whip someday. In breast-cancer treatment, after a radical mastectomy, it already is obsolete—except as a painkiller."

Dr. Johnston said that this is his personal opinion, which is shared by many oncologists, but that some do feel radiotherapy —not drugs—is the treatment of choice for spots of cancer on the bones and for invasion of the internal mammary chain (the nodes along the breastbone under the ribs) and the supraclavicular nodes (at the base of the throat). "I think that once the bone and these nodes are involved," Dr. Johnston told me, "the disease is probably systemic—in other places in the body. That's why I feel chemotherapy is indicated in these cases. But that's just an opinion at this time. There's nothing proven one way or the other yet."

"But postmastectomy prophylactic irradiation is still routine after radical mastectomy in most hospitals in the country, isn't it?" I asked. "Even if all the nodes are negative . . ."

He sighed. "Well, we sit here in our ivory tower in Bethesda, outside Washington, and plot the ideal. It takes a while for the word to filter down. Sometimes it take a pretty long while. There's nothing we can do about that."

NIH research, by the way, is being done, with NIH funding, in institutions all over the United States, and in many other

countries as well. The results are reported to Bethesda and disseminated by publications, conferences, seminars, and various
"outreach" programs. But physicians and surgeons cannot be
force-fed information. So, unfortunately, Dr. Johnston was absolutely right: it can take years for news to "filter down." In addition, under the law that created them, the National Institutes of
Health can only "report the results of research." The most au-
thoritative medical research center in the country may *not* recommend specific kinds of treatment. All it can do is disseminate
results of research and hope they are read by the average family doctor. As far as postradical prophylactic X-ray therapy for
breast cancer is concerned, the word has been sifting with the
speed of a snail.

I had called Dr. Johnston for that telephone interview early
one morning. Not long after, I spoke to a woman who had undergone a radical mastectomy four and a half years before. I began
my ritual questioning. When I reached the query about postmastectomy X-ray, she told me she had had about twenty "shots
of cobalt."

"Did you have a *radical* mastectomy?" I asked. I had to explain that radical means removal of the nodes in the armpit, as
well as the breast itself. Her surgeon had given her no details.

"All I know is the doctor said he took everything out," she
replied.

"Did he tell you whether he found the cancer had spread into
your lymph nodes?"

"All he told me was he was sure he got everything out."

"Then why did he give you X-ray treatments?"

"Is anything wrong with it?" she asked. "He stopped my
monthly periods with X-ray, too. Was that all right?"

"He X-rayed your ovaries?" I could not believe this was still
being done. However, I learned afterward that many physicians
do prefer to destroy ovarian function with X-ray, rather than
surgery. Medical opinion is divided, because some doctors feel
the three needed radiation treatments are more comfortable for
the patient. Others believe the possible unknown aftereffects of
X-ray are potentially dangerous and that surgical removal is
safer—if less comfortable initially.

"But was it all right?" she repeated.

"You've gone more than four years now," I told her cheerfully. "That's a very good sign it was okay." However, I cautioned her to watch for and report certain symptoms.

She sighed and seemed relieved. "I guess new information will keep coming out to show what was done years ago was not the best," she said. "It's been almost five years since my operation, in 1970," she continued. "I'm sure they've learned a lot since then."

In 1946, a medical report, "The Role of Roentgen Therapy in Carcinoma of the Breast," said that, although X-ray treatments might slow local nearby recurrences, metastases to other, often distant, organs occurred more frequently in irradiated women. X-ray had no effect whatever on the ultimate progress of the disease in either group of women; their survival rates were the same.

For the next fifteen years, scientists all over the world continued to compare the recurrence, metastatic, and survival rates of women with breast cancer who had been given postoperative X-ray therapy after a radical mastectomy with the rates of those who had not. All age groups and stages of the disease were studied. The general opinion was that the increased incidence of metastases to other organs after irradiation made postoperative X-ray therapy risky when the axillary nodes had been removed. Preventing recurrences did not warrant the risk, because new local tumors could be treated surgically. On the other hand, metastases might occur far from the original tumor site and thus not be found until too late. This was the opinion of many specialists by the early 1960s.

X-ray was discovered in 1895 by Wilhelm Conrad Roentgen, who was awarded the Nobel Prize in physics in 1901 for this work. Doctors soon found that the invisible force could harm external body tissues while it was photographing the bones inside—and also harm their own bodies while they were taking the films. Scientists studying cancer immediately began to look for the quantity of irradiation that could be tolerated by normal cells, yet would damage or kill malignant tissue.

Early in this century, the precise workings of the phenomenon were not understood. Scientists knew what happened empirically, but without knowing why. They tested the effects of various time

intervals and dosages without understanding the effects the
X-rays were having on cellular operations, normal or malignant.
Only since the invention of the electron microscope have scientists learned why X-ray destroys malignant cells without killing
all the healthy ones around them.

X-rays are caused by electromagnetic waves similar to light
and heat waves. They are produced in a vacuum tube, when
speeding electrons hit a metal plate, and the depth to which
they can penetrate depends on the rate of speed at which the
electrons strike the plate. Roentgen's 1895 machine has, naturally,
been made obsolete by new technical know-how, such as the use
of certain "boosters" in linear accelerators and betatrons to increase the speed of the electrons. With their modern equipment,
radiologists can home in on a cancer more precisely, resulting in
two important advances: healthy tissue is more easily avoided;
X-rays can more safely be aimed at deep-seated organs, like the
pancreas.

X-ray destroys malignant cells by attacking them while they are
reproducing, during that vulnerable period when their DNA
molecules are twinning. Since they reproduce more frequently
than healthy cells, they have more of these vulnerable periods,
and thus more of them are destroyed. In other words, malignant
cells are more "radiosensitive" than normal ones. In addition,
some cancers are more radiosensitive than others. This is directly
related to the rapidity of cell growth.

The electron microscope was also needed to learn why X-rays
that destroyed cancer could cause it as well. It was observed
that sometimes a dose of radiation will only damage the DNA
molecule during the duplication process, without destroying the
cell. If the growth gene is the part of the molecule affected, a
healthy cell will probably become a malignant one.

To kill a cancer cell, the dosage of X-ray given must be enormous. Diagnostic X-rays, on the other hand, use relatively tiny
doses. A chest X-ray gives an exposure of about one-tenth of a
rad; a set of mammograms, about four rads, two to each breast.
X-ray and radioactive irradiation (whose unit of measurement is
the rem) both have effects on living tissues that are cumulative,
that is, they build up over long periods of time. For example, two
rads given daily for six months can have the same effect as a

single dose of 360 rads. Ignorance of radiation's cumulative effect explains why, in the earliest days of experimentation. many scientists working with X-ray developed cancer. Even today, no one knows the maximum dose that can be absorbed without harm.

Palliative radiotherapy exposes the patient to a few hundred rads. A therapeutic dose for breast cancer, as administered in cancer clinics or centers where simple (or total) mastectomy is followed by irradiation, can be as high as 5,000 rads. Exposure time is also longer for therapy than for diagnosis or pain relief. Malignancies are irradiated either by X-ray or by radioactive isotopes of certain chemicals. Certain cancers are more likely to be destroyed by radioactive isotopes, but for most of them X-ray treatment—radiotherapy—is the more conventional weapon.

When radiotherapists calculate how much X-ray to give a patient and what the length of exposure should be, they take into account the kind of cancer it is and where it is located in the body. A great deal of expertise is required to be certain the normal tissues around, above, or below the malignancy receive as little irradiation as possible. This is a very tricky process, and radiotherapy is not to be entrusted to anyone except a physician who has received additional training in the subspecialty of radiology. Similarly, the technicians who operate the equipment should be specially trained. Therapeutic radiotherapy is far more complex than diagnostic radiology (mammograms or X-rays to find bone fractures) and a technician who is trained only to snap the shutter of a sophisticated camera has no business giving X-ray treatments to cancer patients.

Some kinds of cancer cannot be destroyed by any dose of X-ray that would not also be lethal to surrounding normal tissues. These are radioresistant, as opposed to radiosensitive, and X-ray therapy is ineffective against them. Muscle, heart, and nerve cells, for example, never duplicate. However, these nonreproducing cells are often overlaid by cancers metastasizing from other organs. They may also develop primary cancers arising from neighboring cells that do reproduce—that is, are *not* nerve, muscle, or heart cells *per se*. The radiosensitivity of these cancers would be that of the cells constituting the tumor, and such cancers might, therefore, benefit from X-ray. Cells that divide rapidly— those of the intestines, blood, bone marrow, skin, and hair—are the most radiosensitive because their DNA molecules are constantly twinning. Since they are so fast-growing, their healthy cells are easily damaged during radiotherapy. This explains why the first side effects of X-ray treatment are usually intestinal upsets, reduction of white blood cells, peeling skin, and baldness.

Not all the cancer cells in a tumor will be in the twinning stage at the same time. Only those in the process of splitting will be affected by an X-ray treatment, and therefore only a small percentage of the cancer cells are destroyed during a single therapy session. Timing is as important in radiotherapy as it is in all cancer therapies.

Some tumors may be so deep in the body that even the most modern X-ray equipment has difficulty penetrating to them without harming organs in between, or harming the skin. X-ray equipment is always being improved, however, and so are exposure techniques. It is now possible to treat some deep internal cancers with very high-intensity rays, which can be focused more directly on the tumor. Also, the patient can be rotated during therapy, so that the same healthy organs are not always exposed. A technique called crossfiring prevents the same healthy tissue from being bombarded repeatedly; rays are aimed at the tumor's site from various angles.

Most breast cancers are relatively slow-growing. But this virtue also means that most of them are relatively radioresistant. On a ranking of thirteen cancers in descending order of radiosensitivity, breast cancer was fifth from the bottom: X-ray treatments were far more effective in destroying eight other kinds of cancer. What this means is that before a mammary carcinoma is touched by radiotherapy, the fast-growing skin, blood, bone marrow, and other tissues near it are bound to have been damaged.

It would seem that this basic fact of cellular life, as soon as it was discovered, should have stopped X-ray treatment for primary breast cancer after radical mastectomy. But it did not. Prophylactic irradiation after radical mastectomy is still routine in many hospitals, by many doctors, in the United States and elsewhere.

A Dr. Emil Grubbe is credited with being the first person to treat breast cancer with X-ray, in 1896. In 1960, about a million patients later in the United States alone, a medical paper asked a question. "Now 64 years . . . later, it is established

custom to offer prophylactic radiotherapy in combination with
radical mastectomy. While continuing the custom, the question
is repeatedly raised whether this improves the results over surgery alone."

In the sixty-four years during which X-ray was routinely used
after radical mastectomy, many studies here and abroad supported the combination. The reason for the favorable results
was obvious. In those decades, a cure was defined as survival
for five years after surgery. Since X-ray after radical mastectomy
did reduce local recurrences, more women were alive after five
years. But metastatic disease can take years longer to appear.
When this time lag was finally acknowledged and survival rates
were checked again after ten years, the irradiated women did
not fare as well. There were many more skin, marrow, lung, and
liver metastases in this group than in nonirradiated women.

In 1961, the National Cancer Institute's National Surgical Adjuvant Breast Project (NSABP) began a randomized trial to
finally assess the value of postoperative radiotherapy. After almost ten years and more than 1,000 women, Dr. Bernard Fisher,
chairman of the NSABP, reported, "The survival rate of patients
receiving irradiation was slightly less than that observed in the
[nonirradiated] controls." Dr. Fisher continued. "As the result
of this study, which I consider to be the most definitive investigation yet carried out to evaluate the worth of post-operative irradiation, there seems to be no justification for its further use in
any circumstances as an adjunct to radical mastectomy in the *primary* treatment of breast cancer" (the emphasis is Dr. Fisher's).

The report was published by NCI in 1970. Reporting results,
remember, is all the institute is permitted to do. Dr. Fisher cannot
go into every hospital and force general practitioners and general surgeons to read the reports.

In 1962, Dr. Dao and an associate at Roswell Park, Dr. John
Kovaric, published an account of 354 women they had treated
postoperatively, some with radiation, some without. In 48 per
cent of the nonirradiated women, lung and skin metastases developed later; within the same period, 89 per cent of those who
had had radical mastectomies followed by irradiation developed
distant secondary cancers. The irradiated women survived the

same number of years as the others, but they suffered more bouts of cancer after their surgery.

Although the report was criticized at the time, Dr. Dao has not given X-ray therapy after radical mastectomy since 1962. And since then, there has been a growing body of data—including the NSABP's—in support of his practice. But still the X-ray habit continues around the country.

In a medical journal dated January 13, 1975, obstetricians and gynecologists in the United States were given some stunning "news" from Lausanne, Switzerland. "A Swiss investigator," the bulletin said, "reports that the routine use of local post-operative irradiation of early breast cancer should be seriously questioned. 'In the six controlled trials that have been published so far,' says Dr. Jan Stjernesward of the Swiss Institute for Experimental Cancer Research, 'survival rates were significantly lower among those women who were irradiated than among those who were treated by mastectomy alone.'" The news announcement said, "Dr. Stjernesward concludes that stopping the routine use of prophylactic local radio-therapy after radical mastectomy not only could increase the survival rate but also save resources." Perhaps having the word handed down from Switzerland will finally succeed in making doctors in this country pay attention.

Dr. Johnston has many colleagues around the world who agree that radiotherapy should not be used for breast cancer except to relieve pain. Dr. Dao uses X-ray for spots of metastatic bone cancer, as well as for palliation. But Dr. Johnston and Dr. Dao also believe in removing the axillary lymph nodes during mastectomy.

Many studies are going on in the United States on the long-term results of simple (or total) mastectomies followed by irradiation. So far, in patients whose axillary nodes were left intact and then X-rayed, the recurrence rates have been the same as for women treated by radical mastectomy, either the Halsted or the modified. Of course, it will take many more years to see if the rate of metastases is different. One controlled trial of about 1,700 closely matched women, now in its fourth year, is being conducted by NSABP. The preliminary results announced at the end of the first three years showed no difference in recurrence rates between the women who had simple (or total) mastectomy with X-ray and those who had radicals.

Several specialists here have gone even further. With patients who either refused to have mastectomies or could not tolerate the massive surgery for other reasons, they removed only the tumor and then irradiated the breast and nodes—lumpectomy followed by radiotherapy. Dr. Leonard R. Prosnitz, a Yale Medical School radiology professor, and Dr. Ira S. Goldenberg, a professor of surgery there, even reported, in early 1975, that this technique "may be more effective than mastectomy for treating early stage breast carcinoma." At about the same time, M. D. Anderson's Dr. Eleanor Montague, a professor of radiation therapy at the University of Texas, told the Radiological Society of North America that less extensive surgery followed by irradiation, in her study, had a recurrence rate of only 4 per cent, while women who had undergone radical mastectomies had recurrence rates ranging from 35 to 50 per cent.

All emphasized the very preliminary nature of their short-term results and the fact that distant metastases would take many more years to appear. Nonetheless, they felt that women who wanted to keep their breasts should have the option of trying such treatments.

Since the simple (or total) mastectomy plus irradiation is what Professor Mustakallio, Dr. McWhirter, and Professor Forrest have been doing for many years in Europe, their survival rates may prove something. Only time will tell if they are as good as those with radical mastectomy alone.

It is important to stress again that X-ray treatments after surgery in which the axillary nodes *were not removed* is different from the prophylactic radiotherapy given after radical mastectomy. When the lymph nodes are gone, there is nothing to irradiate but healthy skin, blood, bone, and other tissues. It is this kind of X-ray treatment that must be abolished—the prophylactic "drying-up" shots after radical mastectomy.

The patient is likely to remember postoperative X-ray treatments as being much worse than the mastectomy itself. All the women I interviewed who had had such treatments—some thirty-five—complained bitterly about them. None escaped side effects. They were nauseated—sometimes unable to keep anything down for days. Most were temporarily bald. The irradiated skin became red and scaly (the medical term is dry epidermis), and then the area began to "weep." Some women, I learned, also have complete paralysis of the nervous system of the shoulder region (the brachial plexus), due to the damaging of nerves by radiation. According to warnings in medical books, the risk of infection is high while undergoing radiotherapy.

In Edinburgh, Dr. Roberts assured me that a special "four-field" X-ray technique leaves few such symptoms. Perhaps. I found the morbidity following X-ray therapy to be so common in the United States that I would have to see the Scottish women with my own eyes to believe they were escaping Scot-free. If the Edinburgh method does indeed prevent the terrible after-effects of irradiation, it should be used everywhere.

X-ray can leave a woman with another appallingly morbid problem. Even if she has been spared milk arm caused by severed lymphatic vessels, the irradiation can cause lymphedema too. X-rays burn; if they are not expertly administered, some of the minuscule vessels can be sealed as if by a soldering iron. Then, as is true when any tissue is burned, the body rushes a repair crew of immunological cells to the area, via the blood stream and lymph, to help heal the damage. The fluid, trapped in the arm by the blocked lymphatic vessels, builds up and can cause severe lymphedema. Dr. Dao told me of one woman who came to him with such a bulging, gargantuan arm from post-operative irradiation (given elsewhere) that it had to be amputated to prevent gangrene.

Within the past few years, advances in immunological knowledge have added to the evidence against the use of X-ray for breast-cancer treatment. Irradiation does evil things to components of the body's immune system called T-cells, B-cells, lymphocytes, and macrophages. So, while X-rays may destroy a cancer cell or even an entire tumor, as they do this killing they may also be weakening the body's ability to fight bacteria, viruses, or other invaders. Immunology is in its infancy, and no one really knows much yet about what it signifies for cancer research. However, it is known that X-ray has a powerful effect on the immune system. Most of this information came out of the experimentation and research that preceded organ transplantation.

Before it will accept a kidney or a heart, the recipient's body must be treated with immunosuppressants that will prevent its various defense cells from rejecting the transplant. The donor organ must also be treated to make it as neutral as possible. In testing drugs and other techniques to accomplish these goals, irradiation was found to be a powerful immunosuppressant. Then it was theorized that anything strong enough to reduce the body's resistance to a strange kidney or heart might also lower its defenses against an invading cancer cell.

Theory became proof when many of the patients receiving immunosuppressants subsequently developed cancer. The Human Renal Transplant Registry of the American College of Surgeons reported that, among 629 transplant patients, the appearance of lymphoma was thirty-five times higher than in the normal population and the risk of reticulum-cell sarcomas was 350 times higher than expected. Other cancers were 2.5 times more common among transplant patients, but in men only. Often, the transplanted kidney itself became malignant. This kind of knowledge is relatively new, and more will certainly be flowing from immunological labs in the next years.

There are occasions when X-ray is useful in the treatment of breast cancer. One is palliation. Low doses of radiation help to relieve the pain of advanced metastatic disease, especially of the bone. When a patient has reached the stage where she has little chance of living much longer, it is ridiculous to worry that irradiation may cause another tumor or two. Why withhold anything that will make her more comfortable?

Another occasion is debated by experts. In the case of a breast tumor so large it has been diagnosed "inoperable," dooming the woman to die anyhow, irradiation of the breast might shrink the cancer enough for a mastectomy to be performed. While the prognosis is not good for this woman, she might perhaps gain a few more years of life. As a matter of fact, it may even be possible, in many cases, to control such cancers with irradiation alone. The decision should be left to the patient. Are the slim odds worth the ordeal?

Obviously, postoperative radiotherapy for women whose breast cancers were not stopped by mastectomy is not yet in the "buggy whip" category Dr. Johnson predicts. But it is well on the way to obsolescence.

IMMUNOTHERAPY

On December 3, 1967, Dr. Christiaan Barnard, the South African surgeon, performed the first human heart transplant in history. He removed the healthy heart of a twenty-five-year-old woman who had died after an automobile accident and put it into the chest of a fifty-five-year-old man, Lewis Washkansky. The patient appeared to do very well, and within a few days television screens around the world were showing him walking around with other patients and giving his wife a long, loving kiss. Eighteen days later, Washkansky was dead of a lung infection.

Less than a month later, on January 2, 1968, Dr. Barnard again transplanted a heart, to a man named Philip Blaiberg. This time, however, the patient was kept in isolation. There was no walking around and chatting, and no long, loving kisses. In a few short weeks, Dr. Barnard had drastically changed his postoperative procedure. What had happened?

I don't know what went on in Dr. Barnard's mind, but I suspect he got some very strong mail from immunologists who saw Washkansky visiting with germ-infested patients and kissing his bacteria-laden wife. This kind of socializing simply cannot be permitted by a patient who has been given immunosuppressants so that his body will accept a foreign organ as its own. Every immunosuppressant known weakens the body's resistance to all disease.

Most people are familiar with immunology in the form of the various vaccinations they have had all their lives. The science was born one day in 1796, when Dr. Edward Jenner scratched his son's arm with secretions from a pustule of a cow suffering from cowpox. This first vaccination immunized the boy against the smallpox epidemic then raging throughout England. In 1796, Dr. Jenner knew nothing about T-cells, B-cells, macrophages, antigens, or antibodies. But he did know that anyone who survived an attack of smallpox was somehow able to resist catching the disease again for the rest of his life. He theorized that if a person could be given a mild case of a similar disease, the protective system of the body might be fooled into conferring immunity to the more virulent disease. Medical history shows that Dr. Jenner's theory was correct.

All living things have built-in defense systems to fight off disease, and that is why life has continued on earth as long as it has. Building on this theory of bodily immunity and on the first successful smallpox vaccination, scientists have developed vaccines against many diseases that were once fatal to millions. Most of these are infectious diseases, however, which are passed from one person to another, not diseases that are caused by the kinds of carcinogenic agents suspected of causing cancer.

Dr. Paul Ehrlich, a bacteriologist by training, whose work has been a forerunner for so much cancer research, first proposed a general theory of immunity, in 1885, in Germany. He suggested that the blood stream carried antibodies—proteins manufactured by various cells—that searched for and either neutralized or destroyed bacterial invaders. He called the invaders antigens. But he and his followers worked on the assumption that cancer, like infectious diseases, was caused by a bacteriumlike parasite. So, although Dr. Ehrlich's hypothesis about the existence of an immune system was later proved correct, he and the scientists who continued his research made no progress against cancer because they were attacking it in the same way they attacked bacterial diseases. This was long before anyone suspected that a cancer virus might be something quite different—an agent that merged into the cell and disappeared entirely, except for a submicroscopic dot of chromosome.

In the years that followed, doctors found that cancer patients who developed diseases with very high fevers, like malaria and erysipelas, frequently improved considerably afterward or even had their cancers disappear entirely. Such phenomena led researchers to believe that the antibodies being produced to fight the infections were also effective against cancer. Essentially, 1896 —the year this evidence was accepted—marks the year when real research in immunology began, although adequate financial support did not come until almost seven decades later, when kidney transplantation became a surgical reality.

As was said in the discussion of irradiation, to avoid rejection of a kidney or other foreign organ, the body and the organ to be transplanted must first be treated with immunosuppressant drugs or irradiation. By suppressing the immune system artificially before surgery, instances of rejection were dramatically reduced. Then, when it was realized that a disproportionate number of kidney-transplant patients were developing cancer, scientists felt this was proof of some relationship between cancer and the immune system. More research was initiated to study the possible link, and immunology became an established branch of cancer investigation.

But what is the exact role played by the immune system? After reading reams of scientific reports and questioning many researchers, I discovered that—at least as far as breast cancer is concerned—no one really knows. There are many theories, of course, and for every theory there seems to be a countertheory. There is also much agreement, however.

The immune system is made up of the thymus gland, the spleen, bone marrow, and the regional lymph nodes, and they produce such things as T-cells (from the thymus), white corpuscles (also called leukocytes), B-cells (from bone marrow), macrophages (the Greek word for "large eater"), and lymphocytes (from the lymph nodes). There may be others, as yet unknown. In dealing with breast cancer, the most important parts of the immune system are the axillary lymph nodes and their lymphocytes.

All these are killer cells, which work in different ways as they wander through the blood stream and lymphatic system searching for and destroying foreign invaders. And all these defenders can be damaged or destroyed by X-ray and some of the anticancer drugs.

The fact that people with metastatic disease usually have live cancer cells in their blood streams that never "take" in other parts of the body has been accepted as proof that something in the body is killing them, weakening them, or otherwise preventing them from colonizing. Another piece of evidence evokes general agreement. Carcinomas induced in mice by irradiation, chemicals, or other carcinogens can be changed by various immunological manipulations of the animals' systems, and this would not be possible if the immune system played no role in cancer development.

Then there are well-documented cases of cancers that have spontaneously disappeared, without treatment (presumed miracles and superstitious cures not included). Not many, but enough to prove such phenomena do occur. Scientists feel these spontaneous remissions or regressions are due to something in the body that destroyed the tumor without outside help. Autopsy rooms have also contributed data. Often old people have been found to have cancers that were stopped at a very early stage, never spreading elsewhere. Many immunologists feel this, too, is proof that the body's defense system arrested the malignancy. Others do not—just one very minor example of the differences of immunological opinion. And there are lots of such differences.

For example, some scientists agree with Dr. Crile that removing the axillary lymph nodes during radical mastectomy is wrong and that, if left in place, these nodes will be free, once the primary tumor is gone, to kill stray bits of residual cancer or "centricles" in other parts of the breast. Other experts say the idea is nonsense, since the body has thousands of other lymph nodes, which begin working overtime to compensate for those lost in surgery. Another possible clue may be found in the cases on record where, after the original breast cancers alone were removed by surgery, there were no recurrences, with or without postoperative irradiation. While it is possible that the tumor was all the cancer present in the breast, many scientists—citing multicentricity as their reason—feel this phenomenon, too, is due to some action by the woman's defense militia. Other experts say such cases are too rare to prove anything.

Some researchers support the notion that cancer cells have tumor-specific transplantation antigens on their surfaces. If a few of these harmless particles could be kept active long enough, it is theorized, it might be possible to develop a vaccine by using them instead of potentially dangerous weak or dead cancer cells —the conventional process for making a vaccine. This theory was described to me by Dr. Ernest Plata, a virologist, who also thinks "antigen banks" could be used to store lymphocytes "educated" to attack and destroy a cancer in another person's body.

But Dr. Tibor Borsos, a National Cancer Institute immunologist, told me he thought neither idea was practical. "How can anyone know for certain that a part of a cancer cell in a vaccine is harmless?" he asked. "And who can be sure antigens injected in a healthy body would not create a breast cancer, especially if a virus is found to˙ be the cause?"

Then there is the argument that cancers occur more commonly at the two extremes of life—in the very young and the very old—when the defense system is either immature or failing. Thus, the theory says, an immunodeficient body is more vulnerable. (However, this is certainly not true of breast cancer, which attacks women in their prime, when, according to the immunological yardsticks now available, they are fully immunocompetent.) Supporters of the immunodeficiency school point out that when pieces of a malignant tumor are implanted in "nude mice" (a specially bred strain having no thymus gland, which leaves them artificially without any self-defense system), the cancers almost invariably "take" and grow. Dr. Borsos argued that this has happened only when living cancers are implanted. When the immunodeficient mice are treated with chemical carcinogens or irradiation, in doses that cause breast cancer in healthy mice, the nude animals are no more vulnerable than the others. He added that the deficiency controversy probably has nothing to do with breast cancer, anyhow, since none of the malignancies that developed in the immunosuppressed transplant patients occurred in the breast.

Another disputed point is the surveillance theory, which states that some normal body cells are always in the process of becoming malignant and that the immune system is constantly at work searching for and destroying them. If malignant cells manage to establish a colony somewhere, according to this theory, it is a sign that the defense system has been damaged. It would therefore follow that by adding certain immunoboosting drugs, the system would recover. There is also much debate about a cell-mediated immune reaction. Does each healthy cell in the body have its own ability to defend itself? Both the surveillance theory and cell-mediated immunity are being investigated intensively at this time.

Many cancer researchers believe that some malignant cells have such strong membranes that drugs cannot penetrate them. They hope that certain substances, like an enzyme called neuroaminidase, if given along with chemotherapy, will strip away whatever barrier the tough membrane imposes. Other experts I questioned put little faith in the idea, although they thought it worth investigating further.

The biggest controversy I encountered in immunology concerned the definitions of immunological deficiency and immunological competence, and what—if anything—these have to do with cancer. To a layperson, the whole subject is contradictory and confusing, to say the least. Being artificially immunosuppressed (as in the transplant cases) can trigger a cancer, yet all cancer therapy is immunosuppressant. Animals known to be immunodeficient—like those nude mice—are no more susceptible to carcinogens than other mice, while animals—including humans—with apparently fully competent immune systems can and do grow cancers. Fetal tissue, an excellent incubator for keeping cancerous tumors alive and healthy, does not develop cancer from chemical carcinogens or X-ray.

After trying to get to the bottom of the mystery by reading, I finally asked Dr. Borsos for his opinion. It was the familiar refrain of technical know-how. "As far as current tests can now measure," he told me, "we cannot evaluate a body to determine if it is fully immunologically competent." He also described several experiments in which presumably deficient animals did not develop cancer, even when it was implanted. "There is, at this time, no way to evaluate a fully immunologically deficient system, either. We simply do not know how to do this yet."

In the meantime, much of the research in immunology now is based on the assumption that a deficient immune system is helpful to cancer growth and that strengthening it somehow will be beneficial.

Using the work of Dr. Ehrlich and his followers as a foundation, scientists are giving various bacteria (BCG, a substance containing weakened tuberculosis bacilli, is the most popular now, although many others are also being tried) along with anticancer drugs, in the hope that the lymphocytes produced to fight the bacterial invaders will be fooled into attacking the cancer cells, as well. Lymphocytes are not very smart or sophisticated, apparently, because early trials using BCG have shown promising results. The bacteria do, indeed, fool the killer cells into attack.

All in all, to me immunology was the most complex and incomprehensible area of cancer research I explored. The more I learned, the more questions I had.

For example, there is evidence that some parts of the body's immunological system actually help the growth of many diseases, including cancer; somehow, the invaders are not recognized as being illegal aliens and are assisted, not attacked. Why? In experiments using human volunteers, cancerous implants have not "taken," although this transplantation technique is used regularly to grow cancers in laboratory animals of the same species. Why? The list could go on forever.

In addition, there are the conflicting and contradictory points of view held by acknowledged experts in the field. I concluded that immunology is still too new to be certain of very much, especially where cancer is concerned. The only unanimous agreement I found is that the immune system does play some role in the cause of cancer and, it is hoped, will play a role in curing the disease.

New data are constantly pouring out of laboratories all over the world. For this reason, it is impossible to give specific details about what is being done today. Anything I write may be obsolete tomorrow. Basically, immunological research is trying to answer the following questions: (1) How does the immunological system work? (2) How can a person's immunological deficiency or competence be measured? (3) Are there any drugs or other substances that can assist or boost a weak or deficient system besides bacteria, which can themselves be dangerous? These concern all diseases, not just cancer.

In cancer research, the long-term goals are some kind of safe vaccine, for prevention, and some way of strengthening the patient's immune system, for treatment. Dr. Plata's hope that harmless surface antigens can be used to deceive lymphocytes into attacking cancer is not shared by everyone, as I have indicated, and, at this stage, is purely academic, anyhow. Antigens from breast-cancer cells cannot be kept active longer than a few weeks at this time.

No immunologist I interviewed saw any light shining yet at the far-off end of the tunnel. But they are looking for it. Even marijuana researchers have found that grass has a substance—tetrahydrocannabinol—that affects the growth of breast cancer in mice. At the Medical College of Virginia, animals with mammary carcinoma who were on pot lived longer than mice in the control group. Because the substance was found to be an immunosuppressant, the scientists involved in this study concluded that the effect on the cancers had something to do with the substance's action on the immune system of the mice, rather than any direct action on the tumors themselves.

In early 1975, Dr. Ben W. Papermaster, a Galveston, Texas, biochemist and microbiologist, reported remissions in six of eight breast cancers through the use of substances called lymphokines, extracted from cultures of human lymphocytes. The culturing process is very difficult, and further advances must await advances in technical know-how. Dr. Borsos pointed out that it was only one of many such experimental studies. They may all be stabs in the dark. But who knows?

Some immunological treatments are really experimental at this time, and for this reason are given only to patients for whom all hope is lost. In Bristol, England, for example, twenty-five patients with a very malignant kind of bladder cancer had chunks of their tumors inoculated into pigs. When tests showed that the animals had developed antibodies against the malignancies, samples of their blood were injected into the patients. The doctors managing the experiment hoped that the antibodies produced by the pigs would unite with the patients' own killer cells to fight off the cancer. Of the twenty-five patients—none of whom would have lived longer than a year from the time of diagnosis—one-third were still alive after more than a year. In other cases, the bladder tumors disappeared, but the patients died of metastases already established before the pig-cell treatment. One patient was still alive two and a half years afterward.

This cross-inoculation method seemed to be most effective when combined with X-ray treatment given about six weeks after injection of the antibodies. The Bristol team was very cautious in its report and emphasized the extremely small size of the sample, but the experiment could be a milestone. If cross-inoculation using an animal as the intermediary incubator should be successful with bladder cancer, the same kind of procedure might also be useful against breast cancer.

Along the same line, some success—*very limited* success, but *some*—has been achieved in cross-transplantation of cancers. Patients with different kinds of cancer exchange bits of their tumors with each other. Where this has been tried, the immune systems have manufactured large numbers of lymphocytes, which have reacted strongly to the new, strange invaders, and the donated cancers did not "take." While the added boost of lymphocytes in the recipients' blood streams did not destroy their own tumors, there was enough improvement to convince some scientists that cross-transplantation merits further trials. Opponents fear that exchanging cancers is almost "Hitlerian."

It must be remembered that all such experiments are being done on patients with very advanced disease. As was the case ten years ago with chemotherapy, when drugs were a last resort for patients already in poor physical condition, these are not really fair trials. If people are deteriorated because of cancer—or any other disease—their immunological systems are deteriorated, too. Perhaps if such trials could be done with patients having early cancer—while they were still in good over-all physical condition—the outcome would tell us more. However, it is legally, morally, and ethically impossible to conduct such trials on the basis of what is now known.

In April 1975, it also became illegal to try new procedures on tissues from fetuses aborted after the twentieth week of pregnancy. Experts have written extensively about the valuable knowledge regarding other diseases that has been acquired from fetal research. For cancer research, such tissue is vital, because of the disease's species-specificity, which makes extrapolation from mouse to man unreliable. Fetal tissue is the *only tissue* whose reactions can be related to human cancers. For some research, twenty weeks may be enough; for other investigations, older fetuses are needed.

While I am not arguing for or against such late abortions, it is legal in the United States to terminate pregnancies until twenty-six weeks. It is incomprehensible to me—a cancer victim—that we cannot benefit from research that requires those additional six weeks. During the so-called moratorium on fetal research that followed the manslaughter conviction of Dr. Kenneth Edelin in Boston (for not having done more to save a fetus alleged to have been born alive), research in this field was halted. Even with a presidential commission's recommendation that research be resumed with fetuses less than twenty weeks old, Dr. Edelin's conviction has "chilled" hospitals and doctors all over the country, and many are refusing to perform abortions on women who have advanced pregnancies, even though the operations are perfectly legal. If this fear continues—and reports indicate it will—what will happen to the vital cancer research that depends on fetal (not embryonic) tissue?

At this time, everything being done by immunologists—from the search for a preventative vaccine of some kind to the search for a cure—is exploration of new territory. Little work has been done specifically on breast cancer. There has been some success with other kinds of cancer, and this gives us good reason to hope. But it is nowhere near enough to count on yet.

As I said in beginning this discussion, the field of immunology is so dynamic that wonderful results may be forthcoming in the next few days, and what I have written here may be ancient history. I know the work will go on, however, and there must be progress.

Everything published about new anticancer treatments and every expert I talked to about either chemotherapy or immunology had one constant, common refrain: "Science does not promise miracles."

A miracle, by definition, is "an event or effect in the physical world deviating from the laws of nature." The "laws of nature" I have described here are those that involve breast cancer and a cure would be a deviant event. What I want is this kind of deviation from the laws, something like a Salk vaccine, some "white magic" from the research laboratories. But experts are sensitive to any talk of miracles or magic. Understandably, nothing in medicine is more cruel than fostering false hope. A way either to prevent or to cure breast cancer is impossible to predict, and we cancer patients know that well enough. We also shy away from talk—or even thoughts—of miracles.

But still, we expect them.

14

Male Chauvinism, Sex, and Breast Cancer

There is a patron saint of breasts. She is Saint Agatha, an early Christian martyr. Born in third-century Italy, when the Christians were still being persecuted by the Romans, she was so beautiful, according to legend, that Quintianus, the pagan governor of Sicily, fell madly in love with her. The only way he could manage to meet the young beauty was to have her arrested and brought to him for trial. The charge was her religious beliefs.

Quintianus made it quite clear that the case would be dropped if Agatha let him make love to her. However, she had no use for a man who felt the way Quintianus did about her God. She refused. Unable to get Agatha to submit, the governor found her guilty and sentenced her to a brothel. A term in the House of Aphrodisia (named for a "wicked woman of unsavory fame and wanton reputation") was supposed to convince the young virgin that she should mend her ways and give up not only her church but also her chastity. Somehow, Agatha was able to keep both, even after a month of Aphrodisia, and when Quintianus called back to see if she had changed her mind, he found her still "pure and undefiled."

Hell hath no fury like a man scorned. Agatha was tortured mercilessly, and several harrowing versions exist of how Quintianus took his revenge for her rejection of him. According to some records, he ordered that she "be bound to a pillar and her

breasts be torn off with iron shears." Another description tells
how Agatha was stretched on a rack and red-hot iron plates were
put on her body. Then her breasts were ripped off.

Breasts were so important—even then—that Agatha's reward
for her martyrdom was their miraculous restoration. Saint
Agatha's ordeal has been immortalized by artists, Anthony Van-
dyke among them, through the centuries since, and poems have
been written about her suffering. Even in Sicily, over a millen-
nium ago, breasts were a very important part of the female
anatomy, and having them hacked off as the price necessary to
keep one's faith was a good reason for sainthood and Divine
intervention. Agatha's story floated as far north as Scandinavia,
where February 5 is Saint Agatha's Day, as it is in the calendar
of the Book of Common Prayer. Hundreds of thousands of women
pray to her if their breasts are too small, too large, or too pendulous, do not produce milk or develop disease.

Breast consciousness is a universal obsession, which probably
began with Adam and Eve in Eden. But why? Why did Atossa
hide her breast tumor from her husband 700 long years before
Saint Agatha? Could she have been afraid that King Darius
would find himself another wife? A mistress? When a modern
woman discovers a lump, does she delay in seeing a doctor for
the same reason?

Whether we liberated women admit it or not, fear of not catching a man or fear of losing one probably is the main reason we
are so "obsessed" with keeping our breasts, even when doing so
could be fatal.

In his book *Early Detection,* Dr. Philip Strax wrote:

We live in a breast-oriented society. To the average woman, her
breast is the badge of femininity, an important part of her allurement
to charm her male. To the man, the breast is a source of excitement,
an erotic stimulation. It has become a bridge between male and female
and is used as a reward to be flaunted before the eyes of the male in
the female's attempt to attract him. This emphasis on the breast as a
sex symbol begins in adolescence and apparently persists throughout
life.

Dr. Strax supports this opinion with some "typical incidents"
he encountered in the course of a day as a physician.

"I'm a school teacher," said an attractive 45-year-old woman. "I first noticed this lump in my left breast 2½ years ago. At first, I thought it would just go away. It didn't hurt or bother me in any way. Then as I watched it get bigger and produce changes in the skin, I thought it was probably serious. I felt strongly about breast surgery and the fear of losing my breast. I simply couldn't bring myself to see a physician. I even wear a bra at night to hide the condition from my husband."

A twentieth-century Atossa. Another conversation between doctor and patient:

Mrs. K. lowered her eyes, clasped her hands, and began shyly. "My husband likes to manipulate my breasts as part of our lovemaking. Sometimes he's rather vigorous and once my breast was black and blue. I've heard that an injury can lead to cancer. Is that true? I've been worrying about our relationship."

Dr. Strax says that the "common thread in all these episodes is the tremendous preoccupation with the female breast that has been developing in the past 30 years. . . . Billboards, movie marquees, newspaper ads, and magazine photos all stress the female breast as the sex symbol of our age."

A successful movie must show a close-up of a woman's breast with the hero looking at it admiringly. Topless waitresses, dancers, and actresses have become a hallmark of our society. The younger female is being stampeded into a bra-less generation. Designers vie with each other in attempting to emphasize the bosom with low-cut or transparent blouses. . . .

This elevation of the female breast as an important sex attribute has brought with it a greater apprehension and anxiety about breast conditions . . . and the totally erroneous idea has been spreading among many women that the loss of a breast is equivalent to loss of sexual attraction or prowess or both.

But, Dr. Strax, who is creating all this apprehension over being sexy and alluring?

Men. Entrepreneurs of machismo like Hugh Hefner and Bob Guccione, that's who!

When I discussed my opinion with a young man, he sneered. "What are you talking about, Rose? The girls do it to us. From the time I was in seventh grade, when only a couple of the girls in my class had anything, they were always sticking them out and practically shoving them in our faces. You've got it all wrong," this budding MCP insisted. "It's not the males who do it to the females. It's the girls who make breasts a sex symbol, not the boys."

"I bet you were sneaking *Playboy* centerfolds into your room long before you were in seventh grade," I said.

"Well, maybe I was," he admitted. "But the girls were the ones who started it."

"How many girls have anything before they're twelve?" I snapped.

He looked down at his hands, as if he were trying to count the number of chesty girls in his elementary-school class. Sheepishly, he conceded there were none. "I guess I didn't know any."

Having two boys and a girl, and having watched their progress through early childhood, adolescence, and now young manhood —my daughter is still very much an adolescent—I feel qualified to say that by the time a girl is old enough to have anything to put into a training bra, little boys have had two or three years to teach her the importance of those small eruptions on her chest.

It does not take much time or effort; it almost seems to be instinctive. But learning experts know that breast consciousness is definitely nurture, not nature. Either way, our culture certainly considers breast loss a sexual deficiency of some dire kind.

Several years ago, one of the mathematicians who works with Harvey lost the tip of one of her middle fingers in a garbage disposal. For months afterward, she worked tirelessly to retrain her other fingers to punch the buttons of the calculating machine she used all day on her job.

"I'm not having as much trouble after my surgery as you did after you lost that little piece of your finger," I quipped, when she offered her condolences at an office picnic. "I'd be in the same bad shape as you were if I had lost a part of my finger instead of a breast." We both laughed.

"Yeah," she said. "I never thought of that. You can't hardly do much typing with a breast."

Even though her loss was actually more handicapping than

mine, no one ever asked her if she still felt "attractive and appeal-ing"; nor did anyone ever wonder whether she might lose her husband because a piece of her body had been lost.

Dr. Strax made much ado about the influence of the media—magazines, book jackets, movie billboards, et cetera, *ad nauseam.* I agree. He set the time frame of such media influence within the past thirty years, only dating back to the time when the "boyish" figure went out of style. I do not know about this. I doubt the obsession is so recent. What about the buxom ladies who graced the *Police Gazette* in the 1890s, Lillian Russell, or those cruel girdles designed to pull in the stomachs and push out the chests of our great-grandmothers?

Men dominated the media then and still dominate them today. Obviously, they believed then and believe now that emphasizing the breast is good for business.

Even now, with the Equal Rights Amendment, the Equal Em-ployment Opportunities Commission, women's liberation, and the urgent rush to hire women, there is still only a handful of them in the policy-making echelons of all the media. The Na-tional Broadcasting Company, for example, was brought before the EEOC not long ago because it had no women in the top executive levels. In advertising, where most of the sexy-breast brouhaha is born and nourished, only a faint sprinkling of women is found in the major jobs; when a Mary Wells Lawrence reaches the top, it is so noteworthy that the achievement merits stories in national magazines.

But merely having a woman in a top advertising job or putting one in charge of a national magazine does not necessarily make the difference it should. Look at the exploitation of breastiness in the advertisements in *Cosmopolitan,* edited by Helen Gurley Brown, a major source of journalistic wisdom on how women can win in a world of men.

Dr. Strax is right. The media have made breasts into the ulti-mate erotic symbol, to men and to women, too. The media are responsible for the long hours my sons spend discussing who is 32A or 34B and—wonder of wonders!—the fifteen-year-old who is a 40D. The media are also the main reason my daughter and her girl friends, at the age of twelve or thirteen, stood before

their mirrors trying to make the bumps in their training bras
larger with the help of cotton balls, Kleenex, or ripped nylons
(those worked best, by the way).

Yes, Dr. Strax, you are absolutely right. You men have done
an appalling thing to us with *your* billboards, *your* marquees,
your centerfolds, *your* advertisements. Every time a man leaves
an extra-large tip to a topless waitress or pays to see a Blaze
Starr or a Racquel Welch, a woman is made to believe she must
have two, preferably large, breasts, no matter what the cost—
even death. Girls and women do not want real breasts so they
can show them off to other girls and women.

Male influence has likewise affected the search for treatments
and cures of breast cancer. It is curious that those early Egyptian
medical papyri gave instructions for treating breast tumors only
in men. Today, breast cancer attacks only about 1 per cent of the
male population, many of its victims being older men who develop it from taking estrogens for prostatic cancer. Is it possible
that breast cancer was a more masculine disease in the days of
the pharaohs? Or is it more probable that not as much medical
effort was spent on treating women's ailments?

Although a lot of money and attention is now devoted to
breast cancer, its treatment is still influenced by male opinions
and masculine attitudes. In the United States, the medical profession has always been and still is dominated by men; the American College of Surgeons has a female membership of 3 per cent.
Until recently, all medical schools had strict quotas governing the
admission of women, and those who did succeed in being en-
rolled were discriminated against by being subject to the same
rigid rules and schedules that applied to men. For example, no
provisions were made for maternity leaves, and during their
training periods in hospital clinics women were not permitted to
adjust their schedules to the hours their children were in school.

I do not know why I am using the past tense. Except for a
few progressive medical schools and hospitals, these are still the
common practices in our country. Although admission quotas are
disappearing, because of antidiscrimination laws, there is still a
rigid inflexibility in the demands medical schools and hospitals

make on women students and doctors—a barrier that keeps many capable women out of medicine.

Another obstacle is the tremendous cost of medical training in the United States today. A fairly good undergraduate college costs at least $3,000 or $4,000 annually, including room, board, tuition fees, clothes, travel, and expenses. (The Ivy League schools and the "seven sisters," of course, are considerably more.) After that, the *tuition alone* for a good medical school has risen to about $5,000 a year, usually for a four-year program. In addition to this punishing fee, there are books (expensive in medical school), lab costs, instruments, room, board, clothing, and pocket money.

Bright, enterprising undergraduates often are able to work their way through college, but the heavy workloads of a good medical school do not allow for this. And the heavy amounts of money required necessitate working full-time—impossible while going to medical school.

How does all this affect women who want to study medicine?

Parents who must choose between putting a son or a daughter through medical school will most likely decide the son is the more worth-while investment for their $40,000. "A girl doesn't need a college education to learn how to diaper a baby" was still the slogan when I graduated from high school. I did not go to college until long after my children had outgrown diapers.

Women's liberation and the feminist movement notwithstanding, this hard financial fact of life is something many parents are facing today. I can say so from personal knowledge, because it is true for Harvey and me, and for most of our contemporaries. With the enormous cost of higher education, and with a limited amount of money to be shared, in our case, by two sons and a daughter, who has the priority? I hate to be admitting this, but if all three wanted to go to medical school, I am afraid the boys—who will be the initial, if not the major, breadwinners of their families—would have higher priorities than my daughter. Luckily, Lesley does not have a scientist's DNA molecule in her body and wants to be an artist. So that is one painful quandary we will miss.

But many parents are not so lucky. Unless it is a daughter and not a son who is interested in medicine, they must make the

brutal and unfair decision that most of the available family education funds should be spent on males, rather than females.

What does the small number of women doctors have to do with
breast cancer? I think the exceedingly small number of women
involved in treating the disease in the United States—especially
in the surgical treatment—makes an enormous difference in what
is being done.

There is no way to prove a negative, no way to prove that the
small number of women in medicine here is related to the small
amount of progress made over the last century. But I can compare Professor Sviatukhina's work in Moscow, where she is trying
partial mastectomies, with the work of Professor Melnikov in
Leningrad, who swears by the Halsted radical mastectomy.
Breast-cancer staffs that include many women are generally more
interested in and sympathetic toward saving as much of the
breast as possible. Men just do not understand the importance
of that. A search through the medical literature shows that many
more women are involved in looking for alternatives to mastectomy than would be expected from the small number of them in
the medical profession. Many dedicated male doctors would also
like to do away with mastectomies of all kinds, of course, but
where there are more women, there invariably seems to be a
greater effort to do less chopping and more preserving.

No, I cannot prove that the absence of women doctors has
caused the lag in progress in the treatment of breast cancer in
the United States. But I cannot accept it as mere coincidence,
either.

Nowhere are women doctors as sorely missed as in the surgical
treatment of breast cancer. Premastectomy sympathy and understanding from a woman surgeon are hardly ever available. Afterward, under the care of male surgeons, women were left almost
entirely on their own until Terese Lasser, a mastectomee herself,
began the Reach to Recovery program in 1952. It is now under
the aegis of the American Cancer Society. But that worthy and
noble organization, too—despite its sponsorship and support of
Reach to Recovery—is dominated by men. Only two of its nine
past officer-directors were women; only nine of its forty officers
in 1975 were women; of the 190 members of its House of Dele-

gates, the policy-making board, only twenty-three are women. The entire 1974–1975 Breast Cancer Advisory Committee was male!

It seems as if the United States's entire breast-cancer Establishment is masculine. On September 30, 1974, the National Cancer Institute held an international conference on breast cancer, and, of the twenty scientists who reported on their work, only one was a woman—Dr. Philomena Hegeman, who talked about the virology of breast cancer in mice. I do not mean to disparage laboratory research. The cure or prevention of breast cancer will, I am convinced, be found in a laboratory somewhere. But the reports on all the subjects of most immediate, vital concern to women—detection, the breast-cancer demonstration projects, other ways of finding early cancer, breast cancer's causes, and, of course, surgery and chemotherapy—were given by men.

Nowhere in the course of the all-day conference, including the treatment section, was there any mention of the psychological aspects of mastectomy such as those reported by Michael J. Asken in his *American Journal of Psychiatry* article. As far as the men attending that meeting were concerned, the important areas of breast-cancer investigation were all physical. No mention was made of any past, present, or proposed study of what goes on in a woman's heart and mind when she is faced with the disease. Inevitably, patients are told to take their emotional problems to Reach to Recovery. This is a very useful organization in helping women adjust to the everyday problems they face after a mastectomy. However, the program was created not to give long-term help with individual psychological woes, but to assist with immediate, practical postoperative matters. No agency, not even Reach to Recovery, has published any articles or manuals telling husbands and boyfriends how they can help. If there is such information available, I did not find it anywhere.

In England, Mrs. Betty Westgate, who started the Mastectomy Association there, is trying to do something about this information gap. She has put together and is distributing a leaflet for both the husbands and children of breast-cancer patients. In addition to giving a short list of helpful hints, mainly concerning household chores, she explains that these women suffer from certain disabilities—pain, swelling, and limited movements—and therefore everyone in the family should pitch in to help with housework, shopping, cooking, and so on. This needs saying, especially to the family of a woman accustomed to being considered the do-everything drudge, and something like it should be distributed here.

I must add a short lecture addressed to husbands and/or friends on the subject of what they must do to give their women maximum emotional support in the critical weeks following surgery.

While some women may be eager to resume love-making, most of those who have had some kind of radical mastectomy will be too sore even to think about it for weeks. It may seem too obvious to say, but men must be understanding about this, and often they are not. Also, a mastectomy has those traumatic psychological components that are not present in other surgical procedures. The woman may be reluctant to be seen nude for a while, as I was, for a variety of reasons. In such cases, a man may finally have to rely on his instincts and take some kind of positive action to help her get through this phase. (If the shyness and withdrawal go on too long, they could be signs of a severe disturbance.) For all I know, Harvey may have deliberately come into the bathroom to take something from the medicine cabinet in order to break my pattern of reticence. The strategy was enough for me, and something like it may be enough for other women. But please, for a month or so—patience. The woman must have a little time to get used to the idea.

By all means, a man must go out of his way to be loving and tender, and to show that, whatever physical difference the mastectomy has made, it has not changed his feelings. This is difficult for most undemonstrative American males, but they must somehow learn how to show affection without any sexual connotations, and must try to make the woman feel more precious than she was before.

Marvella Bayh, the wife of the Indiana senator, has told of her anxiety and fear the night before her mastectomy. "I'm only thirty-eight years old," she cried tearfully, "and I have to live the rest of my life with only one breast."

"Honey," Mrs. Bayh recalls her husband saying, "I'm forty-three years old, and I've lived all my life without any breasts at all."

I mention this here because it is the kind of answer every husband should file away in his memory box, to use when and if his wife ever needs it.

Among the women I interviewed, older women—the married and the previously married—were the ones who had the most difficult emotional adjustment to make. Divorced husbands must make a special effort to help their former mates. Few second wives would object if their husbands visited their predecessors in the hospital after surgery, took care of finances and other household problems for a short time, or offered to look after the children. Ex-husbands should read, in the chapter on postsurgery psychological problems, about my conversation with a woman whose first husband gave her no help at all. This kind of cruelty is barbaric. A divorced woman in our family subsequently had a mastectomy, and I am very proud of the cousin who was always at his ex-wife's side in the hospital, has chauffeured her for postoperative treatments, and has probably helped her financially as well. That is the way it ought to be.

Men who are still living with their wives but whose marriages are no longer close need the strongest lecture. It is a difficult enough time for an older woman even if the marriage is fairly good. "Let's face it," one fifty-eight-year-old woman told me. "My husband is sixty, very handsome and distinguished-looking. He can and, I've been told, does get women in their thirties to go out with him. He may even have a mistress, for all I know. Why should he bother with me?"

This woman's attitude, perhaps, was more bitter than usual, because she did apparently have some reason for doubting her husband's fidelity. What an awful additional blow the operation must have been for her! But the difference is only in intensity, not detail. It is a bad time.

So, to husbands of women in this very troubled—physically and psychologically—age group, I make this plea: Be with your wife as much as you can throughout the ordeal, and support her with your presence as well as your checkbook. If you have ever had any feeling for her as a human being, a partner, and perhaps the mother of your children, assure her, above all, that it does not make any difference to you whether she has one breast or two. She may not believe you, but she will nonetheless be happy to hear you say it.

Nowhere is male domination more evident than during the short interval in which the decision is made about the mastectomy—because we patients are usually unconscious! Since most surgeons do not take the time in advance to outline the different surgical alternatives, the patient would not have the knowledge with which to make a decision even if she were awakened and asked—an argument doctors use to defend the system.

Occasionally, however, surgeons bring husbands into the decision-making process. This was apparently the case with both Betty Ford and Happy Rockefeller.

I remember very well the night of September 27, 1974, the night before Mrs. Ford underwent her mastectomy at the Bethesda Naval Hospital. She had entered the hospital earlier that evening. The news broadcasts mentioned the event, but soft-pedaled it by saying she was to have a simple, routine biopsy of a small "nodule" found during her regular gynecological examination. A friend in the White House press corps told me the rumor was that mammograms had already been taken and the diagnosis from them was positive. The Washington news reports indicated that, if the biopsy confirmed this diagnosis, a Halsted radical mastectomy would be done immediately.

Having just gone through my own surgery, I knew such extreme speed was unnecessary. Besides, there could not have been enough time between the discovery of the tumor and the scheduled operation for the doctors to have done any preoperative work-ups—the staging examinations of the bones, lungs, skull, spine, and liver—so necessary before a mastectomy. From the news reports, it did not sound as if these necessary tests had been done.

"The poor woman is being railroaded," I told Harvey at dinner. "To the Bethesda Naval Hospital, in the bargain!" *

Wanting to put some of my hard-learned knowledge to use,

* Later, I asked a veteran cancer specialist who had served many years as a navy doctor what he thought about having a mastectomy in that hospital. "Well," he answered, "I was over there for a long time. Bethesda Naval does a great hernia."

I tried to call Ron Nessen, the President's press secretary, whom I had met briefly once at a press conference. He was not available; no one was available. President Ford, Nessen, and everyone else on the White House staff were attending the "mini-summit" on the economy and a reception for the delegates. Finally, at 11:45 P.M., I was able to reach one of the President's speech writers, to whom two mutual friends had referred me.

Introducing myself quickly, I told him why I was calling. "I'm not a kook," I said, convincingly, I hope. "I've just had a mastectomy myself, and I want to pass along to the President some of the information I've learned."

"What is it?" he asked.

Briefly, and as simply as I could, I told him that the biopsy should be done and that then, if the diagnosis was cancer, certain tests should be completed before a mastectomy was performed. And, I added, the President should not let a general surgeon do the operation, but should find the best breast-cancer specialist in the country. "If the President's wife isn't going to get the best," I asked, "who is?"

There was a silence.

"Are you still there?" I asked.

"Just a minute. I'll see what I can do."

I held the line, feeling like a toenote to history. But that was not to be. In a few minutes, he returned and transmitted what may well be the most memorable line in feminist history.

"I am sorry, Mrs. Kushner," he told me. "The President has made his decision."

I was speechless. I finally blurted out, "The President has made *his* decision? It's not his decision to make. Mrs. Ford should make that decision, don't you think?"

It was his turn to be speechless. Then, in an emotionless monotone, he answered. "I am sorry, Mrs. Kushner, but that is all I am authorized to say. The President has gone to bed, and he has already made his decision."

The next morning I read the paper, heard the news, and learned that the President's decision had indeed been made. Betty Ford, at 8:30 on the morning of September 28, 1974, had been found to have breast cancer, and a naval surgeon, Dr. William Fouty, and a professor of general surgery at the George Washington Medical

School, Dr. Richard Thistlethwaite, were at that moment performing a Halsted radical mastectomy on the wife of the President of the United States.

Harvey was listening to the radio with me. When the broadcast
was over, he turned to me. "Well," he said, "it looks like the wife
of Harvey Kushner got a hell of a lot better treatment than the
wife of Gerald Ford."

It may seem in questionable taste to recount my conversation
with the White House speech writer here. I would prefer to forget
it, for reasons of compassion. But even the President of the United
States is not free of a lifetime of conditioning in our masculine
society. Just as I hope women will learn from reading this book
what they have a right to expect and demand, I hope men will
understand that their wives should not be denied a conscious
voice in their destinies.

A few months later, the absence of "freedom of choice" became public knowledge when Happy Rockefeller's second breast
was removed for a mirror-image carcinoma.

According to Vice President Rockefeller's own statement,
broadcast and telecast live, he had been told immediately after
the first mastectomy that there was a microscopic tumor in the
second breast. (The routine policy at Memorial Sloan-Kettering
is to do a biopsy of the same spot in the opposite breast whenever
a mastectomy is performed, because about 1 per cent of women
with one breast tumor have a mirror-image cancer in the other
breast.) However, Vice President Rockefeller told the millions
in his radio and TV audience, he had withheld this information
from his wife after the first operation because of her emotional
state. In the interim, he, her surgeon, Dr. Jerome Urban, and
other surgical consultants had pondered what should be done.
Among them—all men, probably—they had decided that removing
the second breast was the safest thing to do. Finally, in the middle
of November, Happy Rockefeller was informed of her fate. The
second breast was removed, as the men around her had decided.

Of course, that may be exactly what Mrs. Rockefeller herself
would have chosen, had she been consulted. I know I would
have. Also, she had plenty of time after being told of the decision to say no, and she didn't. Neither would I. But—in her husband's own public words—she had not been told anything for

more than a month, and the decision about treatment was made by her husband, her surgeon, and whatever other specialists had been asked for advice.

Writing about politicians inevitably leads me into the role of politics in breast cancer. Research is not cheap. A lot of money is needed to develop equipment and to hire top-notch people. It is very expensive, and the major source of such huge sums is government. The government means politicians.

Congress, as the world knows, is predominantly male. Nowhere does its masculine orientation show as clearly as in the number of dollars appropriated by that august body to study cancer of the breast.

Cancer of the lung and bronchus has been the top malignant killer since data were first collected. It still is. (Although the breast-cancer *incidence rates* now exceed those of lung cancer, the *death rates* of the latter are higher.) Because men have been smoking cigarettes longer than women, until recently lung cancer has been considered a masculine disease. I could not find an estimate of the millions—perhaps billions—of dollars spent before the tars and nicotines in cigarettes were found to be a major cause of lung cancer, mainly because the money came from so many different sources. Before the early 1960s (when cigarette smoking was officially blamed), the NCI, the National Institute of Heart and Lung Disease, the American Cancer Society, the American Medical Association, anti-lung-disease organizations like the Christmas Seal and emphysema societies, the tobacco companies themselves (at least $10 million spent to prove the reverse), and numerous privately supported foundations poured hundreds of millions of dollars into a search for the cause of this (then) masculine cancer. And, because so much lung cancer is associated with certain jobs, labor unions, insurance companies, and government agencies concerned with occupational hazards spent additional millions for research.

Even now, the costs of the battle against lung cancer can't be counted. Dollars are still flowing to stop smoking in public buildings, elevators, department stores, theaters, on common carriers, and even in certain areas of motels, hotels, and restaurants. Who knows how expensive it was to drive cigarette commercials off radio and television? In addition, miscellaneous environmental agencies, federal, state, local, and private, are spending money to regulate or prohibit the emission of various carcinogenic pollutants into the air. And I am talking only about funding with American dollars. Other countries have also contributed from their treasuries to get rid of lung cancer. With so many millions —probably billions—flowing into anti-lung-cancer budgets, from so many sources, it was and is impossible to calculate, even roughly, the totals spent.

It has been a far different story with breast cancer. This disease, along with uterine and cervical carcinomas, has been the top killer of women in this country for a long time (and, in 1974, its incidence rate leapfrogged over the lung-cancer incidence in *both* sexes together). But Congress did not declare financial war on this specifically female cancer until 1966, several years after cigarettes as a cause of lung cancer had been pinpointed.

I have often wondered what congressman's wife, mother, sister, or mistress developed a breast cancer or died of the disease in 1966. Something like that must have happened, to get the appropriation passed creating the Breast Cancer Task Force. It was not much, but it was a beginning. According to the National Cancer Institute's budget history, less than $500,000 was spent in 1966 on the task force. By 1970, it had about $2.75 million to spend on all federal research studies into the causes, treatment, and cure of breast cancer. A tiny cost-of-living increase was included in the 1971 budget, but the total was still less than $3 million—about enough for eight B-52 sorties over North Vietnam.

But the next year another woman related to a member of Congress (perhaps it was Marvella Bayh) must have developed breast cancer, because in 1972 the task force was given almost $5 million—twelve B-52 raids' worth. In 1973, the budget was increased again, to about $6.5 million, and once again in 1974, to almost $9 million. In 1975, the Breast Cancer Task Force received $9.75 million. Then the largesse of the United States Treasury began to be cut back.

The budget being proposed for the fiscal year 1976 is $582 million for *all* cancer research (President Ford's Pentagon budget request was for $92.8 *billion*), of which $9.75 million will be devoted to breast cancer—the same as for the previous year. Although the Secretary of Health, Education, and Welfare, Caspar W. Weinberger, insisted this was not a cut, inflation meant that the same dollar amount was significantly reduced in value.

Still, almost $10 million is more than the $450,000 of 1966, and we should be grateful, I suppose. But it makes a breast-cancer patient wonder how much progress might have been made in finding the causes, and perhaps even the cure, if breast cancer had been given the same high priority in the 1950s and 1960s as the mostly masculine disease of lung cancer.

I do not begrudge lung-cancer research a penny, and of course I am not proposing that funds to study breast cancer be taken out of the budget for research on any other disease. Every illness—arthritis, diabetes, heart trouble, and so on—should get all the money needed to eradicate it entirely. But, in view of that $92.8 *billion* Congress will doubtless manage to find for the Pentagon, less than $600 *million* for all cancer research seems paltry. There is no reason why this richest country in the world cannot find enough money to cover all its medical needs.

No, I do not want lung cancer to lose a nickel. My reason for comparing the huge expenditures on research into it with the piddling pennies spent on breast cancer is because, again, this cannot be a coincidence. The long and expensive hunt for a cause finally ended with the first official reports linking cigarette smoking and lung cancer in the early 1960s. A few years later, in 1966, a niggardly Congress appropriated less than half a million dollars to begin to do something about breast cancer. The male disease had come first.

I said it was impossible to prove a negative when I discussed the probable role male chauvinism plays in the problem of saving women's breasts. It is equally impossible to prove a negative here. There is no way to correlate the lack of progress in breast-cancer research with the paltry amount of money made available by an almost all-male Congress and by other male-dominated organizations. It is an historical fact, however, that even the weak push given to breast-cancer financing did not begin until 1966, after a major cause of lung cancer had already been found.

Male chauvinism plays an important role in all aspects of breast cancer, from the moment a sixth-grader's budding chest bumps make her popular with pimply-faced boys. Later, the belief that breasts are vital in getting and keeping a boyfriend and then a husband is reinforced by the blatant blandishments of our male-dominated media. Next, there is the malevolent influence of a male-dominated medical profession, specifically in surgery, reinforced by decades of discrimination against women by admissions offices in medical schools, which has perpetuated the medical masculinity to the present. Because of the exorbitant expense of getting a medical education in the United States, this disproportion will doubtless continue, although entrance statistics indicate that the number of women in schools of medicine in the United States is higher now than ten years ago. Those stalwart women who survive and are finally awarded M.D. degrees usually go into pediatrics, obstetrics and gynecology, psychiatry, and dermatology—not surgery. Their reason is not schedules, but another kind of discrimination.

Americans do not accept the notion that women doctors should be in certain fields of medicine, and one of these is surgery; Americans—men and women—just do not cotton to the idea of female surgeons. Naturally, they would not make worth-while incomes, and most women doctors do not even try. The result, of course, is the 3-per-cent-female component in the American College of Surgeons.

Finally, the money for breast-cancer research is voted by a male-dominated and male-oriented Congress. And, in spite of the cancers that struck his wife and his Vice President's wife, and in spite of the rising breast-cancer incidence rates, President Ford decided to keep his request for cancer-research funds low, as a part of his battle of the budget. At the same time, he was insisting that Congress must provide almost the same amount to "rescue" South Vietnam and Cambodia. Somehow, men have their priorities scrambled in strange ways.

Not long before I found my lump, I attended a press conference held to protest the so-called Buckley amendment to the Constitution, which, if passed, would invalidate the Supreme Court decision of January 22, 1974, liberalizing the abortion laws of most states. Several leaders of the women's liberation movement, feminist groups, and the Women's Political Caucus spoke against the amendment. In her remarks, the writer Gloria Steinem

lashed out against male doctors who do unnecessary mastectomies, hinting that there is some kind of male-chauvinist con-
spiracy whose goal is to mutilate women by cutting off their
breasts.

In the research I have done and the conversations I have had,
I did not find any suggestion whatever of such a sadistic con-
spiracy in the present situation where amputation of a breast is
the best first treatment. But other kinds of male chauvinism?
Plenty!

15

Where We Are Now

For weeks I have toyed with the idea of installing an unlisted telephone. It is hard to write a book with that jangling in my ear. But, until Lesley and her friends get out of school, most of the calls are from women who need advice about lumps, biopsies, and mastectomy. There is a paucity of information around, but no lack of problems.

For example, in late February the telephone rang very early one morning. "Are you the Rose Kushner who wrote the article in the *Washington Post* about breast cancer?" a young voice asked. Since I am listed in the phone book under my own name as well as "Mrs. Harvey D.," I was easy to find.

"Yes, I am."

"I have a problem."

"A lump?" I asked, by now routinely.

"No," she replied, a tremolo in her voice. "I already know it's cancer. What I need now is information."

"You sound awfully young to have cancer," I told her, my astonishment, I am certain, apparent.

"I'm only twenty-seven," she acknowledged. "The doctor was so sure it was just a benign cyst that he didn't even ask me to stay in the hospital for the biopsy. He did it as an outpatient."

"And it was cancer?"

"Yes," she answered. "And it was the long lab analysis, not the quick one. The surgeon is sure the pathologist didn't make a mistake."

"Have you been taking the Pill?" It was the first thing that fell into my head.

Her tone was hard and bitter. "For eight years."

"Eight years?" I howled. "Didn't your doctor tell you that's too long?"

"I kept asking him if it was safe, and he kept telling me everything was all right and not to worry," she explained. "Now the surgeon has told me I should have taken a break after three years at most."

Fighting hard and reluctantly, I kept my mouth shut and said nothing about gynecologists who permit young women to take oral contraceptives, without a break, from the age of nineteen to twenty-seven.

"My problem is what to do now."

"You want to keep your breast," I said matter-of-factly.

"You're damned right I do," she snapped. "I'm not married, not settled, nothing. What would life be like for me without two breasts, at my age and in my situation?"

"You know, I suppose, that a modified radical mastectomy is the best thing for you to do?"

"That's what the surgeon said," she replied. "But you're a woman, and he's a man. What would you do in my place?"

What would I have done had I been her age, unmarried and unsettled? I did not know and told her so.

"Can't you try to put yourself in my position?" she begged.

I thought about it. Not married, so very young to be mastectomized, no husband or children to count on for emotional support. What would I do? "How big was the tumor?"

"I don't know. I think he said it was as big as a cherry."

"A cherry? That's pretty big," I said. "Are you sure he didn't say a cherry pit?"

"Now that you mention it, I'm not sure. What difference does it make?"

"If you're going to gamble with your life, you've got to have some information to know the odds. Otherwise, you might just as well flip a coin."

"Okay," she said. "I'll ask him. Is there anything else that might be important?"

"Yes," I told her. "Where was it? Was it in a lobe? Was it in a milk duct? What kind of cancer was it? Some cancers hardly ever spread, but others metastasize like mad."

"I'm writing all this down," she said. "Is there anything else I should ask?"

"Ask if he thinks plastic surgery would be safe for you," I added, explaining that operation briefly. "At your age, not married—I'd look into that, if just taking out the lump or a partial is too risky."

"I see," she said softly.

There was a long pause in the conversation. Then she continued. "You know, I had the biopsy a week ago and have talked to dozens of people by now, a lot of them doctors. Nobody has given me the kind of information you've given me. How come?"

How come? Perhaps because nobody, especially the male members of our 97-per-cent-male surgical profession, has given much thought to such problems.

"Have you talked to any women doctors?" I asked.

"No, they were all men."

"That's your answer."

"You mean male doctors don't give a damn?"

"Not all of them," I stressed. "But most of them only know one kind of mastectomy—the Halsted radical. It's even hard to get a modified radical mastectomy around here, much less a partial or a lumpectomy."

She told me that she had already telephoned Dr. George Crile, at his Cleveland Clinic, and had an appointment with him a few days later.

"Dr. Crile has been very much misquoted in the press," I warned. "Everyone thinks he does lumpectomies and partials on anybody who walks in, but he doesn't. He's very careful about the selection of candidates for those operations."

"No," she said, "I didn't know that. I had the impression he did them all the time." She paused. "But if he says I can have one, what do you think?"

I paused. "I can't put myself in your position," I repeated. "I just don't know."

"I went through the whole university library looking for some information," she continued, "and I couldn't find anything but the Crile book. You may not be able to give me any real advice about what I should do, but you gave me something to go on."

She thanked me, promising to call after seeing Dr. Crile. I reminded her that, since her biopsy had been done a week earlier, she did not have too much time to procrastinate. "The idea that you have to have the mastectomy immediately is ridiculous," I explained, "but you can't wait too long. According to what I've been told, you have about another week before you might have a hard time finding a surgeon to do a mastectomy on you, if that's what you decide to have."

"Why?"

"Because most surgeons in this country believe the wait between biopsy and mastectomy gives the cancer time to spread. There's a lot of evidence that this isn't true, but it hasn't filtered down yet. So as long as surgeons believe in the two-week maximum, you might not get one to take on a patient he believes is such a high risk—it will go on his record as a fatality."

I explained that the length of time between biopsy and mastectomy is still one of the many unknowns of breast cancer. "As a matter of fact, some immunologists feel there *should* be a wait between taking out the primary tumor and doing the mastectomy, to give the body's immune system a chance to stop fighting the big lump, regroup and recoup, and have more strength to attack and kill the microscopic cancers. But," I added, "this is still only a theory. Most doctors—especially surgeons in the United States— don't believe it."

"Do you?"

"I don't know. It has to have more time to be tested, and anything that involves breast cancer takes a long time before the word is final. But," I admitted, "it does seem to make sense. It's just another thing you will have to weigh when you make a decision. But you do have another week, according to what is accepted."

She called me as soon as she returned from Cleveland. Dr. Crile had ruled out anything less than a modified radical mastectomy for her, suggesting reconstructive mammoplasty. After talking to some surgeons, she decided this would also be too dangerous, since her tumor was a very invasive kind of carcinoma.

She had her breast amputated in February 1975, at the age of twenty-seven.

It is preposterous for a young woman to be on the Pill for eight years without a word of warning about its possible dangers. It is even more preposterous that she should have had to travel from Washington to Cleveland to get professional help before she could make an intelligent decision. If a general surgeon does not know enough to help a young woman in this position, he should refer her to someone who can—a breast-cancer specialist. Certainly I am not qualified, legally or medically, to give such advice.

Above all, I really did not know what I would have done if I had been only twenty-seven years old and alone. After thinking about her for hours, I made up my mind—based on what I do know now—about what I would do if her cancer were mine.

If I were her age, unmarried, with a very small tumor, of a type that does not metastasize quickly or easily, and with no visibly affected lymph nodes, I would take a chance on leaving my breast as it was. The tumor, after all, would have been removed in the biopsy. Although it's true that some breasts having one malignant tumor also have microscopic malignant "centricles," the same statistics show that even more do not. I decided I would risk a recurrence and, if necessary, have a mastectomy later if one appeared. It would be a calculated risk to buy time—if I were only twenty-seven and unmarried. This is *not advice*, because it is medically and surgically unwise. It is what I decided I would have done in her place—emotionally, not intellectually.

I am sure my own respected Dr. Dao would advise against any such emotional decision. But he is not an unmarried twenty-seven-year-old woman. Nor am I, for that matter. At least I am a woman. And I do know what it is like to be single-breasted.

Combining hard personal experience with information gleaned, often painfully, from breast-cancer literature and from the experts, I have tried to make this a reference book containing everything a woman should know about breast cancer and all that she has a right to expect. She will probably never learn much of anything from her doctor. Or her government.

Since I have detailed the possible role of the Pill in nourishing breast cancer, I must add that our trusty watchdog, the Food and Drug Administration, issued a statement early in February 1975 warning doctors that oral contraceptives play a role in causing high blood pressure. I do not know, however, whether or not a warning will also be printed on the patient package insert. After all, it has none about cancer. But someday enough very young women may develop mammary carcinoma after prolonged use of oral contraceptives to justify a warning about this disease.

This is as good a time as any to talk about the American Cancer Society—what it does and does not do about breast cancer. Certainly the ACS is indispensable, and a number of its programs, like Reach to Recovery, are essential to many women. If its volunteers did not provide such postmastectomy services, no one would. The millions of dollars raised and spent on research and on massive education programs about cancer would not have been raised or spent without the ACS. Detailing all the good and helpful things the society has done since its founding in 1913 would take a chapter in itself.

On the other hand, the American Cancer Society has become an Establishment, issuing ukases for and against various aspects of all cancer treatment. In breast cancer, the edict is that the Halsted or the modified radical mastectomy is the only appropriate initial treatment. While this is certainly true in most cases, there *are* other procedures available. But when women call their local chapters to ask about surgeons who will do less cutting, they get no such information from the American Cancer Society. I have received countless calls, like the one from the twenty-seven-year-old who had to travel to see Dr. Crile, from patients pleading desperately for the names of surgeons who might help them keep their breasts. "I called the American Cancer Society office," I have been told again and again, "and they won't give me the name of any doctor in the area who will do anything except a radical. Isn't there somebody in town who will?"

I am sure no one has reached this page without knowing that I feel the modified radical mastectomy is the best choice. But it was a decision I made for myself, and I have no right to decide for any other woman. When I am asked—and I have been asked many times—I say point-blank that this operation gives the best chance, with the least mutilation, of getting rid of the cancer, providing it has not already spread beyond the axillary lymph nodes. If women, again like the twenty-seven-year-old, want to take the risks of lumpectomy or partial mastectomy, I try to talk them out of it. But it is, after all, not my life. When I see I am getting nowhere, I try—unlike the good volunteers of the American Cancer Society—to give enough information so that they can make an intelligent decision. The kind of cancer the tumor is, its location, its size, and the presence or absence of palpable nodes in the armpit are all factors that must be weighed. I think the American Cancer Society should make such information available when women call for advice, and not arbitrarily endorse only a radical mastectomy. Decreeing what medical practices should be followed is not in its charter; educating the public is.

It would be helpful if the society would commission a poll of top breast-cancer specialists—including Dr. Crile and other "segmental resectionists"—and publish their criteria for performing lesser surgeries, along with the risks involved. This kind of information would be of inestimable value to American women and their surgeons. In addition, I believe that ACS chapters around the country should keep lists of surgeons who will do the two-stage procedure separating the biopsy from the mastectomy, and also of those who will perform less than a radical mastectomy if that is what the woman wants, which it can give out to desperate women who call and ask for them.

In 1974, the American Cancer Society hired the Gallup organization to conduct a poll on women's attitudes to breast cancer, in which 1,007 women eighteen years old and over were interviewed, mainly concerning the factual information they had about breast cancer. The poll revealed that most either had no real information or had a great deal of misinformation. Had the ACS asked me, I could have reported the same thing, much less expensively.

There was, however, one very significant finding—worth all the money. "Breast loss can affect both a woman's self-image and her relations with men," the poll reported. "This attitude is most common among single women (61%) and those 18 to 34 years of age (66%)."

In spite of this large proportion of young, single women who said that they would feel themselves impaired, the ACS has still refused to back away from its all-out support of radical mastectomy and nothing else. The edict has been handed down by the all-male breast-cancer committee (whose chairman, Dr. Benjamin Byrd, prefers the Halsted radical, by the way), and so the ACS plans to make no effort to assist those who might want to take a chance on one of the lesser surgeries. Yet the American Cancer Society could do a great deal to hasten the demise of the Halsted if it chose to. All it would take is a loud and clear statement condemning the unnecessary excision of the pectoral muscles. In short, the same sort of thing the society did when it condemned lumpectomies.

In the same way, the ACS could also do much to stop the practice of the single-stage biopsy and mastectomy that is customary as soon as a frozen-section pathological diagnosis says "Carcinoma!"

The American Cancer Society exerts strong pressure affecting one other aspect of cancer care. By endorsing or withholding its endorsement from anticancer remedies, it has a great deal to say about which ones are available to patients. I am not referring to obvious quack cures, but to untested substances, like laetrile, hydrazine sulfate, and abscissic acid. While the society has no legal power to keep a substance from being sold, its influence over the Food and Drug Administration, which does, is enormous.

Why should cancer patients whose cases are so advanced that their physicians have made it plain they are "terminal" be forced to go to another country, far from families and friends, to try these substances, just because the ACS has not blessed them with its official sanction? Every anticancer drug known can be deadly. How could laetrile be any more dangerous to a dying person than 5-FU, methotrexate, adriamycin, or any of the other approved drugs used in chemotherapy? If the National Institutes of Health are forbidden by law from recommending specific treatment and can only "report results of research," who has given the American Cancer Society such a right?

I cannot criticize the ACS for its arrogance about surgery and drugs without also praising the society for its work in educating women and doctors about the importance of early breast-cancer detection. Certainly the organization has done a superb job in spreading the word about breast self-examination and mammograms, and in supporting research into newer, safer detection methods through the demonstration projects.

I would like to see the ACS put some of its considerable influence to work on school boards around the country, to get BSE made a part of the regular physical education or health curriculum in high schools. Although breast cancer is rare in anyone under the age of twenty, these school years may well be the last time girls are a captive audience for such a program, and they might learn how to do the BSE properly if their grades were dependent on it.

The ACS and Mrs. Terese Lasser—assisted by prominent women like Mrs. Ford, Mrs. Rockefeller, and Mrs. Bayh—have also made a noble contribution in getting breast cancer out of the closet and into the open, where women can see it is nothing to be hidden. As Mrs. Bayh has said, those who have survived mastectomies and who talk openly about their surgeries have done a great deal to eradicate the dread that has prevented many women from getting to the doctor in time.

The American Cancer Society cannot do everything, however. It can do little or nothing, for example, about the lack of women surgeons in this country—but something must be done, by some agency. There is a great deal of difference in breast-cancer treatment where there are more women on hospital or clinic staffs.

Again, I would like to point out that all the members of the ACS Breast Cancer Committee are male, as are all the members of the Steering Committee of the National Cancer Institute's Breast Cancer Task Force. It is interesting that at a joint ACS-NCI breast-cancer conference held in New York on November 15, 1974, the only report suggesting an alternative to surgery as the preferred treatment for primary breast cancer was presented by a woman. Dr. Eleanor D. Montague, of the M. D. Anderson Hospital and Tumor Institute, in Texas, is conducting trials of partial mastectomy followed by irradiation. Although the results after five or ten years may prove to be bad, at least someone—a woman, of course—is trying to find a way to help women who are willing to take a risk to save their breasts.

There is a special reason to explain surgeons' stubbornness about abandoning the Halsted radical: their training. Most physicians concede, albeit confidentially, that surgery attracts a certain breed of doctor—prima donnas who think the scalpel is the solution for every physical problem. I have made the analogy before between cancer and the war in Vietnam. Surgeons can be compared with the bombardiers, who saw every military problem as something to be overcome by wiping places off the map. If a little was good, then, naturally, more was better. Surgeons, after all, are trained to think of surgical solutions to the problems of disease. Coupled closely with personality and training is surgical arrogance. To stop a century-old procedure in favor of one they have struggled against so long and so vehemently would be an admission that they have been wrong.

"What will a shift to modified radicals do to the thousands of women who have to live with Halsteds?" is a question I have been asked again and again. My reply, by now a ritual litany, is "What do you tell people whose parents died of diabetes before insulin was developed? What about people still suffering the aftereffects of polio they caught before the vaccines were developed?" The argument seems silly and self-serving. It is, nonetheless, a frequently mentioned reason against changing from the anachronistic Halsted. Too many surgeons would rather stonewall than switch.

Not all surgeons fit this description, thank heavens. Those who know the most about breast cancer tend to be the most willing to reject or accept ideas as they are disproven or proven. Dr. Dao is one. Another is Dr. Bernard Fisher, chairman of the National Cancer Institute's National Surgical Adjuvant Breast Project, and a professor of surgery at the University of Pittsburgh School of Medicine. He has been an outspoken, although soft-spoken, critic of the penchant in this country for the Halsted.

"In order to further understand Halsted's rationale for the type of surgery he advocated," Dr. Fisher wrote in 1970, "it is important to appreciate his concept of the biology of cancer—and particularly how he thought tumors were disseminated." Dr. Fisher pointed out that in Halsted's time, at the end of the nineteenth century, no one suspected that breast cancer could be spread by the blood stream; Dr. Halsted believed the lymphatics and the lymph nodes were the main routes for its spread to other parts of the body. To explain the logic of Halsted's massive, extensive surgery, Dr. Fisher quoted from a 1907 scientific report.

We must remove not only a very large amount of skin and a much larger area of subcutaneous fat and fascia [Dr. Halsted wrote] but also strip the sheaths from the upper part of the rectus, the serratus magnus, the subscapularis, and at times from parts of the latissimus dorsi and the teres major [all of these are muscles]. Both pectoral muscles are, of course, removed. A part of the chest wall should, I believe, be excised in certain cases, the surgeon bearing in mind that he is dealing with lymphatic and not blood metastases and that the slightest inattention to detail or attempts to hasten convalescence by such plastic operations as are feasible only when a restricted amount of skin is removed, may sacrifice his patient.

Dr. Fisher summed up the Halsted radical by quoting a comment made in 1965 by a breast-cancer specialist, Dr. R. S. Handley: "To belittle Halsted is to commit the stupidity of judging a man's achievement out of context of his time and his circumstances." But, Dr. Fisher commented, "to continue to endorse uncritically a procedure founded on the principles just described is irrational."

A great deal has been learned about breast cancer since Dr. Halsted wrote his 1907 report. It is a bizarre, unpredictable, idiosyncratic disease. Some women have tiny primary tumors and negative nodes, yet die in less than five years from metastases to the brain, lungs, or liver, because a stray cell or two were carried there by the blood stream. Some women have large tumors and many positive nodes, and never develop a metastasis or even a recurrence. My internist, Dr. Heckman, told me of a woman who had refused to have a mastectomy years ago and is still alive. "For years, she's been growing cancers here and there," he told me. "Whenever she gets one, she goes to the hospital to have it removed. It's what we call living in a symbiotic relationship with cancer."

Since so much more is known now than Dr. Halsted knew, it is ridiculous to continue an operation based on the obsolescent medical knowledge available at the turn of the century.

Since the publicity about Betty Ford's Halsted radical mastectomy and Happy Rockefeller's later modified radical, I have been told, many general surgeons—even older ones—have changed and are no longer routinely removing the pectoral muscles. Surgeons are, after all, businessmen, who want to please their customers. The flood of criticism that followed Mrs. Ford's operation informed many women for the first time that a less mutilating and disabling alternative is available. Apparently, they began insisting that their doctors either do the modified or they would take their surgical business elsewhere.

Stubborn cattle are prodded with electricity, and stubborn doctors react to checkbooks. When enough women stop going to surgeons who insist on performing the Halsted radical and go, instead, to those who do the modified, that surgical antiquity will finally become the museum piece it should have been long ago.

If this happens, anything can. Perhaps we will soon see the day when the good old American practice of combining surgical biopsy in a single stage with mastectomy will join the Halsted on the dusty museum shelf.

In an excellent article, "A Critical Look at Cancer Coverage," in the January-February 1975 issue of the *Columbia Journalism Review*, Daniel S. Greenberg, a science writer, described the pitiful state of the "so-called federal War on cancer," then in its third year. His main theme was that the American people are being doled out false optimistic reports on the war.

He begins by quoting the opening sentence of *The Hopeful Side of Cancer*, a publication of the American Cancer Society: "Cancer is one of the most curable of the major diseases in this country." Like me, Greenberg saw a parallel between this war and the Vietnam war, in the reporting of them. "It is useful to contemplate," he said, "certain curious and gruesome parallels that are beginning to appear between the reporting of this 'War' and the early bulletins from Vietnam. We can quickly pass over the doleful similarities of battlefield body counts and their medical counterparts, survival rates; the exaggerated hopes drawn from limited victories, and forecasts of a long, hard fight beyond which shines light at the end of the tunnel—if only we persevere with the grand design of the bureaucracy in charge."

Greenberg goes on to cite information from the National Cancer Institute's 1974 statistics, which, he points out, are "published periodically under the infelicitous title *End Results in Cancer.*" When analyzed, Greenberg insists, these "end results" show that the war on cancer has not been very successful at all. Unfortunately, I cannot disagree. Few, if any, gains have been made in curing any kind of cancer. With breast cancer, of course, all the progress has been in finding the disease sooner and in extending pain-free years of life, none in curing it.

However, I feel Greenberg was unfair in attacking the "few major cancer centers" that the 1971 National Cancer Act is supporting. "The research-oriented institutions can pick and choose their patients," Greenberg wrote—a comment apparently based on a conversation he had with "one specialist." This specialist had told him, "Clinical researchers don't like to treat dying patients and poor risks can be sent elsewhere to die." Greenberg said he had found success rates at cancer centers difficult to get and "ambiguous."

Since Greenberg lives in the Washington area, I telephoned him immediately. "The low survival rates of places like Roswell Park and M. D. Anderson," I told him, "are due to the fact that most of their patients aren't referred by their doctors until they are already at death's door. Even the best treatment couldn't help them." I went on—angrily, I must confess. "If people went to specialized cancer centers, to cancer clinics, or to oncologists from the very beginning, I bet their survival rates would skyrocket. The problem is that general surgeons and general practitioners want the business and don't send cancer patients to specialists until they have exhausted everything they think they know. And they know very little," I added.

I suggested that Greenberg read the testimony given before the Senate Appropriations subcommittee on Labor and Health, Education, and Welfare, on July 12, 1974, by Roswell Park's director, Dr. Gerald P. Murphy. "Two-thirds of the one million Americans who have serious cancer malignancies today," Dr. Murphy had told the senators, "will die within four years. The slowness of some physicians to accept the newer treatment methods at cancer centers can result in the vast majority of cancer patients not benefiting from treatment advances that have been available for two decades at cancer centers. Approximately 90 per cent of cancer patients are seen first by their own physicians, many of whom are not aware of the progress made in cancer diagnosis and treatment."

Such a public reprimand from one physician to his colleagues, breaking, as it does, the professional code of silence, is rare indeed. Family doctors and general surgeons usually dismiss such criticism as one more sign of the traditional rivalry between them and the "ivory-tower types." Nonsense! This attitude is hurting—killing—patients. Every general practitioner and general surgeon should read Dr. Murphy's testimony with care, and pay attention to it.

I summarized the statement for Greenberg. "The friendly family doctor is the reason cancer's survival rates are as bad as they are," I insisted. "What can a place like Roswell Park or the Cleveland Clinic do if patients aren't referred until they're terminal?" Greenberg admitted that he had not considered this aspect of the problem.

Ann London Scott, who died on February 17, 1975, of metastatic liver disease, is—was—an example of this kind of neglect. She was not given good follow-up care by her physician, and when she finally went to Roswell Park for treatment it was too late.

On August 25, 1974, *Parade* magazine published an article titled "The Cancer Circuit Riders." The author, Theodore Irwin, wrote:

Medical-circuit-riders fanning out from here [Birmingham, Alabama] to other cities and towns in the state are helping to salvage lives of thousands afflicted with cancer. In an NCI-supported program, the University of Alabama Medical Center has been sending specially-trained doctors, nurses and technicians throughout the state to educate general practitioners and general surgeons about the latest methods for treating cancer. Behind this program is the realization that too many unnecessary deaths from cancer occur each year from outdated treatment.

Dr. John R. Durant, director of the university's Cancer Research Training Center, told Irwin, "The time has come for the end of pessimism, procrastination and pain-killers. The greatest detriment to treatment of a cancer patient is a physician's attitude of despair. If he thinks nothing can be done, he sends the patient

home to die. But even if the patient is going to die, the quality
of survival is very important."

Many of the cancer specialists Irwin had interviewed said that
physicians did not keep up with new treatment techniques. "Some
resist using chemotherapy because of past reports of severe
side effects and little benefit," Irwin wrote. "Certain older doctors still rely on what they learned in medical school decades
ago." Dr. Sidney Arje, of the American Cancer Society, had told
him that the average doctor is not equipped to deal with the
"full therapeutic approach" to cancer. Too often, Dr. Arje said,
these doctors begin treatment and do not refer patients to cancer
centers until they have begun to deteriorate—too late. "Studies
reveal that only a low percentage of our population, particularly
in small towns and cities, receive proper treatment for cancer,"
Irwin said. He continued to cite specific examples of such mis-
and maltreatment. Here is the "economic incentive" in the medical, as opposed to the surgical, treatment of cancer. Family doctors just will not give up a customer until it is obvious they have
failed.

The "economic incentive" is as prominent at the very beginning of breast-cancer management as it is at the end. A
pamphlet on breast-cancer detection and self-examination was
published by the American College of Obstetricians and Gynecologists in January 1975 (printed first in *Redbook*). "It has
been suggested that mammograms, like Pap smears, be performed as a matter of routine," the text states. "However, the
detection rate above and beyond that obtained by a good physical
examination is very low, and the time and expense involved make
its use impractical for most large, mass-screening programs."

In the large, mass-screening program sponsored by the American Cancer Society and the National Cancer Institute, physical
examination was inaccurate in detecting 57 per cent of the early
breast cancers found; mammograms found 92 per cent of them.
As Dr. Robert L. Shirley, a Boston specialist, wrote, "Physical
examination alone is like flipping a coin."

How can our fee-for-service medical system and its economic
motivation be incorporated into a lifesaving system of excellent
cancer care? By the creation of specialized cancer clinics and
hospitals, using the latest techniques and the leading experts to

treat all cancers correctly. Such cancer centers do not have to be government-subsidized to do the job that is needed.

In all the European countries I visited, of course, they are subsidized by the government. In the United Kingdom, for example, Dr. Gordon Taylor, who directs administration at the Royal Marsden Cancer Hospital, told me that England now has four regional cancer centers. Royal Marsden cares for part of London and its environs; the others are in Manchester, Leeds, and Birmingham. These are pilot projects, and after four years their survival rates will be compared with those from areas that do not have cancer centers. When I talked with Dr. Taylor, in December 1974, the Royal Marsden program had been in operation for about one year. This hospital is responsible for over 3 million people—all of Surrey, all of Sussex, part of Hampshire, and part of London. The budget appropriated by Parliament is small, but some of the deficit is made up by contributions and private fund-raising campaigns.

Dr. Taylor told me the British general surgeons had been difficult to deal with at the beginning. "They do like to follow their patients." He smiled. "But they have been coming around." The four regional centers are especially interested in whole-body scanning and preoperative staging, as well as in early detection. Dr. Taylor is confident their survival rates will be much higher than those elsewhere. If he is right, ten more regional centers will be established in England alone, and others in Wales, Scotland, and Northern Ireland.

A small, economically declining country like England is planning fourteen specialized cancer centers, while the government of the rich United States, with five times the population, is planning a total of seventeen!

In Sweden, Dr. Westerberg told me that general practitioners there refer cancer patients to oncology clinics immediately.

In the Soviet Union, I learned, each of the fifteen republics has its own oncology hospital, and, in addition, twenty-two cancer-research institutes take patients whose diseases are being studied. For those who do not require hospitalization, 242 specialized oncology clinics give outpatient treatment. Professor N. P. Napalkov, director of Leningrad's Petrov Institute of Oncology, told me that some of the cancer centers concentrate on specific kinds of carcinomas, and that if patients can be treated best in one of them, they are taken there, no matter how far distant. "And we have just sent a group of our doctors to treat a patient who was too ill to be brought here, even by jet. We do this for just average citizens," Professor Napalkov emphasized. "It does not have to be anyone of high position. This is the procedure in our country with everyone."

Professor Sviatukhina described for me the routine a Russian woman goes through after finding a breast growth. She would first go to her own doctor, in a clinic near her home. If the growth is suspicious, she is sent to the local oncology clinic or hospital—no woman lives far from one, the professor added. The first medical step there, as elsewhere, is to make a diagnosis of malignant or benign, but not by surgical biopsy unless all methods short of it have failed to give a definitive diagnosis. When the tumor is malignant, the various staging examinations determine how far, if at all, the cancer has already spread, and if it seems to be confined to the breast and axilla, a mastectomy is performed. The patient continues to return to the oncology clinic for follow-up examinations.

My internist laughed when I told him how cancer is handled in the socialized-medicine countries I had visited. "I don't care what you tell me about those other countries," he said. "What we have in the United States is the best. No question."

"Then why aren't our survival rates better than theirs?" I snapped back. "If what we do is so much better, then we should have more patients living a heck of a lot longer than they do in those other countries. We should be curing breast cancer, not just treating it."

He had no reply.

In this day and age, when we go not to a dentist but to an orthodontist to have our teeth straightened, to a periodontist for gum treatments, and to miscellaneous other -dontists for other dental problems, I cannot understand why, in the United States, a cancer patient is not sent immediately to an oncologist. A detached retina is an excellent example of a medical problem that is—as it should be—referred at once to a specialist by the general practitioner. No family doctor would attempt to treat such a problem. Why is this not done with cancer patients?

"Our general men are more highly trained in cancer than even the specialists in Europe are," one surgeon told me. "If you saw all the oncology I had to handle during my residency, you would understand." This is not a sensible explanation. If our training is so superior, if we spend so much more money and have so much more sophisticated equipment, why are our breast-cancer survival rates no better than they were in 1950?

There is a term in religious debate known as "invincible igno- rance." If people err in their faith because they do not know any better, that is taken into account by the Almighty when the de- cision is made between heaven and hell. Is it possible that it is invincible ignorance on the part of general practitioners and general surgeons in the United States, and not greed? Is it pos- sible that they simply do not know?

I would like to be generous and give "invincible ignorance," not the "economic incentive," as the reason ordinary doctors con- tinue to manage cancer cases in this country. But the evidence is against such generosity. There has been too much publicity in the medical literature for too long a time stressing the importance of expertise in cancer treatment. For example, the magisterial *Journal of the American Medical Association* (no rebellious un- derground tabloid, in anyone's opinion) has said: "We have been forced to conclude that the treatment of many major forms of cancer can no longer be wisely entrusted to the unattached general physician or a surgeon or to the general hospital as ordi- narily equipped, but must be recognized as a specialty requiring special training, equipment, and experience. It would be indeed dangerous to entrust these responsibilities to amateur specialists."

That was in 1929. Almost five decades later, 90 per cent of all cancer patients in the United States are still being treated by "amateur specialists."

Perhaps we do not have enough oncologists in the United States to handle all our cancer patients. Dr. Heckman told me that I had done the right thing in going to Roswell Park, if I wanted to benefit from the latest advances. "But," he pointed out, "there are only a couple of places like that in the country. If everybody went up to Buffalo, or to M. D. Anderson or Sloan- Kettering, there just wouldn't be enough beds or staff to take care of them."

Unfortunately, he is right. Under the 1971 National Cancer Act—the "Conquest of Cancer" act—money was appropriated to establish eighteen new comprehensive cancer centers around the country. Some of these are already built, staffed, and functioning; others are in various stages of completion. Some are exclusively devoted to cancer; others are affiliated with general hospitals. *All*, however, are oncology centers. These are the eighteen, in addition to the four centers already established:

Sidney Farber Cancer Center, Boston, Massachusetts
Yale University Cancer Research Center, New Haven, Connecticut
Roswell Park Memorial Institute, Buffalo, New York
Memorial Sloan-Kettering Institute, New York, New York
Fox Chase Cancer Center, Philadelphia, Pennsylvania
University of Pennsylvania Cancer Center, Philadelphia
Johns Hopkins Hospital, Baltimore, Maryland
Vincent Lombardi Cancer Center, Georgetown University Hospital and Cancer Research Center, Howard University, Washington, D.C.
Duke University Comprehensive Cancer Center, Durham, North Carolina
Cancer Research and Training Center, Birmingham, Alabama
University of Miami School of Medicine, Miami, Florida
Mayo Clinic, Rochester, Minnesota
Wisconsin Clinical Center, Madison, Wisconsin
Illinois Cancer Council, comprising Presbyterian-St. Luke's Hospital, University of Chicago Cancer Center, and Northwestern University Cancer Center, Chicago
Colorado Regional Cancer Center, Denver, Colorado
M. D. Anderson Hospital and Tumor Institute, Houston, Texas
Fred Hutchinson Cancer Research Center, Seattle, Washington
USC-LAC Cancer Center of UCLA, Los Angeles, California

Twenty-two centers are certainly not enough for 200 million people.

If the United States ever reaches the stage at which all cancer patients are treated only in cancer clinics or hospitals or by private oncologists, the survival rates will reflect the change. I remember my fellow patients at Roswell Park, who had been going there periodically for "chemo" for more than a decade, and living normal, pain-free lives in between. My solution is to have more oncologists and more cancer clinics and public or private centers. If little England can be planning fourteen, we should have at least one in every state.

But cancer clinics and centers, even where they exist, are not always used as they should be, for one reason—fear. Many patients, and their physicians, are afraid of research hospitals, and all the specialized institutions are engaged in cancer research of one kind or another. This prejudice had first been mentioned to me by my internist, when I told him I was going to one and he made that remark about "if you like a research setup."

The "latest advances," he told me then, might be experimental. "In a research setup," he said, "you're liable to wind up in a control group or random sample or some kind of experiment they're doing over there. You don't want that, do you?"

That had not been the moment to argue about the benefits of private hospitals versus research centers. We have discussed it since, but I am afraid I made no headway in convincing him. He is positive that too many unnecessary tests, X-rays, and so on are done at Roswell Park "because they're collecting data." While I believe that only a research center offers the best possible care, I cannot change his mind.

I know I am a statistic at Roswell Park, as well as at the National Cancer Institute, where I am a sample in that "marker" study. But if such samples are useful in any kind of research, why not be one? It makes no difference to me if my blood and urine are distributed to different laboratories doing different studies. After all, everyone in a private hospital is a statistic, too. It may be only a calculation of the birth rate of twenty-year-old Caucasian women, or a study of breast cancer in sixty-year-old Japanese women, but these are statistics, nonetheless.

As far as being a "random sample" in a clinical trial, I found that informed consent is taken very seriously at Roswell Park and at the National Cancer Institute. No patient is "experimented on" unless she or he—or the family, if the patient is too ill—is told exactly what is to be done. Moreover, few doctors will participate in "experiments" with drugs or surgeries that they believe to be harmful when there is a tried alternative, that is, when it is a matter of comparing something known to be harmful with something else known to be helpful. Usually, in random-sample trials, little is known about any of the treatments, and comparisons must be made between procedures that are equally risky. But this is only when doing nothing is even more dangerous, and someone must take a chance—with informed consent.

As for getting extra, unnecessary tests and examinations to "collect data," that is nonsense. I have done enough research by now to know what kinds of examinations must be done during the critical first years after a mastectomy, and I am *not* getting unnecessary tests at Roswell Park. On the contrary, other post-operative women are being neglected if their private physicians are not giving them the same follow-up examinations. I was amused that, immediately after telling me how research hospitals do so many more tests because they are "collecting data," my careful and thorough internist proceeded to describe his own postmastectomy examinations during the first two years. Had I not gone to Roswell Park for my checkups, I would have received exactly the same examinations and tests from him.

Of course, patients in research hospitals are at the disposal of everyone on the professional staff. This is so in all teaching hospitals, and it did not bother me, although I know many women do not like it. Anyone who has strong feelings about being constantly stared at by interns, residents, student nurses, and all and sundry on the hospital's staff would be very unhappy in a place like Roswell Park. I would advise her to find a well-trained oncologist who practices in a private clinic or hospital, where this kind of co-operation is not required. The important factor is the competence of her physician, not the institution, so long as it is well equipped.

Another personal aspect of being in a cancer clinic or hospital is that all the patients have cancer. As I have said, once I had accepted the inevitable, I found it supportive to be in such a place. But my attitude is probably not typical, and this must be taken into account. While it helped my psyche, another woman might find it depressing. If this is so, she, too, should find an oncologist and go to a private clinic or hospital. Again, it is the doctor that is important, not the institution.

Before leaving the subject of cancer clinics and centers and their virtues, I must describe a unique advisory system offered by

Roswell Park, as well as by a few other centers around the country. This is a toll-free cancer "hot line," on which any doctor, dentist, or osteopath in the state of New York can call the hospital and discuss a case directly with a specialist working in that area, thus gaining the benefit of the latest advances.

I wondered why the National Cancer Institute could not set up such a program nationally. But I was reminded that the law creating the National Institutes of Health says that their specialists may only report on the results of research and are not legally permitted to recommend specific kinds of treatment. I was told that some experts at NCI talk to doctors who call about their patients, but this is not supposed to be done. NCI does have an information office (301-496-6641), but its director, Betty Mc-Vickers, may only refer patients to NCI-supported doctors or institutions around the country. She cannot legally refer a caller to, for example, a surgeon in a particular city who is willing to do a lumpectomy or some kind of modified radical instead of a Halsted radical. Physicians can sometimes find ways to get around the information barrier, but patients who call get no specific advice. Usually, all Ms. McVickers can do is send a stack of the latest publications about their diseases.

And, of course, there is always the matter of money. In spite of Daniel Greenberg's allegations about a wasteful bureaucracy (perhaps true), the total budget of the National Cancer Institute is not much more than the total that was requested in early 1975 for South Vietnam and Cambodia. Having seen both of the battles from the front lines, I know firsthand that there was far more waste in Saigon and Phnom Penh than in Bethesda, and certainly a great deal was gross theft.

Who can possibly measure in dollars the value of the children saved by the leukemia break-throughs of the past few years? How much are the lives of the women saved by Dr. George Papanicolaou's cervical-cancer test worth? No computer can calculate the value of the progress—however little it is, in Daniel Greenberg's eyes—that has resulted from the war against cancer.

On a local television program explaining the proposed cancer budget for 1976, Secretary of Health, Education, and Welfare Caspar W. Weinberger tried to convince his audience that the $582 million being asked by President Ford for 1976 federal cancer research was not any less than the same amount requested for 1975, in spite of more inflation. Secretary Weinberger was not convincing. Of this sum, the proposed budget for the Breast Cancer Task Force was $9.75 million for 1976—also the same as it was for 1975. The cut—with the dollar so eroded, it is a definite cut—will be felt primarily in less money for basic research and for fellowships and grants to the young scientists on whom the future rests.

Without basic research, there would be no penicillin. Dr. (later Sir) Alexander Fleming was not looking for an antibiotic when he discovered that a strange mold had destroyed the bacteria in a Petri dish. In fact, I could find no mention anywhere of exactly what he was working on at the time, except that it was not penicillin. To take another example, the laboratory at the Medical College of Virginia was not doing breast-cancer research when it found that something in "grass" affected the growth of breast cancer. The goal of that particular experiment was to see if the long-term use of marijuana had a harmful effect on the DNA in the cells of pot smokers. Whether or not the substance in marijuana turns out to have any significance in relation to breast cancer is not yet known. One of the laboratories that found the oncogene was funded for research in metabolic, digestive, and infectious diseases. Such serendipity—accidental discovery—has always played a major role in scientific progress.

For the government to cut money from basic research budgets and try to harness scientists' talents and abilities to achieve particular specified objectives would be catastrophic. The final cure for breast cancer—for all cancer—may well come from an esoteric, seemingly useless piece of research in an area totally unrelated to that disease.

By the same token, withdrawing government financial support from graduate students and young physicians who have chosen to do research in universities and hospitals is penny-wise and pound-foolish. Grants, fellowships, or other subsidies are almost the only way such young scientists have of earning a living while they continue their work. Cutting off the relatively small amount of dollars that has, in the past, enabled young scientists to get additional training is as good an example as I can imagine of cutting off our noses to spite our faces. If researchers cannot earn

enough to support themselves and their families while learning
more about cancer, they will naturally leave the field and go
where they can. Where is our next generation of cancer experts
supposed to come from?

Breast-cancer research and treatment suffer from what I call
the "double-helix syndrome." The reference is to the best-selling
book by Dr. John D. Watson, who won a Nobel Prize for helping
to unravel the complex chemistry of the DNA molecule. In *The
Double Helix,* Dr. Watson recalled the intense, often hilarious,
professional rivalry among the various laboratories working toward the same goal. The secrecy enshrouding all the preliminary
findings in the DNA experiments could never be matched by the
Pentagon or by any of our intelligence agencies. While a similar
information blackout is found in all scientific fields, for obvious
reasons I am most interested in its effect on breast-cancer research.

Discoveries are constantly being made in laboratories and hospitals all over the world, but no woman can benefit from them
until the results have been presented publicly in some medical
forum and then published in a medical journal. This can take
many long months—often years. Scientific journals are notorious
for the length of time that elapses between the acceptance of an
article and its publication. On the other hand, many researchers
delay publication in order to place their articles in one journal
rather than another.

I find myself wondering if, at this very moment, some investigator or publication somewhere has information that could help
me. There is no way for me to find out, and nothing I could do
about it even if there were.

Occasionally, I gnash my teeth.

"You just lucked into it," I've been told many times. "You were
able to understand medicalese, and you had friends who could
help you get the treatment you wanted."

I know I have been lucky. But it should not need a stroke of
luck or an accident of education to get excellent medical treatment. It is every woman's right to have the best care medicine
knows how to provide. Of course, I am not out of the woods yet.
Breast cancer is, as I have said, bizarre, idiosyncratic, and unpre-

dictable. Even with the best treatment, there is no way to be sure the disease will be beaten. But at least I know I have gotten, am getting, and will continue to get the best care there is.

In these United States of America, the richest country in the world, it is inexcusable that any woman should have less.

16

The Future

"I've seen great new ideas come and go for more years than I like to think about," a graying, battle-scarred veteran of the war against cancer told me.

Now retired, Dr. Erwin Vollmer was the chief of the Breast Cancer Project's Coordinating Branch at the National Cancer Institute for years. But he began his career as a working endocrinologist, "back in the years when hormones were 'it,'" he explained, smiling. "After a while," he continued, "we found out hormones alone weren't it, at all. They weren't the whole answer to breast cancer—just another clue."

He shook his head. "Then, after the A-bomb was developed, we were sure that somehow nuclear medicine would have an answer for curing breast cancer. But no soap. Radioisotopes and supervoltage X-ray just became extra tools, not cures. Then it was chemotherapy, and I guess it still is," Dr. Vollmer went on. "Certainly, some day soon, I hope, a tumorcidal drug will be found that doesn't have to kill the patient to cure the cancer.

"After Joe Bittner discovered the mouse mammary-tumor virus, back in '36, the big push was to find a human virus. Now all the younger research people think immunology is it." He smiled. "As soon as they find the little bug, they're positive they'll be able to put together some kind of vaccine to prevent breast cancer or a serum to cure it."

A slender, slight man, Dr. Vollmer stared above my head at nothing, his Paul-Newman-blue eyes looking, perhaps, to the future. "I hope they're right. In all these years, after spending so much money, it's incredible that we're still losing as many women from breast cancer as we did forty years ago. There has just got to be a break-through soon."

Dr. Robert Love, another long-time fighter in the cancer wars, was angry, not philosophical. In a Scottish accent as rolling as that country's Highlands, he asked—expecting no answer—"We've really accomplished a lot, haven't we, when we find a cancerous tumor in a woman's breast two years earlier, so that—on survival-rate charts—she has lived another two years? That's where all our progress has been in breast cancer. Earlier detection, not cures."

"As far as I'm concerned," Dr. Love continued, pounding his desk, "that's not enough. So we excise a woman's breast years sooner, have her on record as being diagnosed years sooner, and she has had a prolonged life. What has that accomplished as far as saving her life?"

As the newly appointed director of Programs and Analyses at the National Cancer Institute, Dr. Love is busy finding out exactly who is doing what research, where it is being done, then seeing to it that the data are put into a computer for quick and easy retrieval. While having a data bank of all the NCI-supported cancer research may not directly affect the search for a cure for breast cancer, it will prevent much duplication, repetition, and overlapping, saving not only money but also talent, energy, and time. In cancer, saving time means saving lives.

Time. Everywhere I went, the constant refrain was "It's just a matter of time now."

"I am absolutely positive that more will be done toward finding a cure for breast cancer in the next ten years," Dr. Maureen Roberts told me in Edinburgh, "than there has been in all of prior history. There simply must be. We have learned so very much about the disease and know so much more about its nature. Before all this very basic research, surgeons were simply cutting away in the dark, with no real idea of why they were doing what they did. We have ever so much more knowledge now."

The younger the doctors, and the fewer the years they had spent in the frustrating war, the more optimistic they were. Old-timers like Dr. Vollmer and Dr. Love were cautious about predicting anything. They had been through it all many times before. "The sad part of the whole breast-cancer story," Dr. Love repeated, "is that we must count so much on finding the cancer earlier. It seems that no matter what is done afterward, half the women diagnosed with breast cancer die from the disease before their lives should be over. Finding their tumors earlier just buys a few more years, not a cure."

Luckily, I and most of the women I interviewed are less gloomy than the doctors seem to be. Moreover, in the time between now and definitive cure there is a great deal that can be done with the knowledge already acquired.

For starters, the Halsted radical will soon, I am confident, become obsolete.

Also, I hope that the information has by now sifted down to general practitioners and general hospitals around the world that post-radical-mastectomy prophylactic X-ray treatments do little, if any, good, and a lot of harm. This practice should join the Halsted in the museum of medical antiquities.

Every breast tumor should be assayed immediately after its removal to determine its hormone dependency. Since this information is so important later, if a decision must be made about future treatment, the analysis should become routine everywhere. Hospitals that do not have the equipment and personnel to do these assays should not do mastectomies at all, unless they can arrange to have the assays done by another institution, which can report the results to the surgeon involved.

Another routine practice in the United States that should be discarded, along with the Halsted and prophylactic X-ray therapy, is the one-stage procedure combining diagnostic biopsy with the mastectomy. This is imperative, and the only reason I did not put it in bold-face print at the top of the following list is that I want to repeat the advantages in a single, short list so that women and their surgeons can see them quickly and easily.

The Five Imperative Reasons
Why Biopsy and Mastectomy Should Be Separated
into a Two-Stage Procedure

1. Medically, biopsy and mastectomy must be separated so that women whose diagnoses are positive can benefit from the *vital pre-mastectomy staging examinations*. If these show that the cancer has already spread beyond the axillary nodes, the woman should have no mastectomy at all.

2. Mastectomy is major surgery, requiring inhalation anesthesia. *Pre-operative chest X-rays* must be taken to be certain the patient's lungs are healthy enough to undergo such anesthesia safely.

3. All worry about an error in the quick *frozen-section diagnosis* would evaporate.

4. The *psychological trauma* women experience as a consequence of the now standard one-stage procedure will no longer occur.

5. Separating biopsy from mastectomy gives women *a voice in controlling their own destinies*. Lying unconscious on operating-room tables, they cannot determine or prepare themselves for their surgical fate, which depends on the opinion of the surgeon, usually male. Like me, a woman may want to go elsewhere to find a breast-cancer specialist. Under the current system used in most general hospitals, she does not even have the chance to ask. All women should be permitted to make this profound decision for themselves.

If the custom of doing routine surgical biopsies in a hospital is replaced by diagnostic techniques that can be done on an outpatient basis—and these are available, as I have said—it is true that surgeons in this country would lose a very lucrative source of income. But just think of the immediate effect the abolition of this idiotic practice would have on everyone else!

• Jam-packed operating rooms would be free to handle the more serious, but less urgent, cases now waiting to be scheduled.

• Hospital beds used by postbiopsy patients whose tumors were benign would also be available to patients whose medical needs are more urgent.

• Nurses, technicians, and other hospital personnel would have more time to spend with patients who really need their attention.

• In addition to saving the exorbitant fee paid to surgeons for biopsies—usually by medical insurance—there would be a saving in hospital costs, including laboratory fees, the anesthesiologist, preoperative chest X-rays, medications, room and board. Altogether, a simple biopsy for a benign lump can cost between $350 and $400 in the high CRVS areas. Even when medical insurance pays it, everyone who pays insurance premiums—which, as every policyholder knows, have been skyrocketing—pays in the end.

Of course, for the two of every ten women whose growths are malignant, the benefits of having a separate, earlier biopsy are enormous. In addition to all the advantages just mentioned, there is one other that is particularly vital. If the disease has metastasized and mastectomy would be useless, life-prolonging chemotherapy can be begun immediately, without having to wait for the patient to recuperate from the debilitating effects of major surgery—a delay of at least a month, and usually six weeks.

These are my "hopes for the future" that could be reality today if conventional medical practices were changed.

Another such "future hope" is a complete revamping of the United States medical system under which general practitioners or general surgeons treat breast-cancer patients, rather than referring them to oncologists as soon as a suspicious symptom is found. We do have enough specialists to supervise such patients, even when the direct care is administered by the family doctor. Also, if more patients were referred to oncologists at an early stage of the disease, more young physicians would choose this relatively new specialty, since they, too, necessarily have an economic incentive. Whether the reluctance of general physicians to send women to oncologists or specialized clinics or cancer centers is the result of invincible ignorance or of just plain invincible arrogance, it is a practice that must end, if breast-cancer survival rates are not to remain mired where they were forty years ago.

As Dr. Murphy pointed out in his Senate testimony, 90 per cent of all cancer patients in this country are treated by their family doctors. By now, I have sadly given up hope that the change will be voluntary. The only way to abolish the system is for breast-cancer patients—all cancer patients—to insist on being sent to specialists. We are medical consumers, and we should know by now how much muscle our consumer dollars can give us when properly used.

General physicians should not be dismayed; we do not expect

them to know all there is to know about everything. The human body is a complex and intricate machine, and it is virtually impossible for any one physician to be expert in every disease. Dr. Dao, Dr. Vollmer, Dr. Fisher, and Dr. Carbone, for example, have devoted their entire careers just to breast-cancer research and treatment, yet they would be the first to admit that they are still learning. Why do doctors who treat every disease of every organ think they must act as if they knew it all?

Another hope I have for the future that could be reality today is *more*—not less—government support for qualified young people who cannot afford the stiff tuitions of our graduate schools and medical schools. To become a physician in the United States, a young man or woman must not only be bright and have a lot of physical stamina and endurance, but must also be blessed with wealthy parents. As a result, many young college graduates who would like to go into medicine do not because they just do not have the money. Those who do get through have such a huge investment in their professional educations that they have to recover the money spent as rapidly as possible, often to repay loans. If, as in the countries I visited abroad, medical school were tuition-free and qualified students were given government aid for their living expenses, we would have more and better doctors who would not have such a strong economic motive. Anyone who has invested ten years and about $50,000 wants to get a return on that investment as quickly as possible.

We must remember that it is our free-enterprise "fee-for-service" medical system that is responsible for the "economic incentive" that pays surgeons "by the inch." Today's doctors did not invent the system; they are its products. Until we change our American way of education from the very beginning—substituting paid-for college, graduate school, and medical school—medicine and scientific research will continue to be "businesses" requiring huge investments. First the initial costs must be recovered and then a tidy profit turned. Remember that "the business of America," as President Coolidge once said, "is business."

As for the cutback in government support for basic research, grants, and fellowships, these funds must be restored. There can be no progress without research and without bright young scientists in the field.

Of course, I am referring mainly to breast-cancer research and treatment, but obviously these comments apply to all diseases. A country that can afford to spend billions of dollars for its defense should certainly be able to find the money needed for research and development in medicine to save American lives. The whole budget of the National Cancer Institute is, after all, just petty cash in the Pentagon.

One area where a great deal of work can be done now is in the psychological rehabilitation of the thousands of women who live in hidden misery because of their mastectomies. As I have said, I found twenty-two references to psychiatric studies of this serious problem. Reach to Recovery, while it does a great deal of good immediately after surgery, was never planned to be more than a short-term postoperative program.

If the routine one-stage biopsy-mastectomy is abandoned, Reach to Recovery would have the opportunity to help women before mastectomy, not only for a few weeks afterward. It may be out of the question for the program to assist women beyond the first six or eight weeks. According to nonattributable information I was given, most surgeons would not co-operate, as they do with Reach to Recovery, if volunteers spent too long a time advising patients. Such long-time postoperative assistance, I was told, requires a physician, not a laywoman. But where is the physician six weeks or two months after mastectomy, when the emotional problems really begin? And what good can a male surgeon (the usual physician involved) do for a disturbed woman? Thus, the severe problems some women have in adjusting to a normal life after mastectomy are being met only for those who can bring themselves to see a psychiatrist.

For those patients whose problems of adjustment are less difficult, there must be something else. A promising program, which should be copied widely, has begun at the Georgetown University Hospital, near where I live. Group sessions for women immediately after mastectomy, while they are still in the hospital, and continuing in periodic get-togethers as long afterward as they are needed, have been initiated. How successful this will be in alleviating some of the emotional pain of losing a breast, no one knows now. But at least something will be done.

Getting rid of the Halsted radical mastectomy would go a long way toward erasing some of the emotional scars—for the psychological scars are just as searing on the soul as the physical ones are on the flesh.

As an example, here are some excerpts from an anonymous reply to my questionnaire. The respondent had been forty-five years old when her Halsted was done six years earlier. As usual, she had not known in advance her breast would be missing when she woke up. In reply to my question about the effect the surgery had made in her life, she wrote, "I would have preferred that no one else know, but that was impossible." She was left with ugly, visible scar tissue that could not be hidden. Also, she had a great deal of physical difficulty regaining the use of her arm, and this was demoralizing to her. Six years after surgery, she has still not found a brassiere she can wear longer than eight hours at a time.

"I am very resentful that no matter how hard I try, I cannot find a bathing suit which covers my scar. . . . I like sleeveless dresses [but] my scar must be repulsive to others. . . . I took up tennis last spring, wore sleeveless tennis dresses and no one commented on it. Nevertheless, I am self-conscious, and in my activities, materials rub and chafe that arm. So I am better off [in] sleeveless [dresses]." She continued. "There will always be within me a deep-seated resentment about my mastectomy, but I am thankful that my life has been spared. I feel deeply resentful especially about the high cost of breast prostheses, mastectomy bras, swimsuits, etc. . . . Such essentials should be within everyone's financial reach."

Obviously, as was true in most of the responses I received from disease-free women, this woman's "resentment" and anger were due to the disfigurement and disabling aftereffects of the Halsted radical and not to the loss of the breast.

The Asken report on the psychiatric aspects of mastectomy quoted earlier clearly indicates that there are severe mastectomy-related emotional problems in the United States, problems that have not been touched by any psychiatrist or psychologist. Many women, of course, cannot afford psychiatric treatment. However, from responses I have received and conversations with psychiatrists, I do not believe money is the major obstacle. Most communities and hospitals in the country now have low-cost mental-health centers where troubled women can find help for a small fee or none at all. Making an appointment to see a psychiatrist is an overt, positive acknowledgment that the breast has been taken away, just as getting fitted for a prosthesis is an open admission of the loss. Very disturbed women cannot even take this first step. Healing them requires a positive search, not passive waiting for patients to walk in a door. Psychiatrists, psychologists, and social workers must find a way to bring therapy to them. This step should begin with surgeons and hospital personnel, who should be made acutely aware of the psychological trauma inherent in mastectomy. Moreover, where necessary, professional support should be routinely available in preparation for the operation.

Although they may be anonymous to me, to prosthesis fitters, and to the world at large, somebody, somewhere, knows where these women are. Mastectomies are not done on kitchen tables by husbands; they are done in hospitals by surgeons. Thus, there are hospital admissions records and doctors' files to help find the hundreds of thousands of women hiding in closets.

According to the responses I have received, Betty Ford and Happy Rockefeller did a great deal to bring some of these women out of their closets. There were at least a dozen questionnaires in my survey saying, in one way or another, that no one had known about the respondents' mastectomies until the operation became newsworthy and, therefore, mentionable. However, for every one that has emerged, there are dozens who have not. NCI records indicate there are about 677,000 women in the United States now alive and living with one or no breasts. This number, published by the Biometry Branch, is based on hospital admissions and death certificates. Yet, as I said earlier, the number of living mastectomees that is usually quoted is at most 350,000— probably the ones who never buy prostheses, who will have nothing to do with Reach to Recovery, and who are in the greatest need of psychological therapy.

Certainly, the time has long passed when there should be any discrimination against cancer patients in general, and breast-cancer patients specifically, in hiring and firing. The personnel practices of government and private industry are so preposterous that I hate even to take the time and space to mention them. All personnel managers should realize that the chances of a well-trained secretary's getting married or becoming pregnant and quitting her job are much higher than are the odds that a former breast-cancer patient will have a recurrence of the disease. The idiocy of this kind of discrimination is apparent and needs no explanation. All it needs is someone to figure out a way to get around insurance-company restrictions. The root of the problem, I was told, lies with insurance companies and pension plans that exclude high-risk people, even if they are willing to pay higher rates.

Perhaps the government will have to step in and underwrite this kind of insurance, as it has underwritten insurance policies for businesses in high-crime areas, and for homes in flood and earthquake territory. The precedent has already been set with these awful natural disasters. Why can't the government intervene to help insure victims of personal natural disasters like cancer?

I have some other future hopes that could be realized right now. It would be a great step forward if the National Institutes of Health charter were changed so that the specialists could give recommendations for treatment. This is a restriction that was imposed because of pressure from the powerful medical lobby present in Washington decades ago. The entire concept of government versus private medical care has changed considerably since that law was passed in 1944. The time has come for medical practice to follow the times. The top national medical research center should be obliged to share its expensively gained knowledge—as quickly as possible—directly for the benefit of the citizens who paid for it. If this anachronistic prohibition in the law were rescinded, a national cancer "hot line" like those in existence at state cancer hospitals such as Roswell Park and M. D. Anderson could be set up.

Women's liberation and feminist groups have done a great deal to cut down on all advertising that uses the female body as a lure. But there is still much to be done with the media.

One point I had designated as a "hope for the future" is already a reality: more international co-operation and communication, especially with large areas of the world that have been medically inaccessible for far too long. In mid-February 1975, a Soviet delegation of cancer experts, led by Academician Professor N. N. Blokhin, signed a "mini-détente" at NCI vowing complete co-operation and communication in cancer research between our two countries. My host in Moscow, Professor Blokhin, and his colleague in Leningrad, Professor Napalkov, were most helpful to me when I visited their oncology institutes. All members of their staffs extended me every possible courtesy and took much of their valuable time to help me. It is a good sign, I think, pointing to an excellent future for this humanitarian détente.

But these are all administrative, legal, and logistic hopes. What do I want to see happen medically? An immediate cure for me and for all women with breast cancer, of course. But, knowing this is still a dream, I must be more practical.

In London, I had asked Professor Symington, who struck me as being a visionary sort of scientist, what he would wish for the future of breast-cancer research.

"My first wish," he replied instantly, "would be for a miraculous, harmless drug that would eradicate breast cancer—all cancer —by simply giving a patient some tablets or an injection. That would be my foremost desire."

He looked at me somberly. "But you know, of course, that is entirely out of the question in the foreseeable future. Until such a miracle comes about, we have no alternative but to rely on mastectomy of some kind to remove localized tumors, and here is where my second wish can be found. I hope, within the very near future, we will have found some kind of indicator in the blood stream or urine of women to tell us if a malignancy is growing in those twenty generations of preclinical life—before the tumor is palpable."

The search for an indicator—a "marker" or "discriminant"—is going on in laboratories all over the world. So far, the carcinoembryonic antigen (CEA) level in the blood and urine seems to offer some promise of success. Professor Symington and some mathematicians at the Chester Beatty Research Institute in the Royal Marsden Hospital are using computers to assist in the search for a difference in the CEA levels that accompany breast cancer and the levels found with other diseases. He is hopeful the computer will be able to pinpoint absolute quantities of

CEA that would be a symptom of breast cancer alone. Professor Symington is optimistic that the electronic brain will be able to do this soon.

For women who find that awful lump, it would be miraculous if scientists could develop a way to inspect the rest of the breast and the axillary nodes by means of some harmless substance that settles in malignant tissue. If a radioactive tag were put on this substance that settles in such malignant tissue, the way iodine settles in the thyroid, it could be injected and the diagnosis made by camera, instead of by needle or knife. Who knows? The substance might even show the presence of cancerous multicentricles and the status of the axillary nodes.

If this ever becomes possible, most mastectomies of any kind will be unnecessary.

Of course, any diagnostic technique that exposes a patient to radioactivity cannot be used for routine checkups. And even such a substance would not solve the problem of very early detection, during those twenty preclinical generations when it is most likely that a cancer can be destroyed entirely.

What we most need is a reliable, safe technique that can be used as often as once a month by high-risk women, and as frequently as desired by others. This may be the thermograph; it may be the sonograph. Whichever succeeds first in being the closest to 100 per cent accurate will make a fortune for its inventor and be a blessing for women everywhere. So far, neither is practical enough.

I talked to GE's Regional Director of the Medical Systems Division, Chuck Henkel, about the thermograph's future. "We're investing a lot of money and effort in making the Spectrotherm as close to 100 per cent accurate as any machine can be," he told me. "But we're not there yet." Somehow, knowing that private industry, with a real economic incentive, is investing money to develop this potentially lifesaving machine is encouraging.

As I said earlier, sonography, is still quite new and too dependent on the training and experience of the reader. As for the analysis of breast fluid, I doubt many women would subject themselves to the painful ordeal of having their nipples aspirated every few months.

These are only examples of research into early-detection devices that I personally know about. There may be studies, experiments, and trials going on of techniques that have not been publicized at all. I do hope there are, because we women need all the help we can get.

Not everything that can be done today with the available techniques is yet being done, however. The American Cancer Society and women's organizations all over the country have provided yeowoman service in trying to spread the word about monthly breast self-examination and periodic mammograms for all women over forty—high-risk women over thirty-five, if their doctors approve. Mobile vans carrying X-ray equipment tour slum areas in the centers of our major cities, as well as rural farm districts. But how long will all this interest last? Is it only a temporary response to panic?

I asked Dr. Sidney Cutler, one of NCI's top biometricians, his opinion.

"It's too soon to predict now whether the current panic will be more than just another big hook in the graph, a permanent change in the attention women pay to themselves. It's just too soon to know. In the past," Dr. Cutler cautioned, "the curve dropped back to normal levels within about a year after a lot of publicity. Let's hope this one will be different."

This one *must* be different. Until the fall of 1974, the American Cancer Society was doing the job of breast-cancer education virtually singlehandedly. Afterward, numerous organizations—public and private—pitched in to help. BSE demonstrations were given on TV news and talk shows; lessons in BSE were given in libraries, schools, churches, and community centers all over the country. These programs should continue.

Hopes for the future about treatment? The major hope, as Professor Symington said, is a magic drug that will cure a woman of cancer with a few tablets or injections.

Far out? Unrealistic? Impossible? Maybe. But I remember not too many years ago when every parent of young children lived in dread of the polio plague. When my older son was a little boy, I carefully followed every mother's summertime instructions: do not expose young children to large crowds; be sure they have

daily naps and plenty of rest; avoid this; do that. By the time
my daughter was the same age, a quick and painless inoculation
had made the annual summer scourge just another dreadful
memory.

If this could happen in my experience with one disease, why
not with breast cancer? This is my hope. Perhaps I am being
unrealistic and overly optimistic, but I do think it will happen.
Although, as Dr. Vollmer said, immunology may not prove to be
"it"—the be-all and end-all of breast-cancer cause and cure—the
information coming from immunology labs around the world
seems to be, at this time, the most exciting and promising.

True, Dr. Plata at NCI's virology laboratory was discouraging
about the development of an anti-breast-cancer vaccine. "It will
not happen in the near future," he repeated several times. But,
on the other hand, he also did not rule it out. Although there are
many kinds of breast cancers, more than 50 per cent are adeno-
carcinomas in the milk ducts. If a single vaccine could be developed to prevent just that one common kind of breast cancer,
the incidence rates would immediately be cut in half.

Immunology has also given clues about the roles played by
a woman's own immune system and, as more is learned, more
"boosters" will be developed to strengthen a weak or deficient
internal defense militia. This whole field is so new and dynamic
that it is impossible to predict or even to speculate on its progress.
Old-timers refused to become enthusiastic about immunology's
plans, however. "I've been through all this before," one expert
explained. "It's like *déjà vu.* I've gotten excited before, gotten
my hopes built up and then knocked back."

Most younger researchers, however, were more confident. Like
Dr. Roberts in Edinburgh, they felt that there will be a major
breakthrough in the treatment of breast cancer within the next
five or, at most, ten years.

In the meantime, while I wait for the break-through, along
with thousands of other women, I know we do not have to give
up and die of breast cancer—even without dramatic new advances. With what is available now, women can live symbiotically
with the disease while scientists continue their search.

Such success—the only kind there is now—depends, however,

on the average American physician and his willingness to learn the new treatments and to use them. With the kind of medical care given in specialized clinics and centers by oncologists, we women can live a long, long time—even with our "incurable" breast cancers.

Bibliography and Chapter Notes

Since *Breast Cancer* was written as a guide for women and not as a contribution to the professional literature, I had not at first intended to include a bibliography. A great deal of the information presented here has either not yet been published or is available only as "papers" in scientific journals (researchers do not write articles in magazines, but papers in journals), not kept by most libraries. Also, I obtained much of the data from personal interviews (known in jargon as "personal communications").

However, many women do live near medical schools or hospitals having excellent libraries, and for those who will want to go into the subject more deeply, I have decided to add a list of some of my sources. Personal communications are in every case described as such in the text, and the names and affiliations of the scientists are given there. Where I consulted and summarized several papers by the same investigator, I have indicated in the bibliography that "research reports" about that subject were read. The *Index Medicus*—a valuable scientific reference guide—has the titles listed as well as the names of the journals in which the papers appeared.

The bibliography is divided by chapter, with the pertinent references to specific topics clearly stated. The subject discussed in a paper is usually indicated in the title. Where this was not possible, I have said that a particular scientist has written on

certain aspects of breast cancer (*e.g.*, Henry T. Lynch works on
a hereditary role). The institution where these investigators can
be reached is added to the citation, should readers want more
data.

There were some publications that were invaluable throughout
the writing of *Breast Cancer*. One, *Report to the Profession*, is the
transcript of the research presented orally at the National Cancer
Institute's international conference on September 30, 1974. This
has been published by the Division of Cancer Biology and Diagnosis and can be obtained from the National Cancer Institute,
Department of Public Information, Bethesda, Md. 20014.

Other sources used for almost every chapter were:

Ackerman, Lauren V., and del Regato, Juan A. *Cancer Diagnosis,
    Treatment and Prognosis.* 4th ed. St. Louis: C. V. Mosby, 1970.
Atkins, Hedley, ed. *The Treatment of Breast Cancer.* Baltimore:
    University Park Press, 1974.
Breast Cancer, Early and Late. Proceedings of the Thirteenth
    Clinical Conference on Cancer, 1968, University of Texas,
    M. D. Anderson Hospital and Tumor Institute at Houston. Chi-
    cago: Yearbook Medical Publishers, 1970.
Crile, George, Jr. *What Women Should Know About the Breast
    Cancer Controversy.* New York: Macmillan, 1973.
Cutler, Max. *Tumors of the Breast.* Philadelphia and Montreal:
    J. B. Lippincott, 1962.
Fisher, Bernard, Professor of Surgery, University of Pittsburgh
    School of Medicine; Chairman, National Surgical Adjuvant
    Breast Project, Pittsburgh, Pa. *The Surgical Dilemma in the
    Primary Therapy of Invasive Breast Cancer: A Critical Ap-
    praisal.*
Haagensen, Cushman Davis. *Carcinoma of the Breast.* New York:
    American Cancer Society, 1950.
Hayward, J. L., and Bulbrook, R. D. *Clinical Evaluation in Breast
    Cancer.* London and New York: Academic Press, 1966.
Lewison, Edward F. *Breast Cancer and Its Diagnosis and Treat-
    ment.* Baltimore: Williams and Wilkins, 1955.
Moore, Francis D., *et al. Cancer of the Breast.* Boston: Little,
    Brown, 1967–68.

Papaioannou, A. N. *The Etiology of Human Breast Cancer.* New York, Heidelberg, and Berlin: Springer-Verlag, 1974.

Prognostic Factors in Breast Cancer. Proceedings of the First Tenovus Symposium, edited by A. P. M. Forrest and P. B. Kunkler. Edinburgh and London: E. and S. Livingstone, 1967.

Segaloff, Albert; Meyer, Kenneth K.; and De Bakey, Selma, eds. *Current Concepts in Breast Cancer.* Baltimore: Williams and Wilkins, 1967.

These publications were extensively used:

Cancer: Journal of the American Cancer Society. Philadelphia and Toronto: J. B. Lippincott.

Oncology. Chicago: Yearbook Medical Publishers.

Memorial Sloan-Kettering Hospital for Cancer and Allied Diseases, New York, research and clinical reports.

National Adjuvant Surgical Breast Project, National Cancer Institute, Bethesda, Md. 20014, research reports.

National Institutes of Health, Department of Health, Education, and Welfare, Bethesda, Md. 20014, research reports on progress in cancer.

In addition, certain interviews, articles in scientific journals, and unpublished manuscripts served as my sources for specific sections of the book. To cite them all would make *Breast Cancer* a book for doctors, not lay persons, and therefore I am listing here only the more important.

CHAPTER I

Crile, George, Jr., "The Smaller the Cancer, the Bigger the Operation?" *Journal of the American Medical Association*, v. 199, no. 10, Mar. 6, 1967.

Dao, Thomas L., "Can a Clinical Trial End Controversies over Local Therapies for Breast Cancer?" *New York State Journal of Medicine*, v. 71, no. 3, Feb. 1, 1971.

Fisher, Bernard, "Breast Surgery: Analyzing the Debate," *Modern Medicine*, Sept. 17, 1973.

————, "Cooperative Clinical Trials in Primary Breast Cancer: A Critical Appraisal," *Cancer*, v. 31, no. 5, May 1973.

Handley, Richard S., "Indications and Contraindications for Mastectomy," *Journal of the American Medical Association*, v. 199, no. 10, Mar. 6, 1967.

Kaae, Sigvard, "Does Simple Mastectomy Followed by Irradiation Offer Survival Comparable to Radical Procedures?" *ibid.*

Rosemond, George P., *et al.*, "Needle Aspiration of Breast Cysts," *Cancer*, v. 23, Jan.-Feb. 1973.

Rubin, Philip, "Carcinoma of the Breast, Stage I: Surgical Spectrum," *Journal of the American Medical Association*, v. 199, no. 10, Mar. 6, 1967.

Thomas, Louis, National Cancer Institute, personal communication.

Zimmerman, David R., "Medicine Today: Breast Cancer," *Ladies' Home Journal*, June 1974.

CHAPTER II

Cowdry, E. V. *Cancer Cells*. New York: W. B. Saunders, 1955.

Grieshaber, Charles K., National Cancer Institute, personal communication.

Prescott, David M. *Cancer: The Misguided Cell*. Indianapolis and New York: Pegasus, 1973.

Thomas, Lewis. *Lives of a Cell*. New York: Viking, 1974.

Watson, James D. *The Double Helix*. New York: Atheneum, 1968.

————, *The Molecular Biology of the Gene*. New York: W. A. Benjamin, 1965.

CHAPTER III

Burk, Dean, Bethesda Naval Medical Research Center, personal communication.

Cameron, C. S. *The Truth About Cancer*. Englewood Cliffs, N.J.: Prentice-Hall, 1956.

Campbell-Hurd, Kate. *A History of Women in Medicine*. Haddam, Conn.: Haddam Press, 1938.

Fountain, H. L., "HEW Should Ascertain If Laetrile Is Effective for Treatment of Cancer," speech in U.S. House of Representatives, *Congressional Record*, Mar. 25, 1971.

Gold, Joseph, *Use of Hydrazine Sulfate in Advanced Cancer Patients: Preliminary Results,* Syracuse Cancer Research Institute, Syracuse, N.Y.

Matchan, Don C., "Laetrile: High Politics Blamed for Refusal to Test Anti-cancer Agent," *National Health Federation Bulletin,* October 1970.

Sigerist, Henry E. *A History of Medicine.* Vols. 1-2. London: Oxford University Press, 1951–61.

CHAPTER IV

Sources for this and the following chapter are presented in more detail, because a large part of the information is in scattered bits and pieces and much of it is not generally known even among scientists. The interviews in Europe were, of course, in the nature of personal communications, and the sources are named in the text.

Berg, John W., *et al.*, "The Unique Association Between Salivary Gland Cancer and Breast Cancer," *Journal of the American Medical Association,* v. 204, no. 9, May 27, 1968.

"Cancer Around the World," *World Health Statistics Annual,* World Health Organization, Geneva, 1968–1969.

Cancer Incidence in Finland, 1971, Publication No. 20, Cancer Society of Finland, Helsinki, 1974.

Cole, Philip, "Epidemiology of Breast Cancer: An Overview," *Report to the Profession,* National Cancer Institute, Bethesda, Md. 20014, Sept. 30, 1974.

Craig, Thomas J., *et al.*, "Epidemiologic Comparison of Breast Cancer Patients with Early and Late Onset of Malignancy and General Population Controls," *Journal of the National Cancer Institute,* v. 53, no. 6, Dec. 1974.

Cutler, Sidney, *et al.*, National Cancer Institute, reports on breast-cancer biometry; personal communications.

deWaard, Frits, *et al.*, University of Utrecht, The Netherlands, research reports on breast cancer and nutrition; personal communication.

Doll, Richard; Muir, Calum; and Waterhouse, John. *Cancer Incidence in Five Continents.* Vol. 2. Berlin, Heidelberg, and New York: Springer-Verlag, 1972.

Enstrom, James E., "Cancer Incidence in Mormons," School of

Public Health at the University of California at Los Angeles, in press.

Eskin, Bernard A., *et al.*, "Human Breast Uptake of Radioactive Iodine," *Obstetrics and Gynecology*, v. 44, no. 3, Sept. 1974.

Fraumeni, Joseph, *et al.*, "Cancer Mortality Among Nuns: Role of Marital Status in Etiology of Neoplastic Disease in Women," *Journal of the National Cancer Institute*, v. 42, no. 455, 1969; personal communications.

Hakama, Matti, "The Peculiar Age Specific Incidence Curve for Cancer of the Breast: Clemmesen's Hook," *Acta pathologica microbiologica scandinavica*, 75, 1969; personal communication.

Hint, E., "An Epidemiological Study of Breast Cancer in the Soviet Union," *Soviet Estonian Health*, no. 2, March–April 1974.

Jussawalla, D. J., *et al.*, "Differences Observed in the Site Incidence of Breast Cancer Between the Parsi Community and the Total Population of Greater Bombay: A Critical Appraisal," *British Journal of Cancer*, v. 24, no. 56, 1970.

Leffall, L. D., *et al.*, "Cancer of the Breast in Negroes," *Surgery, Gynecology, Obstetrics*, v. 117, no. 97, 1963.

Levin, David L.; Devesa, Susan S.; Godwin, J. David, II; and Silverman, Debra T. *Cancer Rates and Risks*. 2nd ed. Bethesda, Md.: National Cancer Institute, 1974.

Lynch, Henry T., *et al.*, Creighton University School of Medicine, Omaha, Neb. 68108, research reports concerning familial aspects of breast cancer.

MacMahon Brian, *et al.*, Harvard University, research reports on all aspects of breast-cancer epidemiology; personal communication.

Mittra, I.; McNeilly, A. S.; *et al.*, "Endocrine (Thyroid) Activity and Breast Cancer," *Contemporary OB/GYN*, v. 5, Jan. 1975.

Petrakis, Nicholas, *et al.*, University of California at San Francisco, research reports on breast fluid and ear wax in Oriental, American Indian, and Caucasian women and the relationship with breast cancer.

Phillips, Roland L., "Cancer Incidence in Seventh Day Adventists," Loma Linda University, Loma Linda, Calif., in press.

Purde, M., Institute of Oncology, reports on breast cancer in the Estonian S.S.R., Tallinn, Estonia.

Purde, M., and Rahu, M., "Summary: On Cancer Morbidity in Estonian S.S.R. and Scandinavia," Tallinn, *Estonian Geographical Society Yearbook,* 1973.

Ringertz, N., ed. *Cancer Incidence in Finland, Iceland, Norway and Sweden. Acta pathologica microbiologica scandinavica,* section A, 1971, Supplement No. 224, 1971.

Robbin, Jacob, National Institute of Metabolic, Digestive and Infectious Diseases, personal communication.

Schneiderman, Marvin, National Cancer Institute, personal communication.

Serenko, A. F., *et al.,* "Cancer Morbidity and Mortality Data in U.S.S.R.," International Agency for Research in Cancer, Internal Technical Report 70/003, Lyon, France, July 10, 1970.

Third National Cancer Survey, 1969–1971 Incidence. Bethesda, Md. 20014: National Cancer Institute, Feb. 1, 1974.

"The Thyroid and Breast Cancer," editorial, *British Medical Journal,* 1 (906): 472, March 1974.

U.S. Office of International Demographics, personal communication.

Wynder, E. L., *et al.,* "A Comparison of Survival Rates Between American and Japanese Patients with Breast Cancer," *Surgery, Gynecology, Obstetrics,* v. 117, no. 196, 1963. On Japanese-American differences, see also *Prognostic Factors in Breast Cancer.* Edinburgh and London: E. and S. Livingstone, 1967.

CHAPTER V

Bittner, Joseph J., *et al.,* research reports on transmission of susceptibility to breast cancer in mice, via milk.

Bulbrook, R. D., "Endocrine, Genetic and Viral Factors in the Etiology of Breast Cancer," *Proceedings of the Royal Society of Medicine,* v. 65, p. 646, 1972.

Carter, Luther J., "Cancer and the Environment: II," *Science,* v. 186, no. 4160, Oct. 18, 1974.

Cutler M., *et al.,* "Psychosomatic Survey of Cancer of the Breast," *Psychosomatic Medicine,* v. 14, 453, 1952.

Dao, Thomas L., "The Nature of Estrogen and Prolactin Effect on Mammary Tumorigenesis," *Cancer Research,* v. 33, Feb. 1973.

Dao, Thomas L., ed. *Estrogen Target Tissues and Neoplasia.* Chicago and London: University of Chicago Press, 1972.

deWaard, Frits, research reports concerning role of nutrition in breast cancer.

Egan, R., *et al.*, "Report and Commentary: The Carcinogenic Hazard of Radiation to the Breasts," *Cancer*, v. 20, no. 24, 1970.

Jablon, Seymour, "Reports of the Atomic Bomb Casualty Commission, National Academy of Sciences," *Radiation Research*, v. 50, no. 3, 1972.

Jackson, A. W., *et al.*, "Carcinoma of Male Breast in Association with Klinefelter Syndrome," *British Medical Journal*, v. I, no. 223, 1965.

Le Shan, L., "Psychological States as Factors in the Development of Malignant Disease: A Critical Review," *Journal of the National Cancer Institute*, v. 22, no. 1, 1959.

Martin, Robert G., *et al.* (National Institute of Metabolic, Digestive and Infectious Diseases); Brugge, Joanne C., *et al.* (Baylor Medical College); Osborn, Mary, *et al.* (Max Planck Institute, West Germany); and Tegtmayer, Peter G. (Case Western Reserve University), on the role of an oncogene in malignant transformation of tissue, *Journal of Virology*, v. 15, no. 3, March 1975.

Moore, Dan H., and Charney, Jesse, "Breast Cancer: Etiology and Possible Prevention," *American Scientist*, March-April 1975.

Report to the Profession, Bethesda, Md. 20014. Research reports on role of estrogen, estrogen receptors, and other steroids in the cause of breast cancer, Sept. 30, 1974.

Stoll, Basil A., ed. *Mammary Carcinoma and Neuroendocrine Therapy.* London: Butterworth, 1974.

Todaro, G. J., and Huebner, R. J., "The Viral Oncogene Hypothesis: New Evidence," *Proceedings of the National Academy of Sciences*, v. 69, no. 1009, 1972.

Wanebo, C. K., *et al.*, "Breast Cancer After Exposure to the Atomic Bombing of Hiroshima and Nagasaki," *New England Journal of Medicine*, v. 279, no. 667, 1968.

CHAPTER VI

Auchincloss, H., and Haagensen, C. D., "Cancer of the Breast Possibly Induced by Estrogenic Substance," *Journal of the American Medical Association*, v. 114, p. 1517, 1940.

Corfman, Philip A., "Coordinated Studies of the Effects of Oral Contraceptives," *Contraception*, v. 9, no. 109, 1974.

Cutler, Sidney J., *et al. End Results in Cancer.* Bethesda, Md. 20014: National Cancer Institute, 1971.

deWaard, Frits, *et al.*, "The Bimodal Age Distribution of Patients with Mammary Carcinoma: Evidence for the Existence of 2 Types of Human Breast Cancer," *Cancer*, v. 17, Feb. 1964.

Fechner, R. E., "Breast Cancer During Oral Contraceptive Therapy," *Cancer*, v. 26, Dec. 1970.

Food and Drug Administration, *Drug Bulletins*, 5600 Fishers Lane, Rockville, Md. 20852.

Fountain, H. L., correspondence with HEW regarding Depo-Provera, Oct. 1974.

Goodman, Louis S., and Gilman, Alfred. *The Pharmacological Basis of Therapeutics.* 4th ed. New York: Macmillan, 1970.

Hellman, L., *et al.*, "Studies of Estradial Transformation in Women with Breast Cancer," *Journal of Clinical Endocrinology*, v. 27, no. 1087, 1967.

Herbst, Arthur L., *et al.*, Harvard University, reports concerning DES daughters.

Hertz, R., "The Problem of Possible Effects of Oral Contraceptives on Cancer of the Breast," *Cancer*, v. 24, Nov. 1969.

House Committee on Government Operations, Twelfth Report, "Regulation of Diethylstilbestrol (DES) and Other Drugs Used in Food Producing Animals," 93rd Congress, House Report No. 93-708, Dec. 10, 1973.

Howard, R. J., *et al.*, "Bilateral Mammary Carcinoma in the Male Coincident with Prolonged Stilbestrol Therapy," *Surgery*, v. 25, no. 300, 1949.

Lasagna, Louis, "Caution on the Pill," *Saturday Review*, Nov. 2, 1968.

Lewison, E. F., *et al.*, "The Pill, Estrogens and the Breast," *Cancer*, v. 28, Dec. 1971.

Macdonald, Ian, "Carcinoma of the Breast in Pregnancy and Laction," *Journal of the American Medical Association*, v. 200, no. 2, April 10, 1967.

Petrakis, Nicholas, "Relationship Between the Pill and Breast Fluid Changes," unpublished.

U.S. Senate, *Competitive Problems in the Drug Industry*, vols.

1-3, parts 15-17, Hearings of the Subcommittee on Monopoly of the Select Committee of Small Business, 91st Congress, Second Session, Oral Contraceptives, Feb. 24, 25; March 3, 4, 1970.

Vessey, M. P., *et al.*, papers on relationship between oral contraceptives and breast cancer.

References to the role of female hormones, hormone-related receptors in breast tissue, and the two separate age-related kinds of breast cancer will be found in the notes to earlier chapters.

The opinions expressed in this chapter on the role of oral contraceptives in breast cancer are based on personal communications with approximately thirty scientists, clinicians, and statisticians.

CHAPTER VII

American Cancer Society, publications concerning BSE—breast self-examination.

"Breast Cancer—Specialists React to the NCI Data," editorial, *Contemporary OB/GYN*, v. 5, Jan. 1975.

Dodd, Gerald D., *et al.*, M. D. Anderson Hospital and Tumor Institute, Houston, Texas, research reports on thermography.

Egan, Robert L., *et al.*, Department of Radiology, Emory University, Atlanta, Ga., research reports on mammography.

Fisher, Bernard. "The Surgical Dilemma in the Primary Therapy of Invasive Breast Cancer: A Critical Appraisal," Pittsburgh, Pa.: Pittsburgh Medical School, 1970.

Fisher, Edwin R., Pittsburgh Medical School, Pittsburgh, Pa. 15219, research reports on multicentricity of breast cancer.

Lewison, Edward F. *Breast Cancer and Its Diagnosis and Treatment.* Baltimore: Williams and Wilkins, 1955. Data regarding physicians' delay surveys.

Report to the Profession. Bethesda, Md. 20014, Sept. 30, 1974. Also subsequent results of the ACS-NCI national Demonstration Projects, sonography, breast-fluid analysis and hormone-markers.

Rubin, Philip, "Comment: The Effect of Delay in Treatment on Prognosis," *Journal of the American Medical Association,* v. 200, no. 11, June 12, 1967.

Shirley, Robert L., "Diagnosing Breast Cancer Earlier," *Contemporary OB/GYN*, v. 3, no. 6, 1973.

Strax, Philip. *Early Detection*. New York, Evanston, San Francisco, London: Harper & Row, 1974.

Symington, Thomas, personal communication from London, 1974, on carcinoembryonic antigen levels in the blood as an early indicator.

Tormey, Douglass, personal communications on marker research.

CHAPTER VIII

"Breast Cancer, Mirror Image Biopsy," editorial, *Medical World News*, Dec. 20, 1974.

"California Relative Value Scale: A Guide for Payment of Medical Fees in the United States, by Area," Committee on Fees, Commission of Medical Services, California Medical Association, 1964.

Connell, Elizabeth B. *Self-examination for Detecting Breast Cancer*. American College of Obstetricians and Gynecologists.

Crile, George, Jr., "The Surgeon's Dilemma," *Harper's Magazine*, May 1975.

————. *What Women Should Know About the Breast Cancer Controversy*. New York: Macmillan, 1973.

de Groot, Walter P. H., "Diagnosis of Carcinoma and Benign Cysts of the Breast: The Value of Needle Aspiration," *The Western Journal of Medicine*, v. 122, Feb. 1975.

"Detection by Needle and Xeroradiography Leaves Almost No Scar," editorial, *Medical World News*, Nov. 8, 1974.

Gallup, George. *Women's Attitudes Regarding Breast Cancer, a Summary*. New York: American Cancer Society, 1974. On women's fear of one-stage procedure.

Rosemond, George P., *et al.*, "Needle Aspiration of Breast Cysts," *Cancer*, v. 23, Jan.-Feb. 1973.

Rubin, Philip, "Carcinoma of the Breast, Stage I—Surgical Spectrum," *Journal of the American Medical Association*, v. 199, no. 10, March 6, 1967. On definition of TMN code.

Saltzenstein, Edward C., *et al.*, "Breast Biopsy on Outpatient Basis," *Modern Medicine*, Feb. 15, 1975.

Schwartz, Gordon F., "A Plea for Sensible Breast Biopsy," *Medical Opinion*, March 1975.

Shirley, Robert L., "Diagnosing Breast Cancer Earlier," *Contemporary OB/GYN*, v. 3, no. 6, 1973.

CHAPTER IX

Crile, Helga Sandburg, "Let a Joy Keep You," *McCall's*, Nov. 1974.

Fisher, Bernard, and Wolmark, Norman, "New Concepts in the Management of Primary Breast Cancer," in press.

Ravdin, Robert G., *et al.*, "Results of a Clinical Trial Concerning the Worth of Prophylactic Oophorectomy for Breast Carcinoma," *Surgery, Gynecology, Obstetrics*, v. 131, Dec. 1970.

Roosevelt, Selwa, "Breast Cancer Surgery—Are We Overdoing It?" *Family Circle*, Nov. 1974.

Rubin, Philip, "Carcinoma of the Breast, Stage III—Inoperable," *Journal of the American Medical Association*, v. 200, no. 7, May 15, 1967.

———, "Comment: Male Breast Carcinoma," *Journal of the American Medical Association*, v. 200, no. 7, May 15, 1967.

Wang, Chiu-Chen, "Management of Inflammatory Carcinoma of the Breast," *Journal of the American Medical Association*, v. 200, no. 7, May 15, 1967.

Many of the publications cited earlier also concern primary surgical treatment of breast cancer, and apply here.

CHAPTER X

Brody, Jane E., "Parley Scores the Denial of Jobs to Persons Who Have Had Cancer Treatment," *New York Times*, Nov. 28, 1974.

Lasser, Terese. *A Manual for Women Who Have Had Breast Surgery*. New York: American Cancer Society, 1969.

Responses from women by telephone or questionnaire.

Say, C. C., and Donegan, W., "Biostatistical Evaluation of Complications from Mastectomy," *Surgery, Gynecology, Obstetrics*, v. 138, March 1974.

Tecala, Mila, Georgetown University Hospital, Washington, D.C., personal communication regarding job discrimination.

CHAPTER XI

Akehurst, A. C., "Post-Mastectomy Morale," *Lancet*, v. 2, 1972.

Anstice, E. "The Emotional Operation," *Nursing Times*, v. 66, 1970.

Asken, Michael J., "Psychoemotional Aspects of Mastectomy: A

Review of Recent Literature," *American Journal of Psychiatry*, v. 132, no. 1, Jan. 1975.

Beale, Betty, "Mrs. Ford: 'I Have Saved Many Lives,'" *Washington Star-News*, Nov. 17, 1974.

Courtemanche, Dolores, "Artist's 'Anniversary of Life,'" *Worcester Sunday Telegram*, Nov. 10, 1974.

Crowell, Loretta M., The Airway Surgical Co., personal communication.

Daniell, Constance, "When Breast Cancer Strikes," *Milwaukee Journal*, July 7, 1974.

Ervin, C. J., "Psychologic Adjustment to Mastectomy," *Medical Aspects of Human Sexuality*, v. 7, 1973.

Frankfort, Ellen, "What Women Fear Most," *Viva*, Feb. 1975.

Gallup, George. *Women's Attitudes Regarding Breast Cancer.* New York: American Cancer Society, 1974.

Harrell, H. C., "To Lose a Breast," *American Journal of Nursing*, v. 72, April 1972.

Hochfelder, Pat, "There Is Something More to Be Said About Breast Surgery," *Westchester Magazine*, Jan. 1975.

Klemesrud, Judy, "After Breast Cancer Surgery—A Difficult Emotional Adjustment," *New York Times*, Oct. 1, 1974.

Lewison, Edward F., "The Treatment of Advanced Breast Cancer," *American Journal of Nursing*, v. 62, Oct. 1962.

"Problems of Adjustment," *Newsweek*, Oct. 14, 1974.

Responses from women by telephone or questionnaire.

CHAPTER XII

"Adriamycin: All the News Is Good," editorial, *Medical World News*, Jan. 27, 1975.

Carbone, Paul, National Cancer Institute, research reports on drugs and personal communication.

Carter, Stephen K., personal communication.

Dilman, V. M., personal communication on the use of l-Dopa and Dilantin.

Huggins, Charles, "Control of Cancers of Man by Endocrinologic Methods: A Review," *Cancer Research*, v. 16, Oct. 1956, and other papers regarding hormonal manipulation for treatment of breast cancer.

Lewison, Edward F., "Therapeutic vs. Prophylactic Castration,"

Journal of the American Medical Association, v. 200, May 15, 1967.

McElwain, T. J. *Chemotherapy in Treatment: Toward Cures for Cancer*. London: Cancer Research Campaign and British Cancer Council, 1974.

Moore, George E., "Chemotherapy in Stage I Breast Cancer," *Journal of the American Medical Association*, v. 199, March 6, 1967.

National Adjuvant Surgical Breast Project, reports on chemotherapy.

Report to the Profession. Bethesda, Md. 20014, Sept. 30, 1974. On l-PAM.

CHAPTER XIII

RADIOTHERAPY

Chu, F. C., *et al.*, "Does Prophylactic Radiation Therapy Given for Cancer of the Breast Predispose to Metastases?," *American Journal of Roentgenology*, v. 99, 1967.

Dao, Thomas L., and Hsia, T. W., "Postoperative Radiotherapy in the Treatment of Breast Cancer," *Frontiers in Radiation Therapy and Oncology*, v. 5, 1970.

Dao, Thomas L., and Kovaric, John, "Incidence of Pulmonary and Skin Metastases in Women with Breast Cancer Who Received Postoperative Irradiation," *Surgery*, v. 52, no. 1, July 1962.

Easson, E. C., "Postoperative Radiotherapy in Breast Cancer," *Prognostic Factors in Breast Cancer*, A. P. M. Forrest and P. B. Kunkler, eds. Edinburgh and London: E. and S. Livingstone, 1967.

Fletcher, Gilbert H., "The Advantages of Preoperative Irradiation," *Journal of the American Medical Association*, v. 200, April 10, 1967.

Forrest, A. P. M., personal communication.

Guttman, R. J., "Radiotherapy in Locally Advanced Cancer of the Breast: Adjunct to Standard Therapy," *Cancer*, v. 20, July 1967.

"Irradiation for Early Breast Cancer," editorial, *Medical World News*, Feb. 10, 1975.

Johnston, Gerald S., personal communication.

Kaae, Sigvard, "Does Simple Mastectomy Followed by Irradiation Offer Survival Comparable to Radical Procedures?," *Journal of the American Medical Association*, v. 200, April 10, 1967.

Lipworth, L., "Survival of Cases of Surgically Treated Mammary Carcinoma with and without Radiation Therapy," *Lancet*, v. 2, 1965.

McWhirter, R., "Should More Radical Treatment Be Attempted in Breast Cancer?," *American Journal of Roentgenology*, v. 92, 1964.

———, "The Treatment of Cancer of the Breast," *Proceedings of the Royal Society of Medicine*, v. 41, no. 122, 1948.

———, "The Value of Simple Mastectomy and Radiotherapy in the Treatment of Cancer of the Breast," *British Journal of Radiology*, v. 21, 1948.

Montague, Eleanor, M. D. Anderson Hospital and Tumor Institute, Houston, Tex., oral presentation on limited breast surgery followed by irradiation, American Cancer Society Symposium, New York, Dec. 1974.

Mustakallio, S., "Treatment of Breast Cancer by Tumor Extirpation and Roentgen Therapy Instead of Radical Operation?," *Journal of Faculty of Radiologists*, v. 6, 1954.

Nathanson, I. T., *et al.*, "Hormonal Studies in Artificial Menopause Produced by Roentgen Rays," *American Journal of Obstetrics & Gynecology*, v. 40, 1940.

Prosnitz, Leonard R., Yale University School of Medicine, New Haven, Conn., oral presentation, on limited breast surgery followed by irradiation, American Association of Radiologists, Key Biscayne, Fla., Jan. 1975.

Report to the Profession. Bethesda, Md. 20014, Sept. 30, 1974. Controlled trials by NSABP and simple, or total, mastectomy followed by irradiation.

Robbins, G. F., *et al.*, "An Evaluation of Postoperative Prophylactic Radiation Therapy in Breast Cancer," *Surgery, Gynecology, Obstetrics*, v. 122, May 1966.

Rubin, Philip, "Carcinoma of the Breast, Stage II—Radiation Range," *Journal of the American Medical Association*, v. 200, no. 2, April 10, 1967.

Stjernsward, Jan, "Decreased Survival Related to Irradiation Post-

operatively in Early Operable Breast Cancer," *Lancet,* Nov.
30, 1974.

IMMUNOTHERAPY

Black, M. M., *et al.,* "Cellular Hypersensitivity to Breast Cancer—
Assessment by Leukocyte Migration Procedure," *Cancer,* v.
33, April 1974.

Borsos, Tibor, personal communication.

Galton, Lawrence, "Immunotherapy: Medicine's Most Exciting
Frontier," *Reader's Digest,* July 1974.

Gillie, Oliver, "Doctors Use Pigs in New Fight Against Cancer,"
The (London) *Times,* Dec. 1, 1974.

Good, R. A., *et al.,* Memorial Sloan-Kettering Hospital for Cancer and Allied Diseases, New York, research reports on the
immune surveillance system and the role of the immunological
system in the growth of malignancies.

Jacob, François, *et al., Proceedings of the National Academy of
Sciences,* v. 71, March 1974, on the discovery of a substance
that blocks immunological attack upon neoplastic cells.

Kripke, Margaret, and Borsos, Tibor, "Immune Surveillance Re-
visited," *Journal of the National Cancer Institute,* v. 52, no. 5,
May 1974.

Papermaster, B. W., *et al.,* research reports on role of components
of the immune system on treating cancer.

Plata, Ernest, personal communication.

Prehn, R. T., *et al.,* research reports on the immune surveillance
system and the role of the immunological system in the growth
of malignancies.

Waldmann, Thomas A., "Immunodeficiency Disease and Malignancy," *Annals of Internal Medicine,* v. 77, no. 4, Oct. 1972.

CHAPTER XIV

American Board of Surgery, personal communication.

American College of Surgeons, personal communication.

Fact Book, Bethesda, Md.: National Cancer Institute, 1974. On
information regarding funding.

Peters, Vera M., "Wedge Resection and Irradiation," *Journal of
the American Medical Association,* v. 200, April 10, 1967.
Example of woman's approach to breast cancer.

Roster, House of Delegates and Board of Directors, American Cancer Society, 1974.

Strax, Philip. *Early Detection*. New York, Evanston, San Francisco, and London: Harper & Row, 1974.

"Surgeons Back Radical Mastectomy," editorial, *Medical World News*, Nov. 8, 1974.

Westgate, Betty. *Helpful Hints*. Croydon, England: Mastectomy Association, 1974.

CHAPTER XV

Gallup, George. *Women's Attitudes Regarding Breast Cancer*. New York: American Cancer Society, 1974.

Gillette, Robert, "The Continuing Breast Cancer Controversy—Over Ethics and Over Surgery," *Science*, v. 186, Oct. 18, 1974.

Greenberg, Daniel S., "A Critical Look at Cancer Coverage," *Columbia Journalism Review*, Jan.-Feb. 1975.

Hearings on the Conquest of Cancer Act, 1971, before the Subcommittee on Health of the Committee on Labor and Public Welfare, U.S. Senate, 92nd Congress, March 9, 10, and June 10, 1971.

Irwin, Theodore, "The Cancer Circuit Riders," *Parade Magazine*, Aug. 25, 1974.

Maugh, Thomas H., II, "Marihuana: The Grass May No Longer Be Greener," *Science*, v. 185, Aug. 23, 1974.

Murphy, Gerald P., testimony before the Senate Health and Public Welfare Committee, personal transcript, July 12, 1974.

National Program for the Conquest of Cancer, report prepared for the Committee on Labor and Public Welfare, U.S. Senate, 92nd Congress, April 27, 1970. U.S. Government Printing Office, Document No. 92-9, $1.50, Washington, D.C. 20402.

Policy Statement on the Surgical Treatment of Breast Cancer. New York: American Cancer Society, June 8, 1973.

Rauscher, Frank J., Jr., "Budget and the National Cancer Program," *Science*, v. 184, May 24, 1974.

Rosemond, George P., "Progress Against Cancer," *Washington Post*, May 6, 1975.

"What You Should Know About Breast Cancer," editorial, *Business Week*, Oct. 12, 1974.

CHAPTER XVI

Blokhin, Nikolai N., personal communication, on mini-détente.
Cutler, Sidney J., personal communication.
Love, Dr. Robert, personal communication.
Vollmer, Erwin, personal communication.

Acknowledgments

I would like to express my gratitude to the many people who have generously given me time, patience, and assistance in unraveling the knotted yarn of breast cancer's mysteries. To all the women who so selflessly shared their painful experiences with me, my debt is deep. Although several authorities listed read and criticized the chapters related to their fields for technical accuracy, only Dr. Thomas L. Dao has seen the entire manuscript. The points of view taken in advocacy or opposition in *Breast Cancer* are entirely my own. This list of acknowledgments does not imply anyone's approval of my personal opinions.

Dr. Horsley Gantt, Professor Emeritus, the Johns Hopkins School of Medicine and Director of the Pavlovian Laboratory, the Perry Point Veterans' Hospital, Perryville, Maryland: for helping me learn the language of our modern medicine men. Dr. Thomas L. Dao, Director, Department of Breast Surgery and Breast Cancer Research Unit, the Roswell Park Memorial Institute, Buffalo, New York: for his advice and criticism in the writing of this book and for his kindness and compassion as a physician. Dr. Gerald S. Johnston, Chief, Nuclear Medicine, the National Institutes of Health, Bethesda, Maryland: for the many hours he spent giving me personal and professional advice; and to his wife, Dorothy, for her tolerance and understanding. Dr.

Gerald P. Murphy, Director, the Roswell Park Memorial Institute, member of the National Cancer Advisory Committee and Secretary General of the International Union Against Cancer: for his help in arranging my visits to European cancer centers.

Professor N. N. Blokhin, the Moscow Institute of Oncology, U.S.S.R., and Professor O. V. Sviatukhina, Professor A. Chaklin, and other members of the staff of the mammary carcinoma department. Dr. Frits deWaard, the University of Utrecht, The Netherlands. Professor A. P. M. Forrest, the Royal Infirmary, Edinburgh, Scotland, and Dr. Maureen Roberts and the other members of the breast cancer department. Professor B. E. Gustafsson and Dr. Helen Westerberg, the Karolinska Institute, Stockholm, Sweden. Professor Calum Muir, the International Agency for Research in Cancer, Lyon, France. Professor N. P. Napalkov, the Leningrad Institute of Oncology, U.S.S.R., and Professor R. Melnikov, Professor V. M. Dilman, and the other members of the mammary carcinoma department. Professor M. Purde, the Institute of Oncology, Tallinn, Estonian S.S.R. Professor E. Saxen, the University of Helsinki, Finland, and Professor M. Hakama and Professor L. Teppo. Professor Thomas Symington, the Chester Beatty Research Institute, London, England, and Dr. Gordon Taylor and Dr. Trevor Powles, the Royal Marsden Cancer Hospital, Sutton.

Mrs. Marvella Bayh, Washington, D.C. Dr. Heinz Berendes, Dr. Philip Corfman, National Institute of Child Health and Human Development, Bethesda, Maryland. Dr. Nathaniel Berlin, Dr. Tibor Borsos, Dr. Paul Carbone, Dr. Stephen Carter, Dr. Sidney Cutler, Dr. Vincent Da Vita, Dr. Joseph Fraumeni, Dr. Charles Grieshaber, Dr. Robert Love, Ms. Betty McVickers, Dr. Max Meyers, Dr. Mitchell Parver, Dr. Ernest Plata, Dr. William Pomerance, Dr. Marvin Schneiderman, Dr. Louis B. Thomas, Dr. Douglass Tormey, Dr. Erwin Vollmer, Dr. Thomas Waldmann, the National Cancer Institute, Bethesda, Maryland. Dr. Richard Behrman, College of Physicians and Surgeons, Columbia University, New York, New York. Mr. Howard Bray, Executive Director of the Fund for Investigative Journalism, Washington, D.C., for a small grant to support research on the contraceptive pill. Dr. William E. Bunney, the National Institute of Mental Health, Bethesda, Maryland. Dr. Dean Burk, the Bethesda Naval Hospital, Bethesda, Maryland. Dr. Olcay S. Cigtay, the Georgetown University Hospital, Washington, D.C. Mr. Joe Clark and Mr. Herbert Seidman, the American Cancer Society, New York, New York. Mrs. Loretta Marsh Crowell, the Airway Surgical Co., Cincinnati, Ohio. Dr. Bernard Eskin, the Medical College of Pennsylvania, Philadelphia. Dr. Bernard Fisher, the University of Pittsburgh School of Medicine, Pittsburgh, Pennsylvania. Mr. Ronald Goldfarb, Washington, D.C. Mr. Gilbert Goldhammer, consultant, Representative L. H. Fountain, U.S. House of Representatives. Dr. Frederick Glaser and Mr. Benjamin Gordon, assistants to Senator Gaylord Nelson, U.S. Senate. Dr. William Granatir, the Washington Psychoanalytic Society, Washington, D.C. Dr. Bernard Heckman, Silver Spring, Maryland. Dr. Louis Hellman, the Department of Health, Education, and Welfare, Washington, D.C. Dr. Roy Hertz, the George Washington University School of Medicine, Washington, D.C. Dr. Edward Lewison, the Johns Hopkins Hospital, Baltimore, Maryland. Mrs. Alice Roosevelt Longworth, Washington, D.C. Ms. Joan Piemme, the Georgetown University and Sibley Hospital, Washington, D.C. Dr. Thomas Piemme, the George Washington University Hospital, Washington, D.C. Mr. Constantine Prisekin, Rockville, Maryland. Mr. Randolph Rae and Dr. Ralph Stiller, Silver Spring, Maryland. Dr. Gerald Rehert, Atlanta, Georgia. Dr. Jacob Robbin, National Institute of Metabolic and Digestive Diseases, Bethesda, Maryland. Dr. Joseph Sharp, the National Aeronautics and Space Administration, Moffet Field, California. Dr. Edward Soma, Holy Cross Hospital, Silver Spring, Maryland. Dr. Philip Strax, the Guttman Institute, New York, New York.

Ms. Ruth C. Smith, Chief Librarian, the library of the Clinical Center, the National Institutes of Health, and the staff. Dr. Martin M. Cummings, Director, and the staff of the National Library of Medicine, Bethesda, Maryland. Ms. Judith Randall, syndicated medical writer, the *New York Daily News,* Washington Bureau. Victor Cohn, medical writer, the *Washington Post,* Washington, D.C. Mrs. Jane Popores, Gaithersburg, Maryland, for her invaluable assistance in preparation of the manuscript.

Special thanks are due Harcourt Brace Jovanovich, Inc. and my editors there—William B. Goodman, Catherine Fauver, and

Judith Duffy—for understanding that the need for such a book, published quickly, is vital for women all over the world, and for adjusting their schedules and, most of all, their feelings to the problem of what to do about breast cancer.

Index

abortion, 139, 201, 297-98, 316
abscissic acid, 70-72, 325
adrenal glands, 104, 109, 260, 263, 275-76; removal of, 261, 264
Adriamycin, 266-67, 269, 325
Airway Surgical Company, 211
Alkeran, 265
alkylating agents, 264, 265, 266, 267, 269, 270-71, 273; *see also* mustards
American Cancer Society, 5-6, 65, 71, 72, 75, 79, 92, 148, 155, 156, 160, 184, 192-93, 227, 313, 323-26, 329, 332, 355; dominated by men, 306-07, 325, 326; Reach to Recovery, 210-11, 220, 222-24, 256, 306, 307, 323, 349, 351
American College of Obstetricians and Gynecologists, 332
American College of Surgeons, 304, 316; Human Renal Transplant Registry, 288
American Indian women: incidence of cancer in, 86

American Journal of Psychiatry, 256-58, 307
American Medical Association, 71, 144, 313; *Journal* of, 335
American Pharmaceutical Association, 143
Anderson Hospital and Tumor Institute, M. D., Houston, 109, 286, 326, 330, 335, 352
androgen, *see* hormones, male
anesthesia, 209, 346; history of, 56, 57, 60, 61, 62; traumas from, 170, 178-79
antibiotics, 264, 266-67, 269, 325
antigens, 124, 290, 292-93, 295, 353; carcinoembryonic (CEA), 167, 354-55
antimetabolites, 264, 265-66, 267, 269, 270, 325
Argentina: cancer statistics in, 81
Arje, Dr. Sidney, 332
Arkhurst, Joyce, 225, 227
arm, 220-21, 350; milk (lymphedema), 26, 195-96, 217, 219,

381

arm *(cont.)*
221, 287; numbness in, 208-
09; pain in, 208; and pectoral
muscles, 46, 216, 219; shoulder, 208, 217
Asians: incidence of cancer in,
90, 93, 95
Asken, Michael J., 256-58, 307,
350
Atlanta Tumor Registry, 142
atomic bombs: and cancer, 64,
116-17
Atomic Energy Commission, 116
Atossa, 56, 300
Australia: cancer statistics in, 77

bacteria: antigens, 290; and immune system, 294, 295; and
transplants, 289
Barnard, Dr. Christiaan, 289
Bayh, Birch, 216, 237, 308-09
Bayh, Marvella, 4, 216, 237,
308-09, 314, 326
Bé, Major Nguyen, 31-32, 41
Beatson, Sir George, 260
Bellamann, Henry: *Kings Row*,
29, 239
benign tumors, 15, 23, 45, 58,
67, 83, 146-47, 150, 158-59,
173, 204, 346-47
Berendes, Dr. Heinz, 133-34,
135, 136-37
Berkeley studies, 133-35, 137
Bethesda Naval Hospital, 279,
310 and *n.*, 339
biometry, 78, 82, 142, 351, 355
biopsy, 7, 9, 10, 17, 22-25, 29,
51, 63, 68, 75, 156, 158, 160,
169-70, 172, 178-79, 189,
232, 311, 312, 321, 322; economic incentive for, 180, 183,
346-47; excisional, 15, 19,

170, 173, 186; fine-needle,
172 and *n.*, 175; incisional,
15, 16; of nodes, 17-18, 48,
187-88, 194; outpatient, 173,
175, 180, 183, 190, 318, 346-
47; wide-bore-needle, 172-73
Birmingham Tumor Registry,
142
Bittner, Dr. Joseph J., 110, 343
Black, Shirley Temple, 4, 237
black women: incidence of cancer in, 82
bladder cancer, 296
Blaiberg, Philip, 289
Blokhin, Professor Nikolai N.,
190, 353
blood: cancer, 52; cells, 40, 42,
282, 283; circulation, 61, 68
blood stream, 32; immunological
components of, 47, 48-49,
121, 290, 291; and metastases,
49, 163, 177, 192, 196, 199,
291, 327-28
blood tests, 268; for cancer detection, 158, 159, 164, 166-
68, 170, 171, 175, 178, 228,
353
Bobst, Elmer H., 140
Bohne, Larry, 236-37, 238
Bombay: cancer statistics in, 77,
89, 90
bone: cancer, 49, 161-62, 163,
165, 278, 284, 285; cells, 42,
282, 283; marrow, 121, 282,
283, 284, 291; scans, 165, 173
Borsos, Dr. Tibor, 292-93, 294,
296
Boston Collaborative Drug Surveillance Program, 134-35,
137
Boston Hospital for Women, 192
brain: cancer, 163, 328; hy-

chemotherapy (*cont.*)
(combination of drugs), 267,
268-69; clinical trials, 265,
269, 270-74, 337-38; drugs,
63-64, 200, 201, 234, 236,
264-75, 294, 325, 353, 355;
immunosuppressant   drugs,
288, 289, 291, 293, 294, 296;
neurological drugs, 274; by
oncologists, 266; for pain, 267,
275; in postoperative care,
159, 164, 165, 267, 270-74;
relapses, 267; sensitivity to,
268; side effects, 264, 266,
267-68, 269, 270, 273-74, 332;
timing in, 265, 268; treatment
by, 22, 65, 171, 202, 278, 293-
94, 347; *see also* hormones; individual drugs
Chester Beatty Research Institute, London, 167, 205, 353
Child, Julia, 178
Chile: cancer statistics in, 90
Chinese women, 158; incidence
of cancer in, 98
chlorpromazine, 275
Chua, Dr. Thomas Y., 184
Civil Service Commission, 226
Cleveland Clinic, Cleveland,
172 *n.*, 320, 331
Clowes, William, 70
Cole, Dr. Philip, 108
Colombia: cancer statistics in, 89
Colorado Tumor Registry, 142
Columbia Journalism Review,
329
Comstock, Dr. George W., 87
Congress: investigations of, 130,
133, 136-37, 140, 141, 330-
31, 347; lobbies, 115; male-
dominated, 313, 315, 316; and
research funds, 313-15, 316

Connecticut Tumor Registry,
133, 142, 192
Contraception, 137
Coolidge, Calvin, 348
Corfman, Dr. Philip A., 133,
134, 136-37
cortisone, 263
Cosmopolitan, 303
cough and hoarseness, 73, 163,
228
Craig, Dr. Thomas J., 87
Crile, Dr. George, Sr., 63, 244
Crile, Dr. George, Jr., 17-18,
292, 320-21, 323, 324; *What
Women Should Know About
the Breast Cancer Contro-
versy,* 13-14, 181-83, 193,
196, 198, 205, 321
Crowell, Loretta Marsh, 211-12,
224
Curie, Marie, 117
Cutler, Dr. Sidney, 78-79, 86,
142, 355
cyclamates, 141
cyclophosphamide   (Cytoxan),
265, 266, 267, 269
Cytoxan, 265, 266, 267, 269

Dallas-Fort Worth Tumor Registry, 142
Dao, Dr. Thomas L., 26-27, 69,
102-07, 127, 143-44, 152, 164,
173-74, 176, 178, 179, 188,
189, 192, 199-200, 201, 204,
208, 209, 218, 219, 220, 238,
252, 253, 273, 274, 284-85,
287, 322, 327, 348
Davis, Dr. Hugh, 131
De Cosse, Dr. Jerome J., 184
Democedes, 56
Denmark: cancer statistics in,
80, 94; surgery in, 181, 197